The Skeptical Professional's Guide to Psychiatry

This text critically examines the shortcomings of psychiatry; the flawed development of the diagnostic system, including the DSM-5; and the failure to advance the effectiveness of antipsychotics and antidepressants.

Starting with an overview of the evolution of psychiatry, Dean explores the creation, use, and misuse of medications, a process largely driven by drug companies. Other chapters describe the benefits and risks of medications, the problems associated with rational prescribing, and the embrace of so-called novel therapies including hallucinogenic drugs and opioids. Chapters end with a set of clinical notes that provide specific recommendations to clinicians, families, patients, and other providers, emphasizing the risks and benefits of treatment with medications but also stressing alternative approaches.

This book will challenge clinicians to think critically about the DSM-5 and the current systems of diagnosis and treatment of mental illnesses in the hopes of ultimately improving the lives of people with mental illnesses.

Charles E. Dean, M.D., has 47 years of clinical, educational, and research experience. He has taught psychopharmacology and clinical neuroscience at the Minneapolis VA Medical Center and the University of Minnesota.

The Skeptical Professional's Guide to Psychiatry

On the Risks and Benefits of Antipsychotics, Antidepressants, Psychiatric Diagnoses, and Neuromania

Charles E. Dean

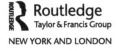
Routledge
Taylor & Francis Group

NEW YORK AND LONDON

First published 2021
by Routledge
52 Vanderbilt Avenue, New York, NY 10017

and by Routledge
2 Park Square, Milton Park, Abingdon, Oxon, OX14 4RN

Routledge is an imprint of the Taylor & Francis Group, an informa business

Library of Congress Cataloging-in-Publication Data
Names: Dean, Charles E., author.
Title: The skeptical professional's guide to psychiatry : on the risks and
    benefits of antipsychotics, antidepressants, psychiatric diagnoses, and
    neuromania / Charles E. Dean.
Description: New York, NY : Routledge, 2021. | Includes
    bibliographical references and index.
Identifiers: LCCN 2020026676 (print) | LCCN 2020026677 (ebook) |
    ISBN 9780367469313 (hardback) | ISBN 9780367469207 (paperback) |
    ISBN 9781003032038 (ebook)
Subjects: MESH: Mental Disorders—drug therapy | Psychotropic
    Drugs | Mental Disorders—diagnosis | Psychiatry—history |
    United States
Classification: LCC RC483 (print) | LCC RC483 (ebook) |
    NLM WM 402 | DDC 616.89/18—dc23
LC record available at https://lccn.loc.gov/2020026676
LC ebook record available at https://lccn.loc.gov/2020026677

ISBN: 978-0-367-46931-3 (hbk)
ISBN: 978-0-367-46920-7 (pbk)
ISBN: 978-1-003-03203-8 (ebk)

Typeset in Bembo
by Apex CoVantage, LLC

To the many thousands of patients, families, and team members with whom I've worked over the decades. A special thanks to William Jepson, M.D., and Joseph Westermeyer, M.D., for their encouragement and providing time for writing and research. Finally, thanks to Stephanie, Jeffrey, Jonathan, Alex, Kelly, and Greg, for their discussions, support, and care.

Contents

Abbreviations

AMA   American Medical Association
APA   American Psychiatric Association
APs   Antipsychotics
ADs   Antidepressants
DSM   *Diagnostic and Statistical Manual*
FGAs   First-generation antipsychotics
JAMA   *Journal of the American Medical Association*
NIH   National Institutes of Health
NIMH   National Institutes of Mental Health
MAOIs   Monoamine oxidase inhibitors
SGAs   Second-generation antipsychotics
SSRIs   Serotonin reuptake inhibitors
SNRIs   Serotonin-norepinephrine reuptake inhibitors
TCAs   Tricyclic antidepressants

Permissions

Edwin Frank, a selection from *In the Dark*. Obtained May 13, 2020.

Allen Wheelis, a selection from *How People Change*, Harper Colophon Books. Permissions Department, General Books Group, HarperCollins Publishers. Agreement HC121094. March 26, 2020.

E.L. Doctorow, a selection from *Andrew's Brain*. Permissions Department, Penguin Random House. The quotation was determined to be fair use by the administrator, May 11, 2020.

Introduction

An excerpt from a poem by Edwin Frank is appropriate to our situation:

we, we have been, we have been waiting now for a very long time for something to become clear, although everything remains unclear.
(Edwin Frank, "In the Dark," *New York Review of Books*, December 2014, p. 24)

What has become clear in psychiatry as of 2020 is our lack of substantial progress in the diagnosis and treatment of those with mental illness—despite 60 years of increasingly complex and elegant studies. Harsh words? Yes, indeed, but I write them out of deep concern for the millions of patients and their families who are being swamped with exaggerated claims of success passed on by their psychiatrists, family physicians, and the pharmaceutical industry.

On the other hand, a few have begun to recognize that what we've accomplished in the past 60 years has fallen far short of expectations, despite the flood of hypotheses, research, and technological advances, not to mention the predictions made by the likes of Dr. Lewis Judd, former director of the National Institutes of Mental Health (NIMH), who, in 1990, predicted "phenomenal progress" in the understanding of mental health.[1] Only two years later, participants in a Neuroscience and Genetics Workshop[2] concluded that psychiatry had yet to identify a single neurobiological phenotypic marker of a gene that is helpful in making a diagnosis of a major psychiatric disorder or predicting response to psychopharmacological treatment. The workgroup added that it was just a matter of time before these efforts would bear fruit, but, here we are in 2020, and we still have no well-replicated or clinically useful biological markers,[3] the lack of which sank the goal of a transcendent diagnostic system for DSM-5.[4]

Contrast Dr. Judd's comments with those made by the past chief of the NIMH, Thomas Insel, who wrote in 2009[5] that "neither genomics or imaging has yet impacted the diagnosis or treatment of the 45 million Americans with serious or moderate mental illness." Even worse, the prospects for recovery have not changed substantially in the past century. Underscoring the lack of progress in achieving recovery, Insel also wrote[6] that despite the heavy use of medications, there is no evidence that the morbidity or mortality of mental disorders has dropped substantially in recent decades. Indeed, mortality rates have risen in many disorders, and the outcome in schizophrenia has worsened.[7] Eric Nestler, a prominent neuroscientist at Mount Sinai, and Steven Hyman, former Provost at Harvard, have deplored the absence of diagnostic tests for mental disorders and noted that diagnoses are still "based solely on phenomenology": that is, observable clinical symptoms.[8] If that weren't enough, they added that psychiatric diagnoses do not "map on to objectively ascertainable abnormalities" in brain structures, with the exception of several neurodegenerative illnesses.

I reached the same conclusions in an essay published in 1991[9] and, in a follow-up piece,[10] had to regretfully conclude that despite another 17 years of research, we still had made no clinically significant advances in diagnosis or treatment, despite the flood of antidepressants, antipsychotics, and genetic studies. This was not the result implicit in the House Joint Resolution 174, which designated the 1990s as the decade of the brain, a proclamation proudly signed by President George H.W. Bush—albeit with no funding.

Well, here we are, two decades into another century, and we see the same pattern of promises. The editor of *Nature*, Philip Campbell,[11] wrote that 2010 would be a decade for psychiatric disorders, in that the science would be much more insightful—a prediction made many times over the past 30 years.[12] We have to give Campbell credit, however, for acknowledging the lack of advances in treatment, the "crudity" of psychiatric diagnoses, and the lack of in-depth exposure of many psychiatrists to recent developments in neurobiology.[11]

But whether the reductionist approach that seeks to clarify the etiology and treatment of mental illness via neuroscience/molecular biology has been of any real value to clinical psychiatry has been sharply debated in the *Canadian Journal of Psychiatry* by Grof[13] and Gold,[14] with Gold arguing that reductionism has not only failed to provide clarity with regard to the mind, but is not capable of providing the answers. This position echoes that of the great southern novelist Walker Percy, who wrote in 1957 that the mind and human needs are not compatible with a biological approach,[15, pp. 251, 275] and the philosopher Isaiah Berlin, who noted in 1991[16, p. 31] that quantitative computation cannot but ignore the hopes and fears of individuals.

Nevertheless, psychiatry is now pinning its hopes on Big Data,[17] despite a scathing critique by Frègnac[18] in the journal *Science* and an admission by Sejnowski et al.,[19] who concluded that massive data sets will make it increasingly difficult to analyze and reach conclusions. Yet that is exactly the direction we are taking, with at least $10 billion aimed at massive brain mapping and genetic studies across the world.[20]

Our lack of progress in advancing the diagnosis, treatment, and indeed the lives of those with mental illness, stands in marked contrast to the optimistic predictions made over the past two decades, predictions that rested largely on improved technology. However, we are experiencing not only *increasing* rates of depression and suicide[21, 22] but also a severe epidemic of opioid addiction, not to mention significant increases in deaths from overdoses of opioids and fentanyl.[23] Yet, oddly enough, we now find psychiatry enthusiastically exploring the use of opioids for depression and hallucinogenic and psychotogenic drugs for a host of disorders, many of which are marked by co-morbid addictive problems!

We also have tens of thousands of the mentally ill languishing in jails and prisons, or in nursing homes and on the street, while funds for psychiatric beds and clinical care have been cut.[24] Indeed, well over half the funding from the National Institutes of Health (NIH) in 2016 went to projects that focused on genes, stem cells, and regenerative medicine, while the number of clinical trials funded by the National Institutes of Mental Health (NIMH) fell by 24% in the years from 2006 to 2014.[25]

The discrepancy between the promises made by psychiatry and the actual results is striking and badly in need of explanation. To that end, I have explored the possibilities in a series of papers, including an essay published in 2017,[7] stressing that poverty, social inequality, and financial inequality are major players affecting the rates of depression, suicidality, and other mental problems. Yet psychiatry, especially those doing research in genetics and brain imaging, seems to have forgotten the impact of social factors on the brain, not to mention the psyche. Indeed, while funding for biotechnology increased at 6% yearly from 1994 to 2004, funding for health services research fell to 0.3% of total health care expenditures.[26]

I am not alone in criticizing our lack of progress. At least 25 books critical of psychiatry have been published in recent years, many of them focusing on the links between Pharma and academic psychiatry, a relationship that has guided research for decades and gave rise to the medical-industrial complex with its financial power and influence.[27] Not surprisingly, this has led to serious misconduct by the industry, which paid out some $3 billion in civil and criminal fines during the years 1999 through 2015, a mere pittance compared with $711 billion in profits![28]

While these reports are disturbing, they fail to answer an important question: What next? How does this information translate into action on the part of clinicians? How do these revelations advance clinical care, whether in outpatient clinics, state hospitals, or the mental health courts? How do they affect individual patients and their families? How can clinicians and patients use the results of a 2020 genome-wide association study[29] that found 111 genetic loci shared by people with schizophrenia, bipolar disorder, major depression, and the body mass index? Why did people in the U.S. between the ages of 16 and 64 experience a 40% increase in suicides during the years from 2000 to 2017?[30] Does the mental health profession have an answer, or will we continue to pin our hopes on worldwide multi-billion dollar projects aimed at developing a supercomputer model of the brain and million-person genetic studies?[31] A recent editorial[32] in the *New England Journal of Medicine* called attention to the unfortunate gap between the biological and social models of disease while Case and Deaton[33] continue to raise alarms about deaths of despair in the United States, but, as we shall see, neuromania is on the rise, both scientifically and culturally. Indeed, some are predicting we will soon be able to upload our conscious selves into a computer and send ourselves off into space, a subject popular in a number of films and novels.

My goal in this book is to provide a highly detailed and critical review of the major developments in psychiatry over the past 60 years, *but with the aim of translating the relevant data into recommendations useful to clinicians, caretakers, and patients*. I will include some technical sections on the biochemistry of antipsychotics and antidepressants and a historical review of the many problems saturating our outmoded diagnostic system, but those with some background in chemistry will find these sections easy. Those without such a background can skip this material, but, again, I hope to make this data clinically relevant.

I have chosen to focus first on antipsychotics, since they have significant potential for serious adverse effects, including movement disorders and the metabolic syndrome (weight gain, hyperlipidemia, diabetes mellitus). I will focus, too, on antidepressants, given their popularity and the increased rates of depression and suicidality in the United States. In addition, the off-label use of both classes of drugs has grown significantly, increasing the risks for the general population, despite the fact that off-label use is legal. This in itself is odd, since, as we shall see, regulatory agencies have long required that medications be used for specific diseases. In the final chapter, I will explore the problems in the new edition of the *Diagnostic and Statistical Manual*, a proposed alternative to the manual, and the growing enthusiasm for neuromania, a highly reductive approach to aesthetics, law, and the brain, as exemplified by the National Institutes of Health Brain Initiative. As of 2018, the NIH has poured over $950 million into 550 projects across the country,[31] sparking concern over the ethics of such projects, both here and in Europe. Will the Brain Initiative and similar projects improve the lives of patients and families?

References

1. Beecher L. A national director of sound mind. *Minnesota Medicine* 1990;73:11–14, for quotations from Dr. Lewis Judd.
2. Psychiatric Research Report. *Neuroscience and Genetics Workshop*, p. 11. American Psychiatric Association, Washington DC, Summer 2002.
3. Gillan CM, Whelan R. What big data can do for treatment in psychiatry. *Current Opinion in Behavioral Sciences* 2017;18:34–42.

4. Kupfer D, First MB, Regier D. Introduction. In: *A Research Agenda for DSM-V*. Editors: Kupfer D, First MB, Regier D. American Psychiatric Association, Washington DC, 2002, xv–xxiii.

5. Insel TR. Translating scientific opportunity into public health impact. *Archives of General Psychiatry* 2009;66:128–133.

6. Insel TR. Disruptive insights in psychiatry: transforming a clinical discipline. *Journal of Clinical Investigation* 2009;119:700–705.

7. Dean CE. Social inequality, scientific inequality, and the future of mental illness. *Philosophy, Ethics, and Humanities in Medicine* 2017;12:10. Doi.10.1186/s13010-017-0052-x.

8. Nestler EJ, Hyman SE. Animal models of neuropsychiatric disorders. *Nature Neuroscience* 2010;13:1161–1169.

9. Dean CE. Diagnosis: the Achilles' heel of biological psychiatry. *Minnesota Medicine* 1991;74:15–17.

10. Dean CE. Psychiatry revisited. *Minnesota Medicine* 2008;91:41–45.

11. Campbell P. A decade for psychiatric disorders. *Nature* 2010;463(7277):9.

12. Jones EM, Mendell LM. Assessing the decade of the brain. *Science* 1999;284:739.

13. Grof P. Psychiatry and neuroscience: reduction of pluralism. *Canadian Journal of Psychiatry* 2009;54:503–505.

14. Gold I. Reduction in psychiatry. *Canadian Journal of Psychiatry* 2009;54:506–512.

15. Percy W. The coming crisis in psychiatry. In: *Signposts in a Strange Land*. Picador, Farrar, Straus, and Giroux, New York, 1991.

16. Berlin I. The bent twig. In: *The Crooked Timber of Humanity: Chapters in the History of Ideas*. Alfred A. Knopf, New York, 1991.

17. Gillan CM, Whelan R. What big data can do for treatment in psychiatry. *Current Opinion in Behavioral Sciences* 2017;18:34–32.

18. Frègnac Y. Big data and the industrialization of neuroscience: a safe roadmap for understanding the brain? *Science* 2017;358:470–477.

19. Sejnowski TJ, Churchland PS, Movshon J. Putting big data to use in neuroscience. *Nature Neuroscience* 2014;17:1440–1441.

20. Huang ZJ, Luo L. It takes the world to understand the brain. International projects discuss how to coordinate efforts. *Science* 2015;350:42–44.

21. Centers for Disease Control. Suicide among adults 35–64 years-United States 1999–2012. *Morbidity and Mortality Weekly Report* 2013;62:321–325.

22. Case A, Deaton A. Rising morbidity and mortality in midlife among white non-Hispanic Americans in the 21st century. *Proceedings of the National Academy of Sciences* 2015;112:15078–15083.

23. Park H, Bloch M. Epidemic of drug overdose deaths ripples across America. *The New York Times*, January 20, 2016, p. A13.

24. Sisti DA, Segal AG, Emanuel EJ. Improving long-term psychiatric care. Bring back the asylum. *JAMA* 2015;313:243–244.

25. Erhardt S, Appel J, Meinert CL. Trends in national institutes of health funding for clinical trials registered in ClinicalTrials.gov. *JAMA* 2015;314:2566–2567.

26. Moses III H, Matheson DHM, Cairns-Smith S, et al. The anatomy of medical research. US and international comparisons. *JAMA* 2015;313:174–189.

27. Angell M. Drug companies and doctors: a story of corruption. *New York Review of Books* January 15, 2009;56(1).

28. Public Citizen. Twenty-seven years of pharmaceutical industry criminal and civil penalties, March 14, 2018. https://citizen.org/our-work/health-and-safety/pharmaceutical-industry-penalties.

29. Bahrami S, Steen NE, Shadrin A, et al. Shared genetic loci between body mass index and major psychiatric disorders. A genome-wide association study. *JAMA Psychiatry*. Doi:10.1001/jamapsychiatry.2019.4188. Published online January 8, 2020.

30. Peterson C, Sussell A, Li J, et al. Suicide rates by industry and occupation—National violent death reporting system, 32 states, 2016. *MMWR Morbidity and Mortality Weekly Report* 2020;69:57–62.

31. Ramos S, Gradyj C, Greely HT, et al. The NIH BRAIN Initiative: integrating neuroethics and neuroscience. *Neuron* 2019;101.

32. Armstrong K, Asch DA. Bridging polarization in medicine—from biology to social causes. *New England Journal of Medicine* 2020;382:888–889.

33. Case A, Deaton A. *Deaths of Despair and the Future of Capitalism*. Princeton University Press, Princeton NJ, 2020.

1   The Biological Revolution in Psychiatry

An Overview of the Dark Ages

Introduction

With the advent of the first antipsychotic and antidepressant into clinical practice in the 1950s, the stage seemed set for a much-needed revolution in the care of the mentally ill. Readers who've viewed the PBS production[1] of *The Lobotomist: The Walter Freeman Story* will no doubt remember the haunting images of patients locked away in the hallways and wards of St. Elizabeth's in Washington, DC, sometimes naked or nearly so, often rocking or lying in a fetal position, forlorn and forgotten. The images of those poor souls immediately stirred memories of a three-month training period at the Longview State Hospital in Cincinnati, a regular rotation for psychiatry residents at the Cincinnati General Hospital in the 1960s. I was on an upper floor of the administration building and happened to look down on a lobby area, where a woman was seated alone on a fountain, half-dressed, appearing motionless and perhaps catatonic. A few days later, I later assisted while she was given electroconvulsive therapy (ECT) without anesthesia or a muscle-paralyzing agent, resulting in a full-blown seizure and a near-faint for me—and this was 30 years after Dr. Freeman roamed the halls of St. Elizabeth's!

What Led to the Snake Pits?

But back to Dr. Freeman and lobotomy. Conditions were so bad in the 19th and early 20th centuries that not even *The Lobotomist* could show the more disturbing acts so common in the asylum: beatings, rape, self-mutilation, and suicide, not to mention the radical and usually toxic therapies inflicted on helpless patients—including lobotomies.[2, pp. 9–13] The era of moral treatment in American psychiatry, begun in the early 1800s and marked by an optimistic approach to treatment involving occupational, work, and group therapies,[3, p. 175] had been badly damaged, not only by the Civil War and its consequences but also by a growing pessimism about treatment outcome.[4, p. 297]

What accounted for that change in attitude? The 1860s and 1870s marked a turning point, with a rapid accumulation of chronically ill patients, severe overcrowding, and an increased emphasis on heredity, racial prejudice, and degeneracy,[3, p. 179] all of which influenced the public view of institutional psychiatry and the mentally ill. This did not occur in a cultural vacuum, but instead in the context of a massive influx of destitute immigrants, who were labeled as not only degenerate but also a threat to the racial purity of the population. Poverty, whether in the immigrant population or among the insane, was viewed as the result of vice, so punitive "therapies" were seen as justified. The term "foreign insane pauperism" became central to the view of immigrants and the mentally ill,[3, p. 179] a view held by many prominent academicians, among them the president of the Rockefeller Institute and a Harvard professor of anthropology, who likened the insane to "malignant growths and poisonous slime."[Cited in 2, p. 56]

Not surprisingly, the patient population expanded dramatically. In 1880, the average state hospital held about 500 patients,[2] but this figure was dwarfed by any number of institutions, including Milledgeville in Georgia, which held some 14,000, and a complex in New York State that housed about 30,000 patients.[5, p. 260] Some 40% of 182 state hospitals held between 1,500 and 4,500 patients,[2] while the number of mental hospitals grew from 18 in 1840 to 139 in 1880. The length of hospital confinement grew as well. In 1904, almost 40% of patients were hospitalized for five years or longer, but by 1923, this had increased to 54%. Money spent on patient care in the asylums began to decrease, while expenditures increased in general hospitals, adding to the stigma experienced by the mentally ill and their caregivers.[2]

In the meantime, the influx of immigrants, the costs of caring for them, and the concerns over pollution of the population led to multiple acts of legislation aimed at stopping the flow of immigrants, including the Chinese Exclusion Act of 1882, the Immigration Act of 1924, and the National Origins Act,[6, 7] further stigmatizing both immigrants and the mentally ill and providing additional rationale for the brutal treatment of those confined in the asylums.

Indeed, what was being done for these patients in the psychiatric dark ages between 1850 and the 1940s? Not much, and what was done was often toxic.[8, pp. 33–40] Many of the drugs were addicting, including opium and barbiturates, while others, such as arsenic and mercury, were clearly neurotoxic. Any number of animal products had been used for years—and not just in the asylums—including sheep brains for insomnia and rabbit testicles for impotence. No approach was too outrageous, so the catalogue of horrors grew quickly. Patients were injected with horse blood and subjected to bleeding, purging, waterboarding, ice baths, and whole-body hyperthermia. They had their skin severely blistered, were made dizzy and nauseous by strapping them into rapidly spinning chairs, and had their teeth pulled to rid them of infectious foci. Virtually every body organ was blamed for their "degenerate state," so out came the ovaries, uterus, colon, thyroid, and testicles.

Despite the mayhem, not even Gerald Grob,[9] in his detailed analysis of mental illness in America, saw a link between these so-called treatments and the high patient mortality rates. For example, he cited a 1931 study of all first admissions to state hospitals in New York where, of every 100 admissions, 42 died in the hospital. He then blamed the high death rate on admission policies rather than the outlandish treatment methods! In fairness, he did acknowledge the mortality rate associated with insulin shock treatment and the high rate of injuries in patients given metrazole-induced convulsive therapy, but the links in those instances were obvious. But Grob wasn't the only contemporary author to gloss over the barbaric treatment methods so characteristic of the asylum. For example, Ross Baldessarini, a prominent psychopharmacologist from the McLean Hospital in Boston, not long ago listed a few of these therapies but said that, by today's standards, such methods appear punitive,[10, p. 373] light criticism indeed.

Despite the lack of convincing evidence that any of these treatment approaches actually worked, the rapid increase in the number of "biological" therapies in the late 1920s and throughout the 1930s did result in a temporary resurgence of therapeutic optimism. Many popular magazines and newspapers ran favorable stories on convulsive therapy, fever therapy, and, eventually, prefrontal lobotomy. The latter became a significant factor in the new wave of treatment methods, due in no small part to the sophisticated use of the media by Walter Freeman and his tireless tours of the country, teaching the technique and lobotomizing patients wherever he found them.

Genetics and Degeneracy in the Early Years

Yet for all these alleged advances, the numbers of patients kept increasing. By 1939, about 425,000 patients were in various institutions, with the majority in state hospitals. Given the emphasis on heredity, states began enacting laws banning marriage in the late 19th century. By 1914, more than 20 states had enacted such laws.[2, p. 36] Taking matters even further, states then began legalizing compulsory sterilization of the mentally ill. In 1927, compulsory sterilization was upheld by the U.S. Supreme Court, making this the first country to support such a practice.[11] About half the 45,000 "defectives" sterilized by 1945 were in mental hospitals.[2, p. 60]

We cannot emphasize enough the fact that these approaches to mental illness—based on the fundamental ideas that the mentally ill were degenerate, beyond hope, and therefore not fully human—were supported by prominent institutions such as the Rockefeller Foundation and prestigious medical journals, including *The New England Journal of Medicine*. Funding of the eugenics movement was provided by luminaries such as Andrew Carnegie, John D. Rockefeller, and Mary Harriman. A number of Ivy League schools began teaching eugenics and writing papers on the subject, yielding some 9,000 articles by 1924.[2, 6, 10] The comments about those with mental illness grew more and more vicious. For example: immigrants and the mentally ill were cancers on the body politic, a bacterial invasion, malignant biological growths, social wastage, viruses, and, of course, a burden on taxpayers.

A semblance of respectability was added by the genetic studies of Franz Kallmann, who in 1938 published a study in *Eugenics News*,[12, p. 105] purporting to show that children of parents with schizophrenia had a 16% chance of becoming schizophrenic, while their full siblings had an 11% chance. He apparently felt comfortable in making the diagnosis in relatives, even if they had died. In 1946, Kallmann published additional sets of data collected from patients in psychiatric hospitals in New York.[13] He included data on monozygotic (identical) and dizygotic (fraternal) twins, demonstrating that monozygotic twins had a concordance rate of 86% compared with 14% in dizygotic twins. This was a very substantial difference and gave a tremendous boost to the notion that genetics must play a major role in the development of mental illnesses.

However, there were serious problems with the data, not the least of which was accuracy of diagnosis, whether in the index patient or the relatives. We have to remember that there were no established sets of diagnostic criteria in 1938 or, for that matter, even in the 1940s and 1950s. In addition, determining zygosity was simply a matter of guesswork. Despite growing concerns about the validity of Kallmann's data, Eliot Slater, another pioneer in genetic research, wrote that "these suspicions had been entirely discredited."[14, p. 22]

What led Slater to that conclusion? The diagnostic criteria cited by Slater included (1) a diagnosis of schizophrenia in a mental hospital at the time when investigated by Kallmann, (2) the patient had a diagnosis of schizophrenia by the end of the stay, and (3) the patient was diagnosed by Kallmann with definite schizophrenia. These criteria are preposterous on their face, since we have no idea of the symptoms or combinations of symptoms used by Kallmann or the hospital psychiatrists. Kallmann's position on the damage allegedly done by people with schizophrenia was clearly supportive of the popular notion that they were degenerate and deserved to be sterilized. Indeed, his view of the character of those with schizophrenia was extraordinarily harsh. He insisted they were asocial eccentrics, criminal offenders, and inferior people.

There is no doubt about the ideological source of Kallmann's work, as well as that of the genetic work of his mentor, Ernst Rüdin, who served on a task force charged with developing the German laws on sterilization, the chair of which was Heinrich Himmler, as noted by Lewontin and his colleagues in their outstanding critique *Not in Our Genes*.[15, p. 207] Lewontin and his co-authors expressed some surprise that so many contemporary studies continued to cite Kallmann's deeply flawed and ideologically biased studies as examples of the scientific foundations of genetic influences in schizophrenia. Yet the data published by Kallmann and others is still cited in texts and papers published in 2008,[16, p. 258] although the methodological flaws have been severely and repeatedly criticized.

It is now abundantly clear that the concordance rate for MZ twins is less than half what Kallmann proposed, and there is no evidence whatsoever that schizophrenia is due to a recessive gene.[17] We shall discuss current work in genetics later, but I will emphasize right now that the pursuit of the genetic basis of schizophrenia and other psychiatric disorders has not only continued but has also greatly intensified with the advent of genome-wide association studies (GWAS). However, there is no evidence at this point that a genetic study can provide external validation of any psychiatric diagnosis or offer a path to prevention or treatment.[18–20] One can only wonder, given the dogged pursuit of the genetic base of this disorder—a pursuit that has required a tremendous amount of money and time with little practical payoff—if there isn't some carry-over from the Kallmann-Rüdin days of viewing these patients as fundamentally degenerate, although no one would dare use the word today.

Paradoxically, a number of studies[21, 22] have shown, contrary to predictions, *that the stigma of mental illness has not decreased with the shift to biological explanations of mental illness; rather, it has increased!*

A Time for Change?

Small wonder that by the late 1940s, the time was ripe for investigations into the horrendous conditions in the state hospitals. Unfortunately, organized medicine was not helpful. Robert Whitake [2, pp. 70–72] noted that the American Medical Association even suppressed the gruesome details of a report submitted by a physician it had hired to look at the state hospitals. As we shall see, this was not the only instance of organized medicine/psychiatry taking years—if not decades—to recognize the damage done to patients: witness the history of prefrontal lobotomy and, more recently, the neurologic side effects of antipsychotics. Nevertheless, other investigations in Ohio and elsewhere convincingly documented the inhumane treatment of the mentally ill. For example, an Ohio grand jury looking into conditions at the Cleveland State Hospital wondered how a civilized society could permit human beings to be treated with methods that were barbaric and inhumane.

Yet the surge of bad publicity failed to dramatically change matters. By the mid-1940s, electroconvulsive therapy (ECT) and prefrontal lobotomies were beginning to supplant insulin coma, but the latter would remain in use for another decade. Lobotomies were becoming increasingly common and were used on a wider array of patients—including children and adolescents—thanks to the tireless crusades of Walter Freeman, who had long since forgotten his own rule that lobotomy should be used as a last resort.[8] However, as reports of lobotomy-associated deaths and brain damage poured in, organized medicine finally said enough is enough. Dr. Freeman was thrown out of St Elizabeth's, but he opened a practice in California. After another patient died during a lobotomy, he was denied further hospital privileges, but he still traveled the country, visiting patients and claiming success. We have to admit, however, that Freeman had been appalled by the conditions at St. Elizabeth's and was determined to find an effective treatment, rather than allowing patients to languish for years. Ironically, lobotomy wound up causing many patients to remain in a permanent childlike state, bereft of motivation and curiosity.

It is clear that much of the first chapter of the biological revolution was founded on bad science, bad judgment, and neglect of the most fundamental rights of patients, including consent to treatment or due process should forced treatment be necessary. With regard to science, there were a few exceptions, including the discovery in the late 1800sof chloral hydrate, which was soon used as a sedative, as were barbiturates, discovered in the early 1900s.[23, pp. 43, 44] By 1940, John Cade was working on lithium.[24] After injecting urine from patients with schizophrenia, mania, or depression into the abdominal cavity of guinea pigs, he noted that the urine from manic patients seemed more toxic, so he developed a hypothesis about the roots of mania lying in the toxicity of urea. He also came to believe that urea toxicity was potentiated by uric acid but that creatinine was protective. However, injections of lithium urate proved to have a significant calming effect on the animals, contrary to his assumptions. After testing lithium urate on himself, he proceeded to test it on patients with mania and published the results in 1949.[24]

Although the results were positive, drug companies had little interest, since lithium is found naturally in the body, albeit in very small amounts.[25] In addition, many were skeptical about its safety, given the fact that lithium had been banned in the United States. Unfortunately, the drug had been used as a diuretic, but the narrow toxic-therapeutic ratio of the drug was not understood, and there was no way to accurately measure blood levels. The end result was a number of deaths.[23] Despite this rather tortuous and prolonged pathway, at least Cade had a reasonable hypothesis and used animal experiments to confirm his ideas, rather than simply hauling the drug off to the nearest state hospital and passing it out to unsuspecting patients.

We should point out, too, that research on brain function was in its infancy. Marcus Raichle, in his review of brain mapping,[26] noted that in the 19th century, one investigator had found that blood flow in the brain increased when patients did some mathematical tests, but these observations were made by looking at changes in the brain seen through defects in the skull! In 1890, other researchers began to look at the relationship between blood flow and brain function, followed by a number of confirmatory observations. However, it wasn't until 1948 that more exact, quantitative methods were published, which eventually led to methods of looking at regional blood flow. By the end of the 1970s, work on CT and MRI scans was well underway, with PET scanning soon to follow, then fMRI and other increasingly sophisticated instruments. However, a meta-analysis and meta-regression of 98 MRI and CT studies of bipolar disorder published in 2008 found only nonspecific changes,[27] a common outcome of imaging studies[28] and a clue that our current goal of developing precision medicines based on structural brain changes and genetic data has not been successful.[29]

References

1. Goodman B, Maggio J. *The Lobotomist*. WGBH Educational Foundation, 2008. www.pbs.org/wbhh.americanexperience/films/lobotomist.
2. Whitaker R. *Mad in America: Bad Science, Bad Medicine, and the Enduring Mistreatment of the Mentally Ill*. Perseus Publishing, Cambridge MA, 2002.
3. Bockoven JS. Moral treatment in American psychiatry. *Journal of Nervous and Mental Disease* 1956;124:167–194.
4. Bockhoven JS. Moral treatment in American psychiatry. *Journal of Nervous and Mental Disease* 1956;124:292–321.
5. Scull A. *Madness in Civilization. A Cultural History of Insanity From the Bible to Freud, From the Madhouse to Modern Medicine*. Princeton University Press, Princeton NJ and Oxford, 2015.
6. Okrent D. *The Guarded Gate; Bigotry, Eugenics, and the Law That Kept Two Generations of Jews, Italians, and Other European Immigrants Out of America*. Scribner, New York, 2019, pp. 98, 99, 293, 333.
7. Lepore J. *These Truths. A History of the United States*. W.W. Norton & Company, New York and London, 2018.
8. Valenstein ES. *Great and Desperate Cures. The Rise and Decline of Psychosurgery and Other Radical Treatments for Mental Illness*. Basic Books, New York, 1986.
9. Grob G. *Mental Illness and American Society, 1875–1940*. Princeton University Press, Princeton NJ, 1983.
10. Baldessarini RJ. American biological psychiatry and psychopharmacology, 1944–1944. In: *American Psychiatry After World War II (1944–1994)*. Editors: Menninger RS, Nemiah JC. American Psychiatric Press, Washington, DC and London, 2000.
11. Cohen A. *Im.be.ciles. The Supreme Court, American Eugenics, and the Sterilization of Carrie Buck*. Penguin Press, New York, 2016.
12. Kallmann F. Heredity, reproduction and eugenic procedure in the field of schizophrenia. *Eugenics News* November–December 23, 1938.
13. Kallmann F. The genetic theory of schizophrenia. An analysis of 691 schizophrenic twin index families. *American Journal of Psychiatry* 1946;151:188–198.
14. Slater ES. A review of earlier evidence in genetic factors in schizophrenia. In: *Transmission of Schizophrenia*. Editors: Rosenthal D, Kety SS. Pergamon Press, LTD, London, 1968.
15. Lewontin RC, Rose S, Kamin LJ. *Not In Our Genes*. Pantheon Press, New York, 1984.
16. Merikangas KR. Genetic epidemiology of mental disorders. In: *Psychiatry*, Third Edition. Editors: Tasman A, et al. Wiley-Blackwell, Chichester, West Sussex, 2008.
17. Gershon ES, Alliey-Rodriguez N, Liu C. After GWAS: searching for genetic risk for schizophrenia and bipolar disorder. *American Journal of Psychiatry* 2011;168:253–256.
18. Hardy H. Psychiatric genetics: are we there yet? *JAMA Psychiatry* 2013;70:569–570.
19. Leo J. The search for schizophrenia genes. *Issues in Science and Technology* Winter 2016;68–71.
20. Schizophrenia Working Group of the Psychiatric Genetics Consortium. Biological insights from 108 schizophrenia-associated loci. *Nature* 2014. Doi:10.1038//nature13595.
21. Angermeyer M, Matschinger H. Causal beliefs and attitudes toward people with schizophrenia. *British Journal of Psychiatry* 2005;186:331–334.

22. Jorm AF, Griffiths KM. The public's stigmatizing attitudes toward people with mental disorders: how important are biomedical conceptualizations? *Acta Psychiatrica Scandinavica* 2008;118:315–321.

23. Healy D. *The Creation of Psychopharmacology*. Harvard University Press, Cambridge MA and London, 2002. Interestingly, Healy predicted that the use of lithium would end with the death of Shou (p. 49), but it remains fairly popular.

24. Cade JF. Lithium salts in the treatment of psychotic excitement. *Medical Journal of Australia* 1949;2:349–352.

25. Schou M. The treatment of manic psychosis by the administration of lithium salts. *Journal of Neurology, Neurosurgery and Psychiatry* 1954;17:250–260.

26. Raichle ME. A brief history of human brain mapping. *Trends in Neurosciences* 2008;32:118–126.

27. Kempton MJ, Geddes JR, Ettinger U, et al. Meta-analysis, data base, and meta-regression of 98 structural imaging studies in bipolar disorder. *Archives of General Psychiatry* 2008;65:1017–1932.

28. Fusar-Poli P, Meyer-Lindeberg A. Forty years of structural neuroimaging in psychosis: promises and truth. *Acta Psychiatrica Scandinavica* 2016;134:204–224.

29. Visscher PM, Wray NR, Zhang Q, et al. 10 years of GWAS discovery: biology, function, and translation. *The American Journal of Human Genetics* 2017;101:5–22.

2 The Biological Revolution

The Middle Years and the Rise of Psychopharmacology

Introduction

Following the collapse of the era of moral treatment in psychiatry, the era of therapeutic optimism collapsed as well. However, the development of insulin coma therapy, electroconvulsive therapy, and prefrontal lobotomies led to a resurgence of optimism, despite the catalogue of horrors inflicted on the patients, including waterboarding, organ removal, and a variety of punitive tactics, including restraints and physical punishment. Yet developments in medicine, including the discovery of the bacterial causes of tuberculosis and syphilis, spurred interest in the possibility of similar advances in psychiatry, although these began with several observations that initially seemed to have few direct connections to mental disorders.

The Rise of Psychopharmacology

In 1952, a report came out of France describing the calming effect of an antihistamine, chlorpromazine, developed by a French company, Rhone-Poulenc.[1, pp. 76–126] This followed an earlier discovery by Henri Laborit of a somewhat different agent, promethazine, which had been targeted as an adjunctive agent for anesthesia. However, chlorpromazine, soon to be marketed in the United States as Thorazine, began to take center stage after two French psychiatrists, Jean Delay and Pierre Deniker, reported that chlorpromazine had not only calmed eight psychotic patients but had also decreased their hallucinations. We should mention that this report dovetailed nicely with studies on the calming effects of reserpine, which, for all the attention given to chlorpromazine, was of even greater interest during the 1950s.

Unfortunately, it was immediately obvious that chlorpromazine was causing neurologic side effects,[2] including motor slowing, tremor, restlessness, and rigidity—hallmarks of Parkinson's disease. These were so severe that psychiatrists used terms such as "apathetic," "immobile," "vegetative," "waxlike," and "indifferent" to describe their patients. Nevertheless, these motor and psychological symptoms were seen as therapeutic goals, as specifically noted by Lehmann and Hanrahan,[3, p. 229] who wrote that "*The aim* [of chlorproma-zine] *is to produce a state of motor retardation, emotional indifference, and somno-lence.*" Further, the dose must be increased as tolerance develops. This in itself is alarming, since one assumes that when the patient was lucky enough to break out of this zombielike state, the doctor would promptly increase the dose! They further noted that when left alone, patients remained largely silent, with motor slowing, but nevertheless were capable of concentrating and reflecting! These symptoms were so profound that Anton-Stephens in 1954 likened the effects to a lobotomy,[4] as did Delay and Deniker.[5]

Since these motor changes were the *primary* goals of treatment, it seems logical that investigators claimed that the side effects of chlorpromazine were minor. At the same time, given the correspondence between the motor effects of encephalitic parkinsonism and those of chlorpromazine, it's easy to under-stand why Delay and Deniker cautioned that the new drugs might cause an epidemic of encephalitis.[5] If that weren't enough, by 1957, papers[6] began to focus on another drug-induced movement disorder, tardive dyskinesia (TD), a condition that haunts us even today. Indeed, the appearance of TD presented a greater problem for biological psychiatry than did antipsychotic-induced parkinsonism, since there was no plausible way of linking TD to a therapeutic effect—but we will have much more to say on this later.

A closer reading of Lehmann and Hanrahan's paper[3] reveals a number of points relevant to our situation today. These include a belief that chlor-promazine could provide a path back to the essential work of understand-ing patients, a goal that had been badly damaged by the use of "comas, shocks, convulsions, confusion and amnesia," all of which severely impaired the patient-psychiatrist relationship."[3, p. 235] Nevertheless, how the goal of understanding patients could be reconciled with the goal of inducing emo-tional indifference and immobility was illogical, but at least the authors acknowledged the pitfalls of insulin coma and the other highly intrusive and sometimes brain-damaging therapies. They also re-emphasized the goals set for psychiatrists a century earlier by the advocates of moral treatment in psychiatry, goals that included the integration of education, work, and play in order to maximize the individual's growth and ability to enjoy life.

Are psychiatrists aiming at these goals today? Sadly, we seem to have reversed course. No wonder that Hobson and Leonard titled their 2001 book *Out of its Mind: Psychiatry in Crisis, a Call for Reform*, with their central tenet being psychiatry's drift into "depersonalized biomedicine,"[7, p. 129] a shift also criticized by Daniel Carlat in his entertaining book *Unhinged*.[8] An all-too-familiar example: the practice of 15-to-30-minute med checks, wherein the psychiatrist reviews drugs, dosing, and side effects; checks on symptoms; and then politely boots the patient out of the office with an appointment three to six months later. This approach was highly recommended by no less than Nancy Andreasen, former editor of the *American Journal of Psychiatry*, who, in her 1984 book[9, p. 31] *The Broken Brain*, accurately predicted "much shorter" office visits and infrequent appointments, with this approach being a primary component of the biological model. Obviously, something had to go, so out went the old focus on early trauma and parental relationships, items of interest to the old-fashioned shrinks. Paradoxically, Dr. Andreasen recommended helping patients with "all aspects" of their lives.[9, p. 31] How that could be accomplished in 15 to 30 minutes is no more obvious today than it was 35 years ago!

Back to Lehmann and Hanrahan, who observed that chlorpromazine could be used in a variety of illnesses, including schizophrenia, mania, mental deficiency, senile psychosis, and post-lobotomy excitement.[3] This, too, is eerily similar to 2020, when antipsychotics (APs) are being widely promoted as effective in a host of conditions, including depression, anxiety, eating disorders, ADHD, and PTSD, as well as other conditions not remotely similar to psychotic states, but much more on this later. Finally, Lehman and Hanrahan cautioned against using chlorpromazine as a sedative, a warning lost on subsequent generations of psychiatrists—including those in 2020, who are fond of prescribing quetiapine (Seroquel) for insomnia, despite the potential metabolic consequences, including severe weight gain, the development of diabetes mellitus (DM), and an increase in blood lipids.

Nevertheless, Lehmann and his associates in Montreal were not the only investigators targeting non-psychotic symptoms with chlorpromazine and similar agents. Kurland et al.,[10] in a widely recognized study, targeted anxiety, restlessness, hostility, and agitation, although the research population was reputedly dominated by those with schizophrenia. While the study scales included ratings of various psychotic symptoms, the ward physician enrolled patients based on whether a "tranquilizer" was indicated, in which case the patient was randomized to one of six chlorpromazine-like drugs (phenothiazines), phenobarbital (used as an active placebo), or an inert placebo over a six-week period. The authors found that phenothiazines were, in general, superior to the active or inert placebos on "total morbidity."

I have to admit that this was a rather sophisticated study, since it was double-blind, utilized both active and inactive placebos, and provided data on inter-rater reliability. Yet the study is also a prime example of problems found in most studies of that era, *including the absence of informed consent.* Patients had no choice with regard to participation, which is all the more disturbing since the protocol called for the drugs to be given by injection three times daily for two days, after which oral medication was used. The patient, of course, had no idea what to expect from these drugs, nor did the authors say what was done if the patient refused. (One can only assume that attendants forced the injections.) One has to admit, however, that such deficiencies were not confined to psychiatry. There was no law or rule with regard to informed consent before 1962, when the Kefauver bill was passed by Congress.[11, p. 162] In fact, the FDA had not set out any rules regarding the conduct of trials or what data had to be submitted with a new drug application. The FDA did not even require that animal studies be done prior to human studies!

Whatever misgivings the patients may have had were borne out by the very high rate at which patients failed to complete the Kurland study.[10] At the end of six weeks, only 24% remained in the study! Of the 33 patients assigned to chlorpromazine, *only* 27.3% completed the study, but this was not different from placebo. The authors are to be commended for their detailed description of the completion rate, but they did not discuss the impact of the low completion rate on study validity. Why were so few patients left at six weeks? Eight no longer required medications, but 33% were removed by the ward physicians due to lack of improvement. Another 11% were removed due to side effects, including neurologic side effects.

Remarkably, *we see similar completion rates today*, even in one of the best contemporary investigations, the CATIE study,[12] published in the *New England Journal of Medicine* in 2005, in which 74% of patients failed to complete the 18-month course of treatment with the first assigned drug! The fail rate in some of the other contemporary trials of atypical APs is somewhat better, but still large. For example, in the two pivotal trials necessary for FDA approval of risperidone (Risperdal), the dropout rates varied from 48%[13] to 25%.[14] In the four pivotal trials of olanzapine (Zyprexa), we find similar figures, with rates averaging 48%.[15]

What are we to make of the failure to retain patients in these trials? I wouldn't argue for a minute that such studies are difficult and that obtaining informed consent is becoming increasingly laborious and complex, but we must remember that given the need for informed consent and the FDA requirements with regard to safety, only competent patients can be enrolled. They cannot be actively suicidal or dangerous and/or have a recent history of illicit drug use. Nevertheless, trial patients are functioning at a higher level than the general patient population yet they still drop out at an alarming rate.

The high fail and dropout rates clearly raise questions about the validity of such trials, be they old or new. This has been addressed to some degree by the Cochrane Collaboration, an independent group of investigators who perform rigorous statistical analyses of treatment studies in all branches of medicine. In their reviews of AP trials, they almost uniformly cite the high dropout rates, noting, for example, that the attrition rate in risperidone trials renders "most of the efficacy and global improvement data unusable."[16] Similar comments can be found about quetiapine.[17] Remarkably, these caveats are often not mentioned in the major textbooks of psychiatry, despite a sometimes-thorough discussion of recent meta-analytic studies and other details.[18, pp. 795–813] I will have much more to say about recent studies of APs in the next chapter.

Chlorpromazine: Mechanisms of Action

What else did the discovery of chlorpromazine bring to the table? I must stress that there were a number of positives, including the search for its neurochemical effects. Given the role of the neurotransmitter dopamine (DA) in the development of Parkinson's disease, investigators began to focus on the role of DA in the action of chlorpromazine and the other early APs. Arvid Carlsson was among the pioneers in this area. Carlsson was aware of earlier work demonstrating that chlorpromazine could block the effects of reserpine, which had been shown to lower brain levels of DA and other monoamines such as norepinephrine (NE) and epinephrine (E). He and Lindqvist therefore began a study[19] on the effects of chlorpromazine and haloperidol (Haldol) on a metabolite of DA, 3-methoxytyramine (MT), and a metabolite of NE, normetanephrine (NM).

The results were fascinating. Both drugs increased brain levels of MT and NM but did not increase brain levels of DA or NE. They went on to propose that chlorpromazine and haloperidol *were blocking the cell receptors for these drugs*, thereby causing a compensatory activation of monoaminergic neurons. In other words, the presynaptic neurons that store neurotransmitters somehow realize that DA and NE are not reaching their target receptors, so they ramp up the outflow of these transmitters, a process that leads to more metabolites. This paper has been cited in virtually every textbook and review of psychopharmacology published to date, but very few have bothered to note that the subjects of this pioneering paper were not patients with schizophrenia, but nine mice.

Several years later, van Rossum[20] also proposed that APs act specifically by blocking DA receptors in the brain, citing as evidence not only the induction of parkinsonian side-effects by APs but also animal studies in which spiramide, a DA antagonist, blocked the DA-induced fall in blood pressure. The hypothesis of DA receptor blockade was correct: even today, *every FDA-approved AP used in the United States blocks certain DA receptors to one degree or another.* However, whether DA receptor blockade *is both necessary and sufficient* for the improvement of psychotic symptoms is another matter, since imaging studies have shown a similar degree of blockade in treatment-responsive and non-responsive patients.[21, 22]

Another boost for the antipsychotic properties of chlorpromazine came about with the discovery that it could block psychotic symptoms induced by LSD and mescaline, two hallucinogenic compounds that were the subject of a great deal of research in the 1950s. Interestingly enough, LSD, despite its hallucinogenic effects, became the subject of multiple papers seeking to demonstrate its therapeutic potential in a variety of psychiatric illnesses. (I shall describe later the resurgence of psychotogenic agents in the treatment of depression, a fascinating about-face for substances that have served as models for psychosis!)

Without doubt, the experimental work of Carlsson, van Rossum, and other pioneers was thought provoking and path breaking, especially compared with theories touting lobotomy, malaria therapy, and organ removal as cures for mental illness. Indeed, this work helped push psychiatry into the realm of science, but so did the work on reserpine, which demonstrated that reserpine could lower levels not only of DA but also of other transmitters, including serotonin (5-HT) and NE. Taken as a whole, these discoveries spawned the development of psychopharmacology and an entire research enterprise aimed at clarifying the relationship between brain chemicals, schizophrenia, mania, and depression.

Indeed, the receptor-blockading effects of APs led to a model of schizophrenia that came to dominate the field, *but* the model was developed by reasoning backward from the proposed mode of action of the drug to the etiology of the illness. Here's the sequence: Since APs block DA receptors and thus block the actions of DA, schizophrenia and perhaps other psychotic disorders might stem from an excess of DA: the first *dopaminergic hypothesis of schizophrenia*. Ironically enough, the Carlssons[23] would later modify their view on the model of excessive dopamine, noting that *even in the absence of dopamine*, a marked increase in behavioral activation can be produced in mice by suppressing glutamatergic transmission, thus paving the way for a theory involving an imbalance between dopamine and glutamine (an excitatory neurotransmitter) in subcortical areas. Others have called attention to the risks of focusing primarily on dopamine,[24] while Nestler and Hyman[25] have stressed the problems with reverse engineering, emphasizing that these abnormalities in schizophrenia are not precisely established.[25, p. 1165, 26] Not surprisingly, these biochemical findings have not been useful as biomarkers of mental disorders.

Small wonder that research has moved on to other areas, including (a) stimulation of so-called immediate early genes (IEGS), so named because they can respond quickly to drugs or environmental changes in the forebrain, thalamus, and other areas;[27, 28] (b) a deficit of alpha-7 nicotinic cholinergic receptors,[29] based on the observation that stimulation of these receptors by smoking seems to correct a defect in sensory gating, thought initially to be specific for schizophrenia; (c) stimulation of metabotropic glutamate receptors,[30] and (d) the potential of some antipsychotics to foster neuronal growth and protect neurons from toxicity.[31]

As with ADs, epigenetic changes are involved since APs can induce demethylation of DNA in the cortex,[32] a process thought to reverse the suppressive effects of hypermethylation on DNA function. Indeed, others[33] have shown that APs can affect chromatin remodeling, with increased transcription of IEGs such as c-fos. Given the ability of atypical, or second-generation, antipsychotics (SGAs) to block certain serotonin receptors, literally hundreds of papers have focused on serotonin as a culprit in the development of psychotic disorders, as well as depression. More recently, the focus has turned to a system of complex signaling pathways in the brain, looking at the effects of APs on glutamatergic, gabanergic, cholinergic, and other pathways[34] in the brain connectome.

Sadly, none of these findings, including well over 1,200 genetic studies of schizophrenia, have been definitive in terms of explaining how these drugs work or whether their associated neurochemical changes underlie the origin of schizophrenia or other psychiatric disorders. Nor have they given us any objective biomarkers of mental illnesses, topics I will return to later. But let's return to chlorpromazine and what it did and did not do for patients, the development of psychiatry, and changes in society.

Did Chlorpromazine Empty the State Hospitals?

Unfortunately, the ascendance of psychopharmacology was boosted by claims that proved to be highly questionable. A prime example: that the introduction of chlorpromazine in 1956 and 1957 was responsible for the massive reduction in the population of state psychiatric hospitals,[35, pp. 1921–1941] which had peaked at 558,000 in 1955. By 1960, the population had fallen to 535,000, and by 1965, it was down to 475,000. Indeed, Davis and Cole wrote in 1975[35, p. 1922] that these numbers were the primary proof of the efficacy of these agents, although 35 of 189 studies had found *no* differences from placebo. They added that about 66% of patients with schizophrenia improved significantly—far more than in current studies—and only 10% failed to be helped.

I shall return to these response rates later, but what about the mass exodus from the state and county hospitals? Was chlorpromazine the most important factor? There is no question that the increase in admissions not only saddled local and state agencies with a huge economic burden but also adversely affected the staffs, patients, and institutions due to severe overcrowding. Several examples: Pilgrim State Hospital on Long Island at one point cared for some 14,000 patients while Creedmoor in Queens housed at least 7,000![36]

The threats—and the possibility of bankruptcy—posed by the rapid increase in admissions was recognized by the Council of State Governments seven years before the introduction of APs. The council had recommended that community resources be developed, including outpatient clinics, and left no doubt that the *goal of state government was to reduce the volume of residential patients*. The same conclusions were reached by the National Governor's Conference on Mental Health, which took place several months before chlorpromazine was introduced.[37, p. 27]

A.B. Johnson, in her book *Out of Bedlam: The Truth About Deinstitutionalization*,[37] has explored in detail the early shift in thinking about the place of the mental hospital, which clearly had tilted toward almost universal condemnation, despite the positives later noted by Oliver Sacks in his essay *The Lost Virtues of the Asylum*.[36] Indeed, some had recommended that mental hospitals be completely phased out. What was to take their place? Community-based treatment.

From One Institution to Another: Another Type of Thorazine Shuffle

The problem, however, was that community treatment for the seriously and persistently mentally ill did not exist. There were no community mental health centers, a deficiency that was supposed to be addressed by the famous Joint Commission on Mental Illness and Health, funded in 1955. The failure of that effort to establish well-functioning community mental health centers is another story, but we know the results of deinstitutionalization: the wholesale transfer of patients to nursing homes, residential treatment centers, prisons, and the street. Johnson cites data from the U.S. General Accounting Office in 1977 noting that nursing homes had become the "largest single place of care for the mentally ill of all ages."[37, p. 119] John Talbott, in his review[38, p. 1113] of this phenomenon cited additional evidence demonstrating that the percentage of patients in institutions didn't change in the period from 1955 to1970; patients had simply moved to different institutions! The more relevant but awkward term for this process is "trans-institutionalization."

Interestingly, this concept crept into a 2005 study,[39] which found that the decline in beds during the 1970s in Europe was accompanied by an increase in forensic psychiatric beds and supported housing, although this varied among the six countries studied. The authors suggested that "reinstitutionalization" might be a suitable term. Another study in Austria[40] found a notable increase in admissions to forensic units following a 50% decline in mental health beds, but, remarkably enough, this surge in forensic admissions occurred *after* community health services were expanded in the 1990s. It appeared that the increase in admissions was dominated by patients who had committed offenses less severe than homicide or other dangerous behaviors but were seen as causing difficulties in the community.

Unfortunately, the maltreatment of the mentally ill has continued, as described by the *New York Times*[41] in 2011. The editorialist noted that Governor Andrew Cuomo had finally settled a lawsuit ending the long-standing practice of transferring patients from state hospitals into prisonlike nursing homes, where they were usually not allowed outside, suffered social isolation, and had little ability to contest their confinement. The settlement included a mandatory review of some 1,000 nursing home residents, with the aim of evaluating their potential for independent living, and the construction of some 200 units of housing. While these steps were badly needed, the editorial serves to remind us that we are still far from providing reasonable care for those most in need.

In any case, there is little doubt that the advent of chlorpromazine fit perfectly with the need to find some way out of the huge economic burden put on the states by the mental hospitals. Yet it appears certain that many patients were destined for discharge, regardless of chlorpromazine. But there is a certain irony to this process, in that the *very drug that fostered the discharge of patients from the state hospitals also hastened their transfer to nursing homes, jails, and the street*—a dubious gain and a disaster entirely ignored by Drs. Davis and Cole,[35, pp. 921–1945] who also neglected to mention the hospital readmission rate, which rose from 27% of intakes in 1956 to 65% in 1975;[37, p. 130] thus, the "revolving door syndrome."

A Model for Antidepressants

In the meantime, the model used for the development of APs was closely replicated by antidepressants (ADs), starting with the discovery of the first tricyclic antidepressant (TCA), imipramine (Tofranil), in the mid-1950s. Rather quickly, it was found that this drug seemed to work by blocking the reuptake of NE into the presynaptic nerve ending and, to a lesser extent, the reuptake of 5-HT (serotonin) and DA. The reuptake blockade prevented the metabolism of these neurotransmitters, which takes place largely in the presynaptic neuron, thus increasing brain levels at the synapse. It therefore seemed reasonable to propose that depression might be caused by a deficiency of these transmitters, so another model was born: the catecholamine hypothesis of depression.[42] As a bonus, one could also explain mania by positing an excess of these same neurotransmitters. Other early hypotheses included a primary deficiency of serotonin;[43] the permissive amine hypothesis, positing a primary derangement of serotonin accompanied by either an excess of amines→ depression or an excess of amines → mania;[44] and the cholinergic hypothesis, featuring an excess of acetylcholine compared with DA.[45]

Given the obvious need for both APs and ADs, the pharmaceutical industry in the late 1950s and 1960s very quickly began an effort to synthesize APs with properties similar to those of chlorpromazine, as well as ADs with properties similar to imipramine. Within a relatively short time, psychiatrists had an array of APs and ADs from which to choose, including trifluoperazine (Stelazine), thioridazine (Mellaril), and its primary metabolite mesoridazine (Serentil), and perphenazine (Trilafon), as well as others. New ADs in this era included amitryptyline (Elavil), nortryptyline (Aventil, Pamelor), desipramine (Pertofrane and Norpramin), and protryptyline (Vivactyl).

We shall have a great deal more to say about ADs later, but I should emphasize that investigators and industry continued to be enamored with the basic biochemical model involved in the development of imipramine, so it is not surprising that the rapid development of these agents was *not* paralleled by an increase in efficacy—which remains true even today. Moreover, TCAs were widely recognized as difficult to tolerate, due to their ability to block multiple brain receptors, including:

- muscarinic cholinergic → constipation, urinary retention, dry mouth, tachycardia, interference with memory;
- histamine-1 → sedation; and
- α-adrenergic → sedation, dizziness, fainting.

Worse, TCAs could be fatal in overdose, partly due to a delay in gastric emptying, such that patients hospitalized in the intensive care unit could deliver a new bolus of drug into the system in an unpredictable fashion, thus setting off a mad scramble to deal with another round of TCA poisoning. Another critical problem: cardiotoxicity with TCAs, including arrthymias and conduction delay with heart block. These problems were intensified by using a combination of TCAs with APs, especially chlorpromazine, thioridazine, and mesoridazine, which were also highly anticholinergic, antihistaminic, anti-adrenergic, and prone to the development of cardiotoxicity. Unfortunately, psychiatrists often felt it necessary to combine these drugs since some patients were psychotically depressed, setting the stage for the later epidemic of polypharmacy, a topic we will address in Chapter 6.

The Shift to High-Potency Antipsychotics

Given the multiple physiologic side effects of the early APs, the scramble was on to find newer drugs with fewer side effects. The result was an era of high-potency APs from about 1978 to the early 90s, during which haloperidol, fluphenazine (Prolixin), and thiothixene (Navane) were widely used. It quickly became apparent that about 2 to 3 milligrams (mg) of these agents were equal in AP potency to about 100 mg of chlorpromazine—a huge increase in potency. Moreover, these agents were considerably less potent at blocking other brain receptors largely responsible for non-neurological side-effects such as sedation, loss of memory, dry mouth, constipation, tachycardia, and dizziness or fainting.

The High-Dose Era With Antipsychotics

The combination of increased AP potency and decreased non-neurologic side effects proved irresistible to investigators and clinicians, who began prescribing these drugs in very high doses. For example, in 1968, Prien and Cole[46] compared patients treated with daily doses of 2,000 mg of chlorpromazine vs 300 mg daily vs a placebo group and a group treated with doctor's choice. The high-dose group had more improvement, but primarily in patients under 40 and in those hospitalized less than ten years. A similar study[47] found 80 mg of trifluoperazine superior to 15 mg daily or placebo. On the other hand, a later study[48] of trifluoperazine in doses of 60 mg vs 600 mg (!) in acutely ill patients with schizophrenia failed to find a significant difference in therapeutic effect.

In a small study[49] of ten highly dysfunctional patients ages 14 (!) to 27 who were said to give "volitional consent," in the form of written consent, fluphenazine was given in doses ranging from 300 mg to 1,200 mg daily for two to nine months. *The reader should know that 1,200 mg of fluphenazine daily is approximately equivalent to 60,000 mg of chlorpromazine,* an unheard of and, I might add, outrageous dose! Five were said to have a good-to-excellent response, while one became worse. The authors claimed that side effects were no worse in the high-dose group than in those taking 15 to 20 mg daily and added that parkinsonian side effects were worse in low doses.

However, this study was uncontrolled and used no rating scales. The clinical reports on each patient consisted of 5 or 6 lines of remarks on symptoms.

In another study published in 1976,[50] 50 chronically ill patients with schizophrenia were treated with 250 mg of the long-acting injectable form of fluphenazine (decanoate) and compared with a group of patients given 12.5 mg weekly. The high-dose group received doses at least 10 to 20 times greater than the standard dose of 25 mg IM every two weeks. The ward staff was free to prescribe additional meds, such as benzodiazepines, and/or ECT (!). These patients had been hospitalized a minimum of 12 months; 29 had been hospitalized for over ten years. The trial was double-blind and used a number of rating scales. All patients were said to have agreed to participation, but there was no mention of a formal consent.

Interestingly, both groups improved, and, while there were no significant differences at 24 weeks on the primary rating scale, the authors noted that the standard dose group had a stormier course, with three patients being withdrawn due to behavioral deterioration and nine others who required benzodiazepines or ECT, vs six in the high-dose group. They concluded that such high doses were unlikely to improve the lot of most patients but went on to recommend trials of up to 150 mg of fluphenazine decanoate every two to three weeks, still six times the standard maintenance treatment! In contrast to others, who had found low rates of neurologic side effects, they found tremor in 35%, oral dyskinesia in 22%, and akathisia in 22%, with lower rates in the standard dosing group.

As study methodology improved, the alleged improvements with high-dose APs began to fade, as they did in a 1991 study of haloperidol, given in doses of 10 mg to 80 mg daily.[51] By 1988, Ross Baldessarini et al., in a massive and highly cited study, concluded that the *evidence did not support the use of high doses of APs*. In addition, high doses not only failed to provide greater benefits, but also tended to yield inferior benefits.[52, p. 88]

Although psychiatrists had grown increasingly enamored with haloperidol—sometimes referred to as "vitamin H"—the patients were not so happy with their parkinsonian side effects. (In short order, the Thorazine shuffle had been replaced by the Haldol shuffle.) We should say, too, that the term "side effects" is more than a little misleading. The casual reader who sees the term might think that a side effect is an unintended result of a drug, and, in some cases, that may be correct. However, I must stress that the early APs were developed using animal models in which the potential value of the experimental drug was judged on the ability of the drug to produce parkinsonism, which, as I noted earlier, depended on the blockade of DA receptors. Thus, the classic symptoms of AP-induced parkinsonism, including tremor, muscle stiffness, and gait disturbances were—and are—*direct consequences of the drug-induced DA-receptor blockade.* As noted previously, some early investigators believed that a correlation existed between the degree of AP-induced parkinsonism and the therapeutic outcome,[53] which is clearly not the case.

In addition, it eventually became clear that DA blockade was inducing what came to be labeled as "neuroleptic dysphoria," a term describing a symptom complex of lethargy, depression, impaired motivation, and foggy thinking.[54, 55] Several of these authors noted the possible consequences: poor compliance, poor quality of life, relapse, and use of street drugs. An editorialist in *Biological Psychiatry*[56] also cited reports of mood swings, despondence, and crying episodes scattered in a number of papers, as well as anxiety and even panic attacks. The authors also called attention to a remarkable study[57] in which two investigators injected themselves with 5 mg of haloperidol and found themselves unable to work for 36 hours after losing energy and motivation. They did not feel sedated but instead experienced severe anxiety, which no doubt was acute-onset akathisia, a condition in which patients develops severe restlessness, anxiety, and a strong compulsion to move, although, in some instances, the patient may not feel subjectively restless.[58] The prevalence of this very disturbing side effect has varied from 8% to 76%,[59] and is still a problem with several of the latest APs, *including risperidone and aripiprazole (Abilify)*. Fortunately, the diagnosis of akathisia and other AP-induced movement disorders has been aided by the development of a number of rating scales[60] and objective instrumental measurements,[61] which we will describe in a later chapter.

Further Development of Antidepressants

In the meantime, development of ADs was proceeding in parallel with APs. Indeed, as with APs, some of the side effects became a bit more tolerable during drug development, since the blockade of histamine, cholinergic, and alpha-adrenergic receptors was weaker with agents such as desipramine and nortryptyline. Interestingly, these two drugs were simply metabolic products of the parent compounds (imipramine and amitryptyline). Obviously, if taking the parent drug, patients actually had both drugs in their systems. Put simply, if taking amitryptyline, the patient is actually taking two ADs, amitryptyline and its metabolite, nortryptyline.

This model of drug development was not exactly innovative but, in fact, set the model for what we see in this decade, when, for example, a metabolite of risperidone has been marketed as paliperidone, and a metabolite of the antidepressant venlafaxine (Effexor) has been marketed as desvenlafaxine (Prestique). I must point out that drug companies never compare the parent drug and metabolite in a controlled study prior to FDA approval and release into the marketplace. *Now here's a surprise: the metabolite is always much more expensive than the parent compound!*

Another, perhaps more subtle, consequence of this path to drug development was an introduction to polypharmacy, wherein two or more drugs of the same or different class are used to treat depression or psychosis. This approach, now the standard of care, received a boost in 2010 with the publication of a study[62] that found significantly greater improvement with combinations of ADs when compared with AD monotherapy. This study was the opening salvo in an effort to treat depression with at least two more ADs, a maneuver similar to that seen with APs, in which drug companies began marketing combinations based on the idea—never proven—that if two drugs could be given in lower doses, this might result in fewer side effects than one drug given in higher doses.

A 2012 review[63] of AD combinations found 3,662 studies, but only 5 met the entry criteria for an RCT in adults, wherein a combination of ADs is given at the start of treatment. The total number of patients was quite limited: 250 for efficacy and 284 for analysis of dropout rates. A combination of mirtazapine (Remeron) plus an SSRI was twice as likely as a single AD to yield remission. A combo of a TCA plus an SSRI was superior to an SSRI alone for both remission and response. The results on the surface looked good, if somewhat odd, but, as the authors pointed out, the number of RCTS was small, and there were a number of methodological problems, including possible publication bias, poor reporting of adverse events, and no placebo arm in any of the studies. In addition, only a limited number of ADs were studied, so the results could not be generalized. Nonetheless, the reader could see what the future would hold. In a later chapter, I will review the growing interest in combining a variety of drugs to treat depression.

Benefits and Costs of the Biological Revolution

By 1980, the biological revolution in psychiatry was well entrenched. We had a dramatic increase in the number of APs and ADs and a significant increase in testable hypotheses of mental disorders, including the catecholamine hypothesis of mood disorders and the DA hypothesis of schizophrenia—although both proved to be highly questionable and were soon replaced by hypotheses involving neuroprotection, cell-signaling mechanisms, genetic changes, and, more recently, epigenetic changes that involve alterations to DNA induced by external events, including stress and the drugs themselves.[64] There was more emphasis on quality of research design, and rating scales were proliferating, lending a semblance of objectivity to outcome studies, despite the fact that clinical rating scales are largely dependent on subjective responses by the patient, coupled with simple observations by the rater. Brain imaging was making considerable progress, with increasingly detailed images of relatively small groups of cells. Psychopharmacology was beginning to supplant psychotherapy as the first-line treatment for many disorders—a debatable development—and Big Pharma was on the way to record profits and a central role in funding research and medical education.

We cannot underestimate what the development of ADs and APs meant to the drug companies. In 1950, the retail cost of all prescription drugs was approximately $0.7 billion. By 1972, this had risen to about $5 billion,[65] but this increase was almost laughable compared with what would soon happen, such that by 2007, $25 billion yearly was being spent on APs and

ADs alone, thanks to the development and marketing of atypical (second-generation) APs, or SGAs, and SSRIs, starting with fluoxetine (Prozac). In 2009, the U.S. spent $15 billion on antipsychotics alone![66] Despite the explosion in costs, and a never-ending parade of additional ADs and APs, *clinicians and patients have seen little improvement in efficacy.* The exception may be clozapine.

The Clozapine Story

There is little question that clozapine (Clozaril) served as perhaps the most important model for the development of the SGAs, including risperidone, olanzapine, ziprasidone (Geodon), quetiapine, aripiprazole, paliperidone, and others, despite its multiple and sometimes very serious side effects. The most worrisome is bone marrow suppression (agranulocytosis) with the risk of death, although agranulocytosis occurs in less than 1% of patients and death in 0.03% of those.[67, 68] However, other problems are much more common,[69] including severe weight gain, adverse effects on blood sugar with the development of diabetes mellitus, an increase in triglycerides and cholesterol, and a host of other problems including seizures, drooling, sedation, pancreatitis, myocarditis, myocardiopathy, dizziness, fainting, and even parkinsonian motor problems and tardive dyskinesia, although the latter two conditions are much less common with clozapine than with conventional or first-generation APs (FGAs). We must emphasize the potential for impairment of gastrointestinal motility, which can lead to bowel obstruction, surgery, and even death.[70] The combination of clozapine with certain agents such as benzodiazepines (Valium [diazepam] and others) seriously increases the risk of fainting and other adverse events. Obviously, giving this drug to people already suffering from DM and/or obesity is not smart, nor can it be given to those with pre-existing bone marrow disease.

Given this nightmarish catalogue of adverse events, including death, why would anyone agree to prescribe clozapine, much less swallow it? Why did the FDA approve it in 1990? Well, the truth is that it *may* be the best AP available for those with treatment-resistant schizophrenia,[71] although some have challenged this assertion.[72, 73] and others have found no evidence that the drug increases levels of functioning.[74] Surprisingly, clozapine has been shown to have lower dropout rates in clinical trials, indicating more tolerability than one might imagine, and it's the only FDA-approved antipsychotic for the treatment of suicidality.

In order to minimize side effects and the risk of seizures, the drug must be started in very low doses (25 mg daily) and increased very gradually. A baseline complete blood count (CBC) is necessary, as is an EKG, and a CBC is needed every week for the first six months, then biweekly for another six months (FDA approval given in 1998) and, if all goes well, monthly until the drug is stopped. Even then, additional CBCs are required in order to be certain that the blood count remains normal.

So what is different about this drug, other than the potential for wrecking the bone marrow? A primary difference is the ability of clozapine to potently block certain post-synaptic serotonin (5-HT) receptors, in contrast to most FGAs such as perphenazine, haloperidol, and fluphenazine. Naturally, the drug companies began to think that a combination of DA and 5-HT blockade might lead to an increase in efficacy and perhaps a decrease in parkinsonian side effects. Janssen Laboratories had been experimenting with several 5-HT antagonists, including setoperone and then risperidone, which is a very potent dopamine D2 and 5-HT blocker. Indeed, every SGA developed since 1990 has been a potent 5-HT and DA-D2 blocker, with the exception of quetiapine and aripiprazole, about which we will say more later. However, clozapine, in contrast to FGAs and most SGAs, is considerably *less potent* in blocking the DA-D2 receptor subtype but more potent in blocking the DA-D1 and DA-D4 receptors.[75]

Another interesting but less well-known difference is the ability of clozapine to increase levels of NE in the frontal cortex,[75] an area where a deficiency of catecholamines (NE, DA) is thought to be important in the genesis of the negative symptoms of schizophrenia (lack of motivation, poverty of speech, and emotional blunting). Finally, this drug separates from DA receptors more rapidly than other APs, with the exception of quetiapine. On the positive side, this may be one reason why it has fewer parkinsonian side effects; on the other hand, skipping doses or suddenly stopping the drug may result in a rapid return of symptoms.[76] However, the notion that clozapine rapidly dissociates from the D2 receptor has been called into question.[77]

The Early History of Clozapine

Despite the early research by Janssen Laboratories on other 5-HT blockers, the biggest splash was made by clozapine—despite reports in Finland in the summer of 1975 of deaths from agranulocytosis, as reported in *The Lancet*[78] on September 27, 1975. (It had been licensed for clinical use in February.) The authors described 18 cases of severe blood disorders, with eight thought to be secondary to agranulocytosis. Another patient reportedly died of leukemia. This was a striking event, since in all of Finland, only 5 to 12 people had developed agranulocytosis annually. Further, some 500 to 2,000 patients had been given clozapine after licensing, and there had been no reports of serious adverse events in the earlier clinical trials.

The National Board of Health in Finland promptly banned the use of clozapine and began an investigation, positing an allergic reaction or perhaps product impurity as causes. On October 4, 1975, Griffith and Saameli from Sandoz LTD, the manufacturer, published a letter in *The Lancet*[79] noting four cases of agranulocytosis in clinical trials but raised doubts about a relationship to the drug in two of the cases. The origin of those four cases was not cited, but David Healy noted a report of four fatalities in 19 patients treated by Deniker, who apparently told the manufacturer the drug was not safe, a common feeling among psychiatrists in Paris.[1, p. 240] Another 12 cases had been reported to Sandoz post marketing. In July 1975, Sandoz notified the various regulatory agencies in countries where clozapine was being sold of the developments in Finland. However, the company pointed out that the frequency of such cases outside Finland was only 0.3/1000 patients. The company then cited earlier studies showing that tricyclic APs had resulted in a frequency of 0.1 to 0.8/1000 cases and concluded that "local factors" were a clear possibility—which was not the case.

Needless to say, research on clozapine almost stopped after the Finnish report, but other factors came into play, especially the fact that parkinsonian side effects were rare with clozapine, leading a number of investigators to conclude, in an echo of the early work on chlorpromazine, that clozapine could not be "a real neuroleptic."[80] Nevertheless, given the growing interest in APs that blocked both DA and 5-HT receptors, and the fact that these agents generally appeared to have a lower potential for neurologic side effects, John Kane and associates undertook a multi-center study of clozapine for the treatment of highly treatment-resistant patients with schizophrenia.[81] Although the authors found that 30% of these patients responded to clozapine, the study is notable for a number of other reasons—both good and bad—so the fine print is worth examining.

We have to say right away that a quality study of non-responders to FGAs among patients with schizophrenia was badly needed since fail rates of FGAs had ranged from 20% to 68%.[82, p. 196] That being the case, Kane et al. deliberately set out to enroll patients who (a) had failed to improve after being treated with at least two different APs from different chemical classes over the previous five years, (b) had experienced at least three treatment episodes, and (c) had been given doses of at least 1,000 mg of "chlorpromazine equivalents" for at least six weeks.

A few words about the term "chlorpromazine equivalents." This is a rough way of describing the clinical potency of an AP compared to the clinical potency found with a 100 mg daily dose of chlorpromazine. Thus, about 2 mg of haloperidol, 8 mg of perphenazine, 2 mg of risperidone, 5 mg of olanzapine, 50 mg of clozapine, etc., are held to be approximately equivalent to a 100 mg daily dose of chlorpromazine. However, these figures are inexact, to say the least. Indeed, the concept of dose equivalencies has been roundly criticized.[83]

The proposed subjects also had to meet DSM-3 criteria for schizophrenia (although no standardized diagnostic interviews were utilized) and had to be capable of giving informed consent. Nevertheless, the subjects were considered to be "beyond the reach of conventional therapy," a criterion not found in recent studies. So far, so good.

But, after some 14 days of baseline placebo, 305 patients began treatment with up to *60 mg daily of haloperidol* for six weeks in order to filter out any patients who were treatment responsive. However, a 60 mg per day dose translates into at least 3,000 mg of chlorpromazine daily, a dose at least nine times higher than the average dose thought to be associated with a clinical response! At no point did the authors justify the massive dose of haloperidol, but one assumes they did not want to be accused of undertreating the patients. But this isn't particularly convincing, given the existence of multiple studies showing that excessive doses of APs are not helpful and, in fact, could lead to higher rates of side effects.[69]

Indeed, the authors clearly expected a high rate of parkinsonism, so they prescribed 6 mg daily of benztropine, an anticholinergic drug used to combat neurologic side effects. This was done in order to level the playing field with clozapine. However, one would also expect significant side effects from benztropine, including dry mouth, constipation, urinary retention, and tachycardia. Indeed, dry mouth was significantly more prominent in the chlorpromazine/benztropine group, as was a drop in blood pressure. Remarkably, 80% completed this phase of the study, but the completion rate may have been largely secondary to the fact that the duration of the current hospitalization averaged 215 weeks.

Only 1.6% responded to haloperidol. Those who failed to respond (including 22 patients who could not tolerate it) entered a seven-day washout period—far too short to clear the massive doses of haloperidol from the brain—and were then randomized to clozapine at an average peak dose of 600 mg daily, or 1,800 mg daily of chlorpromazine, with the average peak dose reached by the fourth or fifth week of the six-week study. Completion rates were again much higher than those of contemporary studies, with 88% of those taking clozapine completing, as did 87% of those treated with chlorpromazine, a startling finding given the very high dose.

Clozapine clearly was superior to chlorpromazine, with significant improvement noted by the end of the first week. On the other hand, *only 30%* of those treated with clozapine responded, but this was significantly higher than the 4% who responded to chlorpromazine. On the face of it, the 30% response rate with clozapine doesn't seem impressive, but the directors of large institutions and health care plans no doubt welcomed the possibility of improvement in another 30% of patients. We should note as well that the effect size of -0.88 found by Kane et al. has *never* been replicated. George Simpson and his co-workers went on to write[84] that this study led to worldwide interest in clozapine and treatment-refractory schizophrenia. Indeed, risperidone (Risperdal) was launched in 1994 and olanzapine (Zyprexa) in 1996, followed by many others.

Yet, for all the positives in this study, important pieces of data were missing. For example: how many of these patients were suitable for discharge? It appears that doses were tapered down at the end of the study, but what happened next? After clozapine was stopped, did they worsen? The reader also had no idea of the cumulative dose of APs given prior to the study, to what extent ECT had been used, or whether—and to what extent—other psychotropic medications or other therapies had been given. It would be surprising indeed if these treatment-refractory patients had not been prescribed

antidepressants, ECT, or lithium. As in many psychopharmacological studies, the patient population was 80% male, and 65% Caucasian, so whether
these results were applicable to other populations could not be determined.
Fortunately, there were no cases of agranulocytosis, although the study was
too brief to fully evaluate the risk.

Moreover, several later studies of clozapine found even lower response
rates of 24% at six weeks vs 13% with haloperidol.[85] At one year, the response
rate with clozapine was 37% vs 32%, not significantly different from haloperidol, but close to the results found in Kane et al. Quality-of-life ratings did
not differ at one year, although clozapine-treated patients spent significantly
fewer days in the hospital and had fewer extrapyramidal side effects. Outpatient costs were significantly higher. Three patients treated with clozapine
developed agranulocytosis, but all recovered. In another controlled one-year
study,[86] *few differences were found between clozapine and chlorpromazine at 12
months*, which is more than surprising.

In a state hospital population, the authors found *no* significant response to
clozapine,[87] while Simpson and his group, who selected patients using the
same criteria used in the Kane study, found *no* responders to haloperidol![84]
Only 8% responded to the initial trial dose with clozapine and 2% with the
next dose. This was a rather complex dosing study, but the point is that of
50 patients, only 5 responded.

The Clozapine Story in Follow-Up: Clozapine vs First-Generation Antipsychotics (FGAs)

Since clozapine was the model for new AP development, not only because
of its possible effectiveness in treatment-resistant schizophrenia but also
because of its rather novel effects on DA and 5-HT receptors, we must ask
if this agent is effective under less-stringent conditions: that is, whether
patients who are less ill also respond. In a meta-analytic study[74] of thirty
trials involving 2,500 patients (both treatment and non-treatment resistant)
who had been randomized to either clozapine or FGAs, clozapine was superior to FGAs, with a number needed to treat (NNT) of 6: that is, 6 patients
would need to be treated with clozapine in order to achieve results superior
to those found with an FGA. (An NNT of less than 10 is generally regarded
as clinically important.) Clinical improvement in the subgroup of treatment-
resistant patients (429 patients), also favored clozapine. Despite these results,
several important caveats remained:

- Clozapine resulted in only a six-point difference in the Brief Psychiatric
  Rating Scale (BPRS), a standardized scale often used in such studies.
  Whether this difference is clinically meaningful—as opposed to statistically significant—is questionable. For example, let's say a patient has
  a BPRS score of 80 at study start, but, at end point, the FGA group
  has dropped to 55 while the clozapine group dropped to 49. Could

clinicians or patients tell the difference? (We shall see this problem again, when talking about antidepressants.)

- Additional analysis revealed that in those studies utilizing explicit diagnostic criteria—adding to the possibility that the patient indeed suffered from schizophrenia—*clozapine did not differ from FGAs in treatment acceptability, dropout rates, or prevention of relapse.* In addition, 21 of 30 studies were short term, lasting 4 to 8 weeks, although clozapine, in keeping with current thinking, has more advantages when given for 26 weeks or longer. The dropout rate with FGAs was 67%, but only 38% with clozapine, despite its side effects.
- Selection bias was thought to be a problem in 24 of the 30 studies and therefore more likely to favor clozapine.
- Finally, data on the practical consequences of treatment was skimpy indeed. Ability to work was assessed in only 6 trials, and *no trial examined the ability of patients to live in the community or how the illness affected the family.* Mortality was not examined in over 60% of the trials, and 24 of the 30 studies took place in a hospital setting. Additionally, there was no difference between the clozapine and FGA groups in readiness for hospital discharge. In the case of those deemed treatment resistant, there was no data at all on social functioning or ability to work.

In view of the many trials comparing clozapine to FGAs, the Cochrane Collaboration did an analysis[88] of 52 trials with 4,746 participants as of November 2008 and found *no significant differences in ability to work, suitability for discharge, or mortality.* However, clozapine was superior for symptom improvement (NNT of six, which is quite good) and fewer relapses and was more acceptable to patients in long-term treatment. Nevertheless, clozapine also led to more sedation, hypersalivation, and problems with temperature control than did FGAs.

Clozapine and Suicide

Among the major selling points for clozapine has been FDA approval for the prevention of suicide in schizophrenia—the only AP to win such a designation.[89] There is no doubt that suicide in schizophrenia is a very significant problem, with a lifetime rate of 9% to 13%.[89] However, in a meta-analysis of 61 studies, another group[90] found a lifetime prevalence of 4.9%, but if followed from illness onset or first admission, the rate jumped to 5.6%, still less than the commonly held rate.[91] Nevertheless, the risk of suicide was at least ten times that of the general population.

In the pivotal study used by the FDA to approve clozapine for the treatment of suicidality,[89] patients were selected on the basis of a high-risk profile, which included an attempt in the previous three years, current suicidality, or command hallucinations urging self-harm. (Note that such patients are almost always excluded from clinical trials, but in this case the institutional review boards gave permission.) Given the clinical risks, only the raters were blinded to the random assignment of patients to clozapine or olanzapine. During the 18-month trial period, 980 patients were enrolled, but 39% discontinued the study.

The study was far too small to accurately examine the rate of completed suicides, a problem recognized by the authors, who had estimated that as many as 20,000 would have been required for adequate statistical power. Note, too, that funding was provided by Novartis, the manufacturer of clozapine; additional funding was provided by several foundations. The authors assured us that the study design and analysis of the data were approved by the FDA. A suicide monitoring board determined the validity of the reported behaviors but note that the board members had been named by Novartis.

Compared with olanzapine, clozapine had a statistically significant advantage with regard to the number of suicide attempts, hospitalizations, and interventions aimed at preventing suicide. In addition, those treated with clozapine required fewer antidepressants and antianxiety agents. *Ironically, however, of the eight completed suicides, five were taking clozapine!* Similarly, the clozapine group also had more deaths (seven) from other causes than olanzapine (five), but these differences were not statistically significant. Overall, there was a 26% decreased risk of suicidality with clozapine.

I must stress that the company had a heavy hand in this study, with its financial support and its role in selecting the monitoring board. There was no comment about how the board was compensated. The lead investigator (H.Y. Meltzer) and a number of the principals had received grants from or were consultants to Novartis.

The Meltzer et al. study,[89] along with several other studies examining the influence of clozapine on suicidality, had several methodological problems, including the lack of a control group of patients not exposed to clozapine, and, where a control group had been used, the demographic data was poor. In contrast, Michael Sernyak and colleagues mounted a very large study[92] using the centralized Veterans Administration database, which enabled them to match patients given clozapine with a non-exposed group. The National Death Index was used to obtain causes of death in both groups. In addition, the data was analyzed using propensity scoring, a technique that maximizes the comparability of the treatment and control groups, thus helping to minimize selection bias. Compared with the Meltzer et al. study, the number of patients was much larger: 1,415 treated with clozapine and 2,830 in the control group, making statistical power considerably greater. The VA provided financial support. Both all-cause and cause-specific mortality rates were examined. Results?

First, those exposed to clozapine for any time period had a *statistically significant lower mortality rate compared to those with no exposure.* Interestingly, those taking clozapine had a significantly lower mortality rate from respiratory disease, probably because those patients with chronic obstructive pulmonary disease were less likely to be given clozapine. *When the respiratory-related deaths were removed from analysis, the rate of completed suicide did not differ in the two groups.* Nevertheless, the rates of completed suicide were high: 175/100,000 patient years in the never-exposed group vs 150/100,000 patient years in the clozapine group.

The authors confessed to several problems with the study, especially the inability to match groups on variables thought to be predictive of suicidality, including previous attempts or current suicidality. In addition, this was a VA population composed primarily of older male patients. Nevertheless, clozapine clearly *did not* protect against completed suicide, a finding that prompted letters to the *American Journal of Psychiatry* in February of 2002, with the writers emphasizing that at least six other studies had found significant reductions in attempts and completions in patients taking clozapine.

Clozapine vs Other SGAs

Given the many side effects of clozapine, it's logical to ask if this agent is superior to the newer SGAs. In an attempt to answer this question, one group[73] examined eight randomized, controlled trials involving 795 patients, most of whom were treatment resistant. There was no difference in clinical response rates between those given clozapine and other SGAs, but the studies did not include ziprasidone, aripiprazole, or quetiapine. While not statistically significant, there was a trend for clozapine to be *less* effective on negative symptoms—much in contrast to some studies—as well as less effective for positive symptoms. *In both groups, lack of improvement was high: 48% with clozapine and 46% for the other SGAs.* The overall dropout rate was 28% but did not differ between groups. The clozapine group had fewer neurologic side effects but more drooling and sedation. No deaths occurred, and there was no difference in blood disorders, but seven of the eight studies were short term; only one lasted 18 weeks. In common with the Wahlbeck et al. study,[74] there were no data on quality of life, ability to work, the burden on families, or cost effectiveness.

In a Cochrane Collaborative study,[93] the authors analyzed 27 blinded and randomized controlled trials comparing clozapine with other SGAs, finding that dropout rates were 30% and, in contrast to smaller studies, higher with clozapine. *Clozapine was not more effective* than other SGAs when examining the total BPRS score, *nor was it better with regard to negative symptoms.* Clozapine had fewer parkinsonian symptoms but more sedation and drooling, lower levels of white blood cells, and more weight gain than was found with risperidone. Other findings were less well documented but included a higher incidence of EKG changes and higher levels of triglycerides but, on the positive side, fewer changes in prolactin levels.

The debate about clozapine continues, as demonstrated by a 2010 editorial[94] in the *British Journal of Psychiatry*, with the provocative title "Clozapine, dangerous orphan of neglected friend?" The authors were clearly on the "friend" side of the equation, recommending that it be used as soon as the patient demonstrates resistance to standard first-line treatment, rather than using the drug as a last resort. However, the authors minimized the multiple side effects and potential metabolic complications of this agent. In the next chapter, we shall continue examining the effects of clozapine but in the context of a broader view of the efficacy and effectiveness of the SGAS in general, with the aim of establishing whether these agents have lived up to their hype.

The key questions: Are SGAs superior to FGAs? If so, in what regard? These are crucial questions, given the rapidity with which SGAs were accepted, the subsequent dramatic increase in their use—even in children—and the explosion in drug costs, now mitigated, at least in part, by the appearance of generic SGAs. In a review of pharmaco-epidemiologic studies, Verdoux and associates in 2010 reported[95] that the rate of AP use in office visits had increased two- to six-fold in adults, children, and adolescents, with expenditures rising correspondingly.

Clinical Notes

The rise of psychopharmacology, with the development of multiple APs and ADs, the use of pseudo-objective rating scales, and improvements in statistical analyses seem to represent a new era in psychiatry. However, the new era also led to markedly shorter clinical visits, less attention to personal histories, the rise of direct-to-consumer advertising, and the related dominance of Big Pharma, with its massive funding of drug studies and research. As we have already indicated, the commercialization of psychopharmacology has led to serious problems with publication bias and fraudulent behavior on the part of the drug companies and physicians.[96-99] So what can clinicians, patients, and families take away from this chapter?

1. First, the dropout rates in many drug studies are quite high, no doubt reflecting the difficulties patients have in tolerating these drugs. Clearly, the lowest possible dose should be used, and careful attention should be given to side effects. Let's face it: These drugs are difficult to tolerate! Strategies for monitoring compliance are rudimentary at best.

2. Systematic monitoring for neurological side effects is mandatory, as is monitoring for the metabolic syndrome. More attention should by paid to the possible cardiac effects of APs. Any patient with a history of cardiac disease should have a baseline EKG before starting an AP. We shall say much more on this in Chapter 3.

3. There is virtually no evidence to support the use of high doses of APs. Instead, we find more side effects, many of which are severe but at least somewhat amenable to treatment. The drugs used to treat neurologic side effects have their own side effects!

4. The usefulness of clozapine in those failing to respond to other agents has come under increased scrutiny. Another meta-analysis published in

2016 of APs in treatment-resistant schizophrenia[100] found "insufficient evidence" for the superiority of clozapine in these patients and, for that matter, "few significant differences in all outcomes" across all APs. Kane and Correll disagreed, however.[101]

5. Similarly, clozapine's effective in preventing suicide is questionable, despite the FDA approval.

6. The mortality rate with clozapine has fallen, making the risk-benefit ratio somewhat more acceptable. The FDA has approved a more relaxed schedule for laboratory studies, but caution is still needed. Agranulocytosis can be fatal but is rare. The drug should not be used with benzodiazepines. The early designation of clozapine as a "miracle drug" was overblown.

7. Remarkably, the debate over the comparative effectiveness of APs continues, despite almost 60 years of research. In 2014, a meta-analysis[102] of 128 controlled trials comparing chlorpromazine to 43 other APs concluded that chlorpromazine was superior to reserpine and 3 rarely used APs but was less effective than clozapine. However, there *were no significant differences* between chlorpromazine and 28 other APs, including several currently used SGAs, including risperidone, quetiapine, and ziprasidone. Again, we see evidence that the advent of multiple APs over the past 50 years has not resulted in consistent, clear-cut advantages over the older drugs, except for lower rates of parkinsonism and tardive dyskinesia. The trade-off, however, has been an increased rate of the metabolic syndrome with many of the SGAs. See the next chapter for more details.

8. The use of APs for non-psychotic conditions is rarely justified. AP polypharmacy should be avoided since we still lack high-quality, controlled evidence that a combination of two APs works better than a single agent, with the possible exception of adding aripiprazole to another AP in cases where negative symptoms are prominent.[103] We will explore this in greater detail in Chapter 6, including recent evidence indicating that combinations may be helpful in some cases.

9. Most studies have found lower relapse rates with long-term use of APs, with greater emphasis on the results found with long-term injectable antipsychotics (LAIs).[104] This is important since non-compliance with oral medications is in the 45% range. (The authors of this study also cited evidence indicating that LAIs should be considered in first-episode patients.) Nevertheless, questions have been raised about the wisdom of long-term maintenance give the side effects, including the loss of brain volume.[105] Yet we need to be concerned about relapse with medicine discontinuation, especially if this is done quickly.

10. Finally, there is evidence that non-drug approaches may be helpful, particularly cognitive therapy, as shown in a 2014 controlled trial.[106] The authors also cite studies indicating a favorable outcome when cognitive therapy is combined with medication.

References

1. Healy D. *The Creation of Psychopharmacology*. Harvard University Press, Cambridge MA and London, 2002, pp. 76–126.
2. Cohen I. Undesirable side-effects and clinical toxicity of chlorpromazine. *Journal of Clinical and Experimental Psychopathology* 1956;17:153–162.
3. Lehmann HE, Hanrahan GE. Chlorpromazine: new inhibiting agent for psychomotor excitement and manic states. *Archives of Neurology and Psychiatry* 1954;71:227–237.
4. Anton-Stephens D. Preliminary observations on the psychiatric uses of chlorpromazine (Largactil). *Journal of Mental Science* 1954;100:543–557.
5. Delay J, Deniker P. Trente-hiute cas de psychoses traits par la cure prolongee et continue de 4568 R. *Annales Medico-Psychologiques* 1952;110:364.
6. Schonecker M. Ein eigentumliches syndrome im oralen bereich bei megaphen applikaton. *Nervenartz* 1957;28:35.
7. Hobson JA, Leonard JA. *Out of Its Mind: Psychiatry in Crisis. A Call for Reform*. Perseus Publishing, Cambridge MA, 2001.
8. Carlat DJ. *Unhinged*. Free Press, New York, 2010.
9. Andreasen NC. *The Broken Brain*. Harper and Row, New York, 1984.
10. Kurland AA, Hanlon TE, Tatom MH, et al. The comparative effectiveness of six phenothiazine compounds, phenobarbital, and inert placebo in the treatment of acutely ill patients: global measures of severity of illness. *Journal of Nervous and Mental Disease* 1961;133:1–18.
11. Hilts PJ. *Protecting America's Health: The FDA, Business, and One Hundred Years of Regulation*. Alfred A. Knopf, New York, 2003.
12. Lieberman JA, Stroup TS, McEvoy JP, et al. Effectiveness of antipsychotic drugs in the treatment of patients with chronic schizophrenia. *New England Journal of Medicine* 2005;353:1209–1223.
13. Chouinard G, Jones B, Remington G, et al. A Canadian multicenter placebo-controlled study of fixed doses of risperidone and haloperidol in the treatment of chronic schizophrenic patients. *Journal of Clinical Psychopharmacology* 1993;13:25–40.
14. Peuskens J, Risperidone Study Group. Risperidone in the treatment of patients with chronic schizophrenia: a multi-national, multi-centre, double-blind, parallel group study vs haloperidol. *British Journal of Psychiatry* 1995;166:712–726.
15. *Psychiatric Times*. Advances in psychopharmacology. Olanzapine: a new atypical antipsychotic, May 1997.
16. Rattehalli RD, Jayaram MB, Smith M. Risperidone versus placebo for schizophrenia. *Cochrane Database of Systematic Reviews* 2010;(1). Art.no: CD006918. Doi:10.1002/14651858. CD006918.pub2.
17. Srisuapanont M, Disayavanish C, Taimkaew K. Quetiapine for schizophrenia (2). Art No. CD000967. Doi:10.1002/14651858.CD000967.pub2.
18. Levenson JL, Crouse EL, Bozymski KM. Psychopharmacology. In: *The American Psychiatric Association Publishing Textbook of Psychiatry*, Seventh Edition. Editor: Roberts LW. American Psychiatric Association Publishing, Washington DC, 2019, pp. 795–813.
19. Carlsson A, Lindqvist M. Effect of chlorpromazine or haloperidol on formation of 3-methoxytyramine and normetanephrine in mouse brain. *Acta Pharmacologica et Toxicologica* 1963;20:140–144.

20. van Rossum JM. The significance of dopamine-receptor blockade for the mechanism of action of neuroleptic drugs. *Archives Int Pharmacodynamics* 1966;160:492–494.

21. Wolkin A, Barouche F, Wolf P, et al. Dopamine blockade and clinical response: evidence for two biological subgroups of schizophrenia. *American Journal of Psychiatry* 1989;146:905–908.

22. Pilowsky LS, Costa DC, Ell PJ, et al. Antipsychotic medication, dopamine receptor blockade and clinical response: a [123] IBZM SPECT (single photon emission tomography) study. *Psychological Medicine* 1993;23:791–797.

23. Carlsson M, Carlsson A. Schizophrenia: a subcortical neurotransmitter imbalance. *Schizophrenia Bulletin* 1990;16:425–432.

24. Kane JM. Towards more effective antipsychotic treatment. *British Journal of Psychiatry* 1994;165(suppl 25):22–31.

25. Nestler EJ, Hyman SE. Animal models of neuropsychiatric disorders. *Nature Neuroscience* 2010;13:1161–1169.

26. Kambeitz J, Abi-Dargham A, Kapur S, et al. Alterations in cortical and extrastriatal dopamine function in schizophrenia: a systematic review and meta-analysis of imaging studies. *British Journal of Psychiatry* 2004. Doi:10.1192.bjp.bp.113.12308.

27. Robertson GS, Fiberger HC. Neuroleptics increase c-fos expression in the rat forebrain: contrasting effects of haloperidol and clozapine. *Neuroscience* 1992;46:315–328.

28. Deutch AY. Identification of the neural systems subserving the action of clozapine: clues from immediate-early gene expression. *Journal of Clinical Psychiatry* 1994;55:9(suppl B):37–42.

29. Freeman R, Adler LE, Bickford P, et al. Schizophrenia and nicotinic receptors. *Harvard Review of Psychiatry* 1994;2:179–192.

30. Patil ST, Zhang L, Martenyi F, et al. Activation of mGlu2/3 receptors as a new approach to treat schizophrenia: a randomized, phase 2 trial. *Nature Medicine* 2007;13:1102–1108.

31. Lieberman JA, Bymaster FP, Meltzer HY, et al. Antipsychotic drugs: comparison in animal models on efficacy, neurotransmitter regulation, and neuroprotection. *Pharmacology Reviews* 2008;60:358–403.

32. Dong E, Agis-Balboa RC, Simonini MV, et al. Clozapine and sulpiride but not haloperidol or olanzapine activate brain DNA demethylation. *Proceedings of the National Academy of Sciences* 2008;105:13614–13619.

33. Li J, Guo Y, Schroeder FA, Youngs RM, et al. Dopamine D2-like antagonists induce chromatin remodeling in striatal neurons through cyclic AMP-protein kinase A and NMDA receptor signaling. *Journal of Neurochemistry* 2004;90:1117–1131.

34. Karam CS, Ballon JS, Bivens NM, et al. Signaling pathways in schizophrenia: emerging targets and therapeutic strategies. *Trends in Pharmacological Sciences* 2010;31:381–390.

35. Davis JM, Cole J. Antipsychotic drugs. In: *Comprehensive Textbook of Psychiatry*, Second Edition. Editors: Freedman AM, Kaplan HI, Sadock BJ. The Williams & Wilkins Company, Baltimore MD, 1975.

36. Sacks O. The lost virtues of the asylum. *New York Review of Books*, September 24, 2009, pp. 50–52.

37. Johnson AB. *Out of Bedlam: The Truth About Deinstitutionalization.* Basic Books, New York, 1990.

38. Talbott JA. Deinstitutionalization: avoiding the disasters of the past. Originally published by *Hospital and Community Psychiatry* 1979;621–624 and reprinted in a tribute to Dr. Talbott in *Psychiatric Services* 2004;55:1112–1115.

39. Priebe S, Badesconyi A, Fioritti A, et al. Reinstitutionalization in mental health care: comparison of data on service provision from six European countries. *British Medical Journal* 2005;30:123–126.

40. Schanda H, Stompe T, Ortwein-Swoboda G. Dangerous or merely difficult? The new population in forensic mental hospitals. *European Psychiatry* 2009;24:365–372.

41. Editorial. Humane housing for the mentally ill. *The New York Times*, September 15, 2011.

42. Schildkraut JJ. The catecholamine hypothesis of affective disorders: a review of supporting evidence. *American Journal of Psychiatry* 1965;122:509–522.

43. Coppen A. Depressive states and indolalkylamines. In: *Advances in Pharmacology, Vol 6.* Editors: Garattini S, Shore PA. Academic Press, New York, 1968, pp. 283–291.

44. Prange AJ. L-Tryptophan in mania. *Archives of General Psychiatry* 1974;30:56–62.

45. Janowski DS, el-Yousef MK, Davis JM, et al. A cholinergic-adrenergic hypothesis of mania and depression. *Lancet* 1972;2(7778):573–577.

46. Prien RF, Cole J. High-dose chlorpromazine therapy in chronic schizophrenia. *Archives of General Psychiatry* 1968;18:482–495.

47. Prien RF, Levine J, Cole JO. High-dose trifluoperazine therapy in chronic schizophrenia. *American Journal of Psychiatry* 1969;126:305–313.

48. Wijsenbeek H, Steiner M, Goldberg SC. Trifluoperazine: a comparison between regular and high doses. *Psyhchopharmacologia* 1974;36:147–150.

49. Rifkin A, Quitkin F, Carrillo C, et al. Very high dosage fluphenazine for nonchronic treatment-refractory patients. *Archives of General Psychiatry* 1971;25:398–403.

50. McClelland HA, Farquharson RG, Leyburn P, et al. Very high dose fluphenazine decanoate: a controlled trial in chronic schizophrenia. *Archives of General Psychiatry* 1976;33:1435–1439.

51. Rifkin A, Doddi S, Basawaraj B, et al. Dosage of haloperidol for schizophrenia. *Archives of General Psychiatry* 1991;48:166–170.

52. Baldessarini RJ, Cohen B, Teicher MH. Significance of neuroleptic dose and plasma levels in the pharmacological treatment of psychosis. *Archives of General Psychiatry* 1988;45:79–91.

53. Hollister L. Complications from the use of tranquilizing drugs. *New England Journal of Medicine* 1957;257:170–177.

54. Caine ED, Polinsky RJ. Haloperidol-induced dysphoria in patients with Tourette Syndrome. *American Journal of Psychiatry* 1979;136:1216–1217.

55. van Putten TV, May PRA, Marder SR, et al. Subjective responses to antipsychotic drugs. *Archives of General Psychiatry* 1981;38:187–191.

56. Emerich DF, Sanberg PR. Neuroleptic dysphoria. *Biological Psychiatry* 1991;29:201–203.

57. Belmaker RH, Wald D. Haloperidol in normals. *British Journal of Psychiatry* 1977;131:222–223.

58. Casey DE. Motor and mental aspects of acute extrapyramidal syndromes. *Acta Psychiatrica Scandinavica* 1994;89(suppl 380):14–20.

59. Sachdev P. The epidemiology of drug-induced akathisia: part I. Acute akathisia. *Schizophrenia Bulletin* 1995;21:431–449.

60. Gervin M, Barnes TRE. Assessment of drug-related movement disorders in schizophrenia. *Advances in Psychiatric Treatment* 2000;6:332–341.

61. Dean CE, Russell JM, Kuskowski MA, et al. Clinical rating scales and instruments: how do they compare in assessing abnormal, involuntary movements? *Journal of Clinical Psychopharmacology* 2004;24:298–304.

62. Blier P, Ward HE, Tremblay P, et al. Combination of antidepressant medications from treatment initiation for major depressive disorder: a double-blind, randomized trial. *American Journal of Psychiatry* 2010;167:281–288.

63. Rocha FL, Fuzikawa C, Riera R, et al. Combination of antidepressants in the treatment of major depressive disorder: a systematic review and meta-analysis. *Journal Clinical of Psychopharmacology* 2012;32:278–281.

64. Dean CE. Psychopharmacology: a house divided. *Progress in Neuro-Psychopharmacology & Biological Psychiatry* 2011;35:1–10.

65. Silverman M, Lee PR. *Pills, Profits and Politics*. University of California Press, Berkeley and Los Angeles CA, 1974.

66. Insel TR. Disruptive insights in psychiatry: transforming a clinical discipline. *Journal of Clinical Investigation* 2009;119:700–705.

67. Honigfeld G, Arellano F, Sethi J, et al. Reducing clozapine-related morbidity and mortality: 5 years experience with the Clozaril national registry. *Journal of Clinical Psychiatry* 1988;59(suppl 3):3–7.

68. Lahdelma L, Appelberg B. Clozapine-induced agranulocytosis in Finland 1982–2007: long-term monitoring of patients is still warranted. *Journal of Clinical Psychiatry* 2012;73:837–842.

69. Baldessarini RJ, Frankenburg FR. Clozapine: a novel antipsychotic agent. *New England Journal of Medicine* 1991;324:746–755.

70. Palmer SE, McClean RM, Ellis PM, et al. Life-threatening clozapine-induced gastrointestinal hypomotility: an analysis of 102 cases. *Journal of Clinical Psychiatry* 2008;69:759–768.

71. Buchanan RW, Breier A, Kirkpatric B, et al. Positive and negative symptom response to clozapine in schizophrenic patients with and without the deficit syndrome. *American Journal of Psychiatry* 1998;155:751–760.

72. Moncrieff J. Clozapine vs conventional antipsychotic drugs for treatment-resistant schizophrenia: a re-examination. *British Journal of Psychiatry* 2003;183:161–166.

73. Schooler NC, Marder SR, Chengappa KNR, et al. Clozapine and risperidone in moderately refractory schizophrenia: a 6-month randomized, double-blind comparison. *Journal of Clinical Psychiatry* 2016;77:628–634.

74. Wahlbeck K, Cheine M, Essali A, et al. Evidence of clozapine's effectiveness in schizophrenia: a systematic review and meta-analysis of randomized trials. *American Journal of Psychiatry* 1999;156:990–999.

75. Meltzer HY. The neuroendocrine profile of clozapine, an atypical antipsychotic agent. *Journal of Clinical Psychiatry Monograph* 1990;8[1]:3–8.

76. Seeman P, Tallerico T. Rapid release of antipsychotic drugs from dopamine D2 receptors: an explanation for low receptor occupancy and early clinical relapse upon withdrawal of clozapine or quetiapine. *American Journal of Psychiatry* 1999;156:876–884.

77. Sahlholm K, Marcellino D, Nisson J, et al. Typical and atypical antipsychotics do not differ markedly in their reversibility of antagonism of the dopamine D2 receptor. *International Journal of Neuropsychopharmacology* January 17, 2014;(1):149–155.

78. Idänpään-Heikkla J, Alhava E, Olkinuora M, et al. Clozapine and agranulocytosis. *Lancet* 1975;2:611.

79. Griffith RW, Saamelli K. Clozapine and agranulocytosis. *Lancet* 1975;2:657.

80. Hippius H. The history of clozapine. *Psychopharmacology* 1989;99:S3–S5.

81. Kane J, Honigfield G, Singer J, et al. Clozapine for the treatment-resistant schizophrenia. *Archives of General Psychiatry* 1988;45:789–796.

82. Cohen D. A critique of the use of neuroleptic drugs. In: *From Placebo to Panacea: Putting Psychiatric Drugs to the Test.* Editors: Fisher S, Greenberg RP. John Wiley & Sons, New York, 1997.

83. Davis JM, Chen N. Dose response and dose equivalence of antipsychotics. *Journal of Clinical Psychopharmacology* 2004;24:192–208.

84. Simpson GM, Josiassen RC, Stanilla JK, et al. Double-blind study of clozapine dose response in chronic schizophrenia. *American Journal of Psychiatry* 1999;156:1744–1750.

85. Rosenheck R, Cramer J, Xu W, et al. A comparison of clozapine and haloperidol in hospitalized patients with chronic schizophrenia. *New England Journal of Medicine* 1997;337:809–815.

86. Lieberman JA, Phillips M, Gu H, et al. Atypical and conventional antipsychotic drugs in treatment-naïve first-episode schizophrenia: a 52-week randomized trial of clozapine vs chlorpromazine. *Neuropsychopharmacology* 2003;28:995–1003.

87. Essock SM, Hargreaves WA, Covell NH, et al. Clozapine's effectiveness for patients in state hospitals: results from a randomized trial. *Psychopharmacology Bulletin* 1996;32:683–697.

88. Essali A, Al-Haj N, Li C, et al. Clozapine versus typical neuroleptics medication for schizophrenia. Published online January 20, 2010. Doi:10.1002/14651858,/CD 000059.pub2.

89. Meltzer HY, Alphs L, Green AI, et al. Clozapine treatment for suicidality in schizophrenia. *Archives of General Psychiatry* 2003;60:82–91.

90. Harris EC, Barraclough B. Suicide as an outcome in mental disorders: a meta-analysis. *British Journal of Psychiatry* 1997;170:205–228.

91. Palmer BA, Pankratz S, Bostwick JM. The lifetime risk of suicide in schizophrenia: a re-examination. *Archives of General Psychiatry* 2005;62:247–253.

92. Sernyak MJ, Desai R, Stolar M, et al. Impact of clozapine on completed suicide. *American Journal of Psychiatry* 2001;158:931–937.

93. Lobos CA, Komossa K, Rummel-Kluge C, et al. Clozapine versus other atypical antipsychotics for schizophrenia. *Cochrane Data Base of Systematic Reviews* 2010;(11). Art No: CD006633. Doi:10.1002/14651858.CD006633.pub2.

94. Farooq S, Taylor M. Clozapine: dangerous orphan or neglected friend? *British Journal of Psychiatry* 2011;198:247–249.

95. Verdoux H, Tournier M, Bégaud B. Antipsychotic prescribing trends: a review of pharmacoepidemiological studies. *Acta Psychiatrica Scandinavica* 2010;121:4–10.

96. Duyx B, Urlings MJE, Swaen GH, et al. Scientific citations favor positive results: a systematic review and meta-analysis. *Journal of Clinical Epidemiology* 2017;88:92–101.

97. Fanelli D, Costas R, Larivière V. Misconduct policies, academic culture and career stage, not gender or pressures to publish, affect scientific integrity. *PLoS One.* Doi:10.1371.pone.0127556.

98. Blumenthal D. Doctors and drug companies. *New England Journal of Medicine* 2004;351:1885.

99. Raven M, Perry P. Psychotropic marketing practices and problems. Implications of DSM-5. *Journal of Nervous and Mental Disease* 2012;200:512–516.

100. Samara MT, Dold M, Gianatsi M, et al. Efficacy, acceptability, and tolerability of antipsychotics in treatment resistant schizophrenia. A network meta-analysis. *JAMA Psychiatry* 2016;73:199–210. Doi:10:1001/jamapsychiatry.2015.2955.

101. Kane JM, Correll CU. The role of clozapine in treatment-resistant schizophrenia. Editorial. *JAMA Psychiatry* 2016;73:187–188.

102. Samara MT, Cao H, Helfer B, et al. Chlorpromazine versus every other antipsychotic for schizophrenia: a systematic review and meta-analysis challenging he dogma of equal efficacy of antipsychotic drugs. *European Neuropsychopharmacology* 2014;24:1046–1055.
103. Galling B, Roldán A, Hagi K, et al. Antipsychotic augmentation vs. monotherapy in schizophrenia: systematic review, meta-analysis, and meta-regression analysis. *World Psychiatry* 2017;16:77–89.
104. Carpenter WT, Buchanan RW. Expanding therapy with long-acting antipsychotic medication in patients with schizophrenia. Editorial. *JAMA Psychiatry* 2015;72:745–746.
105. Moncrieff J. Antipsychotic maintenance treatment: time to rethink? *PLOS Medicine.* Doi:10.1371/journal.pmed.1001861.
106. Morrison AP, Turkington D, Pyle M, et al. Cognitive therapy for people with schizophrenia spectrum disorders not taking antipsychotic drugs; a single-blind randomized controlled trial. *The Lancet* 2014;383:1395–1403.

3 Has the Biological Revolution Delivered? A Focus on Antipsychotics

Introduction

In the previous chapter, I reviewed the discovery of the first antipsychotics and antidepressants, as well as a number of theories and experimental evidence that sought to explain their mechanisms of action. While these investigations resulted in a remarkable expansion of knowledge regarding brain structure and function, the critical question for patients is the extent to which antipsychotics (APs) have improved their symptoms, quality of life, and social/occupational functioning. Given that we were spending some $25 billion yearly on APs and antidepressants (ADs), one would expect that the progressive development of these drugs would have shown a parallel improvement in efficacy with fewer side effects and better outcomes. In this chapter, we will focus on APs, with the transition from first-generation antipsychotics (FGAs) to second-generation antipsychotics (SGAs), also known as atypical antipsychotics.

While there is no question that modern psychotropics represent an improvement over the "therapies" offered in the asylums, has the investment of time and money poured into the ongoing development of SGAs in the early and mid-1990s resulted in significant therapeutic progress? Even prominent critics of psychiatry have been highly optimistic. For example, Hobson and Leonard[1, p. 4] wrote in 2001 that the new drugs offered more hope than any other development in psychiatry, in that they target specific diseases and that most patients will respond well. Nine years later, Daniel Carlat,[2, p. 16] in his entertaining book *Unhinged*, stated that the drugs are remarkably helpful, praise exceeded by that of Nancy Andreasen,[3, p. 32] who in 1984 wrote of the older drugs that "many are almost miraculously effective," although they do not promise a cure.

I will show that these comments are highly questionable and demonstrate that the authors have not done their homework. There is no doubt, however, of the popularity of the SGAs. By 2008 they accounted for 93% of treatment visits for which APs were prescribed.[4] Their use in off-label conditions increased from 4 million visits in 1995 to 9 million in 2008.[5]

(Olanzapine appeared on the market in the early 1990s). By 2010, the estimated costs of all off-label use came to $6 billion in the U.S., but this seemed destined to grow rapidly as off-label use widened[6] and the FDA began to approve SGAs for conditions other than psychotic disorders. While the cost began to lessen with the development of generic formulations, this may be offset by the costs of treating the metabolic syndrome, a topic I will explore in the next chapter.

Schizophrenia and Mortality Rates: Better or Worse?

Before examining the response rates to SGAs, let's take a look at studies that have given us a more general but very disturbing view of mortality rates and outcomes in schizophrenia. Again, it seemed reasonable in the late 1990s to expect that the SGAs would improve matters, but this was too optimistic. Let us first examine a 2007 study[7] of all-cause mortality in schizophrenia. The authors carefully reviewed mortality rates found in 37 studies in 25 countries published from 1980 to 2006. However, they excluded studies that reported only on suicide, as well as those focusing on specific subgroups such as the homeless. What did they find?

Unfortunately, patients with schizophrenia had a standardized mortality ratio (SMR) of 2.5, meaning that their risk of dying was 2.5 times the risk found in the general population—not good news, but not unexpected given previous studies. *However, the stunning news was that the SMR almost doubled from the 1970s to the 1990s*, despite renewed attention to appropriate dosing, minimizing side effects, and a greater emphasis on a variety of psychosocial treatments, including family therapy and rehabilitation. Worse, other studies cited by the authors indicated that SMRs in the general population had fallen in many countries, suggesting that people with schizophrenia had been unable to benefit from advances in health care. The overall economic status of the countries did not play a significant role, although studies were limited. Other research demonstrated similar results, despite the marked increase in the use of SGAs from the mid-1990s on.

In England, for example,[8] a 2012 study found that people with schizophrenia and bipolar disorder who were tracked for one year after discharge died at twice the rate of the general population. Unfortunately, the mortality rate for cardiovascular and respiratory deaths in schizophrenia and bipolar disorder increased during the years 1996 through 2006. Cardiovascular disease and lung cancer led the way in a 2015 study of 1.3 million people with schizophrenia followed from 2001 through 2007,[9] with an all-cause mortality rate over 3.5 times that found in the general population. A 2013 study in Sweden[10] also noted excessive mortality rates from the same illness, but the study period was only six years, so there was no increase over time. By way of contrast, the mortality rate among first-episode patients with psychosis *increased in each decade of a study in the United Kingdom,[11] with a doubling of the SMR for all causes of death.* As we have seen in other investigations, most deaths (84%) were from natural causes, with respiratory, infections, and cardiovascular illnesses leading the way. With regard to unnatural causes, deaths from suicide were 12 times greater than in the general population.

However, a comprehensive analysis[12] in 2015 of mortality rates in mental disorders in 29 countries, found not only a doubling of mortality rates, but a steady increase in the risk over the decades prior to the 1970s and up to 2000 and beyond, echoing the Saha et al. data.[7] Sadly, mental illnesses resulted in a ten-year reduction if life expectancy. We should note, too, that *mortality rates have been increasing across a variety of mental disorders,*[12] in contrast to earlier studies that focused on schizophrenia and bipolar disorder.

The steady increase in mortality rates in schizophrenia and other disorders *contrasts* markedly with an analysis of mortality trends in the U.S. during the years 1969 through 2013.[13] During that era, Ma et al. found a *42% reduction in all-cause mortality*, with significant reductions in the rates for heart disease, stroke, and cancer, although the rate of decline slowed.

I must again stress that the increase in mortality rates occurred in the context of the widespread use of SGAs, as well as an increased focus on psychotherapeutic modalities such as cognitive behavioral therapy, interpersonal psychotherapy, social rehabilitation, and a pronounced shift to outpatient treatment. While the data at this point is disturbing, the disparity between mortality rates in the mentally ill and the general population may well worsen, since the studies just cited did not capture the likely impact of the metabolic syndrome on health, and particularly on cardiac disease.[13] (We shall return to mortality rates in a later chapter and provide additional details, particularly with regard to the induction of the metabolic syndrome by SGAs.)

What lies behind the worsening mortality rates? A number of studies have shown that people with schizophrenia are less likely to receive general medical care and are less likely to be treated with lipids or with medications for diabetes mellitus. Increasing levels of income inequality may play a role, with a steady decrease in life expectancy during the years 1999 through 2014 for those in the lower income brackets.[14] However, for those in the lowest quartile, life expectancy was significantly correlated with geographical differences and health-related behaviors such as smoking. Interestingly, living in cities with highly educated populations and high levels of government expenditures had a positive effect on life expectancy in the lower-income groups.

The progressive rise in mortality rates clearly is at odds with the time and money expended over the last four decades aimed at improving the lives of those with mental disorders. Indeed, patients in the early phases of illness are being affected, as shown by a 2017 study[15] that found a markedly higher risk of death during the first year after discharge from their *first* inpatient psychiatric treatment, compared with patients not admitted. Obviously, those in need of admission are more ill, but it's rather shocking to find that the mortality risk for unnatural deaths—primarily suicide—was 25 times greater than for natural deaths.

It seems obvious that we are in need of more intensive research on the health needs of patients and the reasons underlying their failure to obtain benefits from the advances in medical care. Are lengths of stay too short? Probably. Do we have fewer beds than needed? Yes. Is the gap between inpatient care and outpatient care too long? Probably. Is the rise in socioeconomic inequality so severe that mental health professionals have no answer? Perhaps. (More on these issues later.) Whatever the problems, our lack of progress led one author in 2015 to write a provocative editorial, "Mental disorders and mortality: so many publications, so little change."[16]

An obvious issue is the relationship between mortality and the use of APs, a subject we shall examine in more detail in subsequent chapters. However, we should note that concerns have been raised over the long-term effects of APs on brain volume and cognitive functioning,[17] but a 20-year follow-up of patients with first-episode schizophrenia found that *better long-term survival was associated with continuation of AP treatment*,[18] although the authors did not address cognitive functioning or changes in brain volume.

What About Clinical Outcome? Any Significant Improvement?

In another highly disturbing study, Hegarty et al.[19] analyzed the data on clinical outcome in schizophrenia during the years 1892 through 1992. However, the obvious problem was how to define outcome since definitions varied widely. The authors settled on "improved," essentially meaning substantial freedom from psychotic symptoms and good levels of functioning. Three hundred and twenty studies met the study criteria, representing 51,000 patients from the U.S., Asia, and Europe, who were followed for an average of 5.6 years.

The authors also took care to note the diagnostic systems employed, since as one might expect, the diagnostic criteria for schizophrenia ranged from none to very narrow or very broad. It's worth mentioning that one of the restrictive systems is found in our *American Psychiatric Association Diagnostic and Statistical Manual of Mental Disorders*, which gained fame as the DSM-III in 1980,[20] with revisions issued periodically, including the latest (DSM-5) in 2013.[21] No matter the revision, the DSM has always held that a diagnosis of schizophrenia can be made only if the patient has been ill for at least six months. This, of course, sets up a self-fulfilling prophecy, wherein only chronically ill patients are diagnosed with schizophrenia. The data is then used to prove that schizophrenia is a chronic illness!

Back to Hegarty et al.[19] What were the results? Over the entire century, 40% of patients had a favorable outcome. However, when the authors examined outcome decade by decade and then by era, the results became more interesting and, indeed, shocking:

1895–1955: 35.4% improved.
1956–1985: 48.5 % improved, a positive and statistically significant difference from the first era.
1986–1992: 36.4% improved, *not statistically different from the pre-antipsychotic era.*

What?

How could this be, after all the promises of progress; the millions in research on schizophrenia, APs, and brain function; and more emphasis on social rehabilitation? The authors had two answers. First, there was a clear difference in outcome depending on the diagnostic system, with patients diagnosed according to broader and more inclusive criteria having better outcomes, no matter the decade. This meant that any number of patients meeting the more inclusive diagnostic criteria probably had illnesses other than schizophrenia, including bipolar disorder or psychotic depression. (Whether these diagnostic distinctions have *any* merit is an issue that we will tackle later.) On the other hand, patients meeting criteria under the narrower systems were more likely to have "core" symptoms of schizophrenia, including chronicity and social disability. Second, both diagnostic criteria and treatment with APs were significant predictors of outcome.

Although Hegarty and associates made a persuasive case for the impact of the diagnostic system, we must note that serious questions remain. After all, *APs had been in use for over 25 years before the decline in improvement rates in 1986 through 1992.* Are we to accept that the advent of the DSM-III in 1980, with its narrowly defined diagnostic criteria, was enough to override the putative therapeutic effects of the drugs, or were there other forces at work?

Clinicians may remember that the decade from the late 1970s to the late 1980s was marked by the use of high-potency APs in progressively higher doses,[22] a trend that upped the risk of not only parkinsonism, but also antipsychotic-induced dysphoria and akathisia (motor restlessness). I therefore published a letter in the *American Journal of Psychiatry*,[23] positing that these neurologic "side effects" might have contributed to the fall-off in response rates. The authors disagreed, but as a psychiatrist who has seen the devastating side effects of APs, I still wonder if the prolonged use of high-potency drugs played a role in this phenomenon.

It seems curious that the drop in response rates occurred in the same period as did the increase in mortality. Is this a coincidence, or are these findings linked? As we shall see, there is considerable but conflicting evidence that APs may add to the mortality rate, especially in schizophrenia, but there are other issues as well, including a dramatic increase in the use of street drugs starting in the 1960s, the dissolution of the nuclear family, and a rapid increase in socioeconomic inequality starting in the late 1970s.[24]

With regard to economic issues, these are often ignored or simply mentioned in passing by psychiatry, despite lip service given to the "biopsychosocial" model espoused by George Engel decades ago.[25] As one examines the contemporary literature, it seems as if patients live under a biochemical/genetic dome, untouched by the conditions of the economy and the loss of life savings, jobs, and homes. I'm afraid that too many investigators in psychiatry have failed to take into account the consequences of these losses, perhaps because they feel powerless to alter the course of global events and the downfall of the middle class. (See Chapter 14 for more details and citations.) However, the more likely reason is that socioeconomic factors add many additional variables, thus making analysis much more difficult. As we shall see, very few genetic or brain connectivity studies bother with the socioeconomic status of the subjects. Too messy!

Still, one wonders how many in psychiatry are even aware of the relationship between mental illness, crime, and the rapidly widening gap in income inequality? Wilkinson and Pickett[26] have shown that the *prevalence of mental illness and crime steadily increases with the gap in income equality.* The United States, with the largest gap in equality, has double the rate of mental illness in countries such as Belgium, Germany, Japan, Spain, and Italy, and almost triple the rate of homicides.[26] (Obviously, the availability of guns in the U.S. is another factor, but we cannot visit that here.)

Interestingly, the disparity in income seems to have begun in the 1970s, so one might hypothesize that the impact had gathered steam by the 1980s, the period in which recovery rates fell, the suicide rate in schizophrenia and depression increased, and psychiatry began to overdose patients with high-potency APs—perhaps out of desperation? We should emphasize, too, that John Talbott, in an echo of Dickens, specifically cited the decade from 1985 through 1994 as the "worst and best of times," given the consequences of deinstitutionalization.[27] Indeed, a comparative study of lifetime suicide rates in schizophrenia gives additional cause for concern.[28] The authors compared rates of suicide in two eras: the first from 1875 through 1924 and the second from 1994 through 1998. The early historical data appeared to be unusually reliable, since all British asylums were required to report suicides to the coroner, inquests were held, and autopsies were performed. Extensive case histories (including estimates regarding suicidality) and detailed demographic data were gathered since all admissions were compulsory. The authors made diagnoses based on all the case records. The data from 1994 through 1998 were based on all first admissions in North West Wales. Diagnoses were supplemented by data from a five-year longitudinal follow-up. Interestingly, the ethnic, population, and economic data from that area in the UK seemed to be rather consistent over the span of the study.

As we have seen in the Saha et al.[7] and the Hegarty et al.[19] studies, the results were surprising. *The lifetime rate of suicide in patients with schizophrenia in the pre-chlorpromazine era was less than 0.5%. This contrasts markedly with the rate during the years 1994 through 1998, when it was 20 times higher.* However, caution is warranted when comparing rates of suicide over 100 years, due to changes in social attitudes, stigma, and reasons for admission. Further, the absolute numbers of suicides were low: 1 of 594 patients in the early era and 7 of 133 in the later era. These data were far too small for an epidemiological study, and the fortunately low base rate of suicides continues to plague research and efforts at prediction.

At this point, we need to consider the impact of APs on people with schizophrenia.

Response Rates With Antipsychotics in Schizophrenia

I have already emphasized the free pass given to psychiatric drugs by a number of prominent critics of the field, a view at odds with other investigators, including Seymour Fisher and Roger Greenberg,[29] Elliot Valenstein,[30] and Peter Gøtzsche.[31] Given the ready availability of the data, it's difficult to understand why any serious reader or mental health professional would call these drugs remarkably helpful or miraculous. It seems far more realistic to say that they are modestly helpful and work well to prevent relapse in some patients. Nevertheless, prescribers and investigators who neglect the socioeconomic issues and the benefits of psychosocial treatments are not being realistic.

Early Studies of FGAs

So, let's briefly review response rates in several older but representative studies, utilizing FGAs such as chlorpromazine, fluphenazine (Prolixin), and thioridazine (Mellaril). In 1957, Winkelman published an outpatient study[32] involving 1,000 patients treated with oral chlorpromazine and followed for up to three years. Interestingly, 652 of this group were not schizophrenic, but suffered from anxiety, conversion, and obsessive and phobic disorders. The improvement rate was striking, with 73% showing moderate or better improvement. In a precursor to the current interest in the use of APs for depression, 41% of those with depression had at least a moderate degree of improvement. In those with schizophrenia, 61% had moderate or greater improvement, but 22% failed to respond at all. A smaller double-blind[33] study revealed that chlorpromazine was clearly superior to placebo or phenobarbital. After withdrawal of chlorpromazine, 80% relapsed in six months, but if patients were also treated with psychotherapy, the rate was 40%. The overall response rate to placebo was 35%, *but treatment with chlorpromazine resulted in a response rate of 85%, never duplicated in contemporary studies.*

A collaborative study from the NIMH[34] compared thioridazine, fluphenazine, chlorpromazine, or placebo given to newly admitted patients who had not been hospitalized in the previous year. Of these, 74% completed the allotted six weeks, with 75% showing either "very much" or "much" improvement, vs only 23% on placebo, *yielding a number needed to treat (NNT) of two, almost unheard of today.* As I mentioned earlier, no patient worsened, and only 11 had to be dropped due to significant side effects, results that now seem unrealistic.

The Move to SGAs, but Swimming in the Data Flood: Is Meta-Analysis the Answer?

By 1965, some 200 placebo-controlled studies of APs for schizophrenia had been published. The pace never lessened, such that a 2009 review[35] of head-to-head comparisons of SGAs cited 78 studies with 13,000 participants, while a comparison of the same group of APs against placebo involved 38 controlled trials with 7,300 participants.[36] Given the large number of individual studies and thousands of participants, methods had to be developed that would enable investigators to make sense of the data and summarize it so that clinicians could evaluate whether one drug or one group of drugs was superior to another. Systematic reviews were a first step in this process, but the clear need for better information led to the development of meta-analytic studies, which are becoming increasingly common, given the massive data generated by contemporary studies. The non-clinician can feel free to skip this section.

Methodological Issues and Definitions

Some brief comments about the methods of meta-analysis are needed. In contrast to a systematic review, in which a descriptive review of the literature is undertaken, a meta-analytic study goes a step further, applying a variety of statistical tests such that the results of individual studies can be combined. The results are given in a number of ways, including an effect size (ES), which is a measure of the difference between the drugs or other treatments in the study, and a number that can be more clinically informative than using a p value of <0.05. After all, the p value is an arbitrary number that only denotes statistical significance but does *not* give the reader any idea of the magnitude or precision of the treatment.[37, 38, pp. 95–100]

A small ES is about 0.2, a medium ES is about 0.5, and a large ES is 0.8. Obviously, a treatment with a large ES is more clinically useful. Interestingly, some studies will find a statistically significant ES, but, if the ES is only 0.3 or so, the results may not be clinically helpful. It may be useful to think of an ES of 0.5 as being obvious to the naked eye.[37] Other terms are helpful when the outcome is couched in terms of a "dichotomous variable," e.g., a research question that can be answered yes or no. For example, did the drug prevent relapse? Did the patient die? This type of outcome is described by an odds ratio (OR), in which the number of patients who did not relapse or die is divided by the number who did. Another term is relative risk (RR), wherein the number of patients who relapsed or died is divided by the total number of patients.

For continuous variables, such as weight, blood pressure, height, or a rating scale such as the Brief Psychiatric Rating Scale (BPRS), the difference between the mean values of the experimental groups can be used. But, since different rating scales are often used, the analysis has to combine the results using a common unit called the standardized difference of the mean values (SMD). This is obtained by dividing the mean value of group A minus the mean value of group B, divided by the standard deviation (SD) of the two groups.

In order to further assess the results, two models are often used statistically. One is a fixed-effects model, which assumes that among all the groups being studied, there is a true mean ES, with the mean results of the individual studies being randomly distributed around the true mean. The other is a random-effects model, which assumes that *each* study can have a true mean ES that differs from the others, perhaps due to study conditions.

Meta-analysis also investigates the degree to which publication bias exists: that is, whether negative studies have not been published—a favorite tactic of Big Pharma. This is demonstrated by means of a so-called funnel plot, wherein the effect sizes of studies are plotted against the number of subjects. If all studies have been published, the graphic representation is that of an inverted funnel.

Since I am going to discuss a number of meta-analytic studies, it's only fair that I take note of the criticism of this approach, some of which has been quite strong. Ghaemi,[38] for example, has emphasized the inherent difficulties of lumping disparate studies into a pool, since studies are often quite heterogeneous, but we have to note that virtually all well-done meta-analyses control for the degree of heterogeneity. He further notes that the "statistical alchemy" of meta-analysis might discourage further investigation of the issues at hand, due to the alleged certainty of the results. However, *investigators frequently take a dim view of previous studies*, whether meta-analytic or not, and are more than eager to top whatever was found—part of the rhetoric of science and a pathway to fame and tenure. Ghaemi further makes the controversial point that if an individual study is methodologically sound, the results can be more informative than a meta-analysis. The problem here is that few studies in psychiatry are sufficiently well powered, especially in imaging research,[39] thus making a meta-analytic approach necessary. Nevertheless, Ioannidis has drawn attention to the problems associated with this approach; see his 2016 article[40] on "The mass production of redundant, misleading, and conflicted systematic reviews and meta-analyses," and de Vrieze, who in 2018 analyzed the many problems with meta-analyses.[41]

Meta-Analytic Studies Comparing FGAs and SGAs in Schizophrenia

Given the number of available studies, space doesn't permit a detailed examination of each, so I will provide a brief summary of the largest and more important investigations. But let's begin with a provocative study published in 2000. Geddes and associates[42] analyzed 52 RCTs comparing SGAs with FGAs, limiting the studies to those utilizing licensed therapeutic doses. The comparator drug was usually haloperidol. If the dose of haloperidol was 12 mg a day or less, there were *no differences in efficacy* between SGAs and FGAs, except for a modest advantage for SGAs with regard to parkinsonian side effects. The authors recommended FGAs as first-line agents, unsettling Big Pharma, psychopharmacologists, and any number of clinicians, but this set the stage for a number of subsequent analyses of SGAs vs FGAs and SGAs vs other SGAs in randomized, controlled trials.

To summarize, two additional studies[43, 44] found few differences in efficacy between SGAs and FGAs and only a "modest" advantage of SGAs on relapse prevention in schizophrenia.[45] There were no differences in regard to efficacy for positive symptoms (hallucinations, delusions), but quetiapine was less effective than FGAs for positive symptoms.[46] However, all SGAs were superior to FGAs with regard to parkinsonian side effects, but note that SGAs were *not* superior to low-potency FGAs. All SGAs except aripiprazole and ziprasidone induced more weight gain, but there was little difference in quality of life.[46] In head-to-head comparisons of SGAs, olanzapine appeared superior, but quetiapine was less effective than olanzapine and risperidone.[35]

Unfortunately, the overall response rate with SGAs was 41% vs 24% for placebo,[36] underscoring our lack of progress with regard to efficacy, despite the enormous increase in costs.

Given the criticism of meta-analytical studies by Ghaemi,[38] we should examine two large clinical trials, with the most famous being the CATIE (Clinical Antipsychotic Trials of Intervention Effectiveness) trial published in 2005.[47] The criteria for enrollment were more clinically oriented than most drug studies hoping to provide meaningful data for clinical use. The primary goal was to compare four SGAs against perphenazine (Trilafon), an older FGA, and examine the rates of discontinuation. In keeping with our previous concerns regarding dropout rates, 75% discontinued the drugs! After statistical adjustments, time to discontinuation *did not differ between perphenazine and the SGAs, nor did the rates of neurologic side-effects.* Olanzapine had a lower rate of rehospitalization, but perphenazine was otherwise equivalent to the SGAs and, in fact, demonstrated a *greater degree of improvement in cognitive functioning* and, in a follow-up study, had effects similar to the SGAs![48]

The CUtLASS (Cost utility of the latest antipsychotic drugs in schizophrenia) trial[49] was another clinically oriented but controlled trial of SGAs and FGAs aimed at assessing the quality of life in schizophrenia. Once again, SGAs were *not* superior to FGAs, and there was no disadvantage to beginning treatment with an FGA, with no differences in compliance, effects on positive and negative symptoms, or costs over a 12-month period. Similarly, a multi-center study in the VA of olanzapine vs haloperidol[50] revealed *no significant differences* with regard to improvement in quality of life, positive and negative symptoms, or dropouts due to adverse events, surprising results indeed. Treatment with olanzapine, however, led to more weight gain and higher costs. Not surprisingly, haloperidol led to more akathisia (motor restlessness).

Early-Onset Patients

As we have seen, most of the patients in the studies just reviewed were chronically ill. Are SGAs superior to FGAs in those with first-episode illness? Several groups have provided data that should be of interest to new-onset patients and their families. A double-blind investigation[51] of olanzapine vs haloperidol prescribed to first-episode psychotic patients found that both drugs led to substantial reductions in symptoms, although olanzapine was superior—*depending* on the statistical models and rating scales. More patients taking olanzapine completed the 12-week study (67% vs 54%). While olanzapine-treated patients had fewer neurologic side effects, they also had significantly more weight gain.

In 2008, Sikich et al.[52] compared molindone (Moban), an early FGA, to olanzapine and risperidone in patients ages 8 to 19. Patients randomized to molindone also received benztropine (Cogentin) in order to minimize parkinsonian side effects. Previous APs were cross-tapered over a two-week period, and, perhaps unfortunately, patients taking antidepressants and/or mood stabilizers were allowed to continue those medications throughout the eight-week study period. There were *no statistically significant differences* in response rates, which ranged from 34% to 50%.

In addition, there were no significant differences in study retention; however, consistent with what we've seen in adult studies, the dropout rates were high, with *only 60% of the sample completing treatment.* Remarkably, a Data and Safety Monitoring Board (DSMB) decreed in 2006 that randomization to olanzapine be stopped since it was causing more weight gain than the other drugs and had no advantage with regard to efficacy—an admirable decision. However, patients previously assigned to olanzapine "continued their participation and the integrity of the study blind was maintained."[52] If these findings were that important, *why* were those patients allowed to continue? Were they informed of the DSMB findings? If not, why not? We can say right away that the study was already underpowered, and the removal of the group taking olanzapine no doubt would have severely compromised the original study goals, but what about the safety and health of the participants?

In another study of 400 first-episode patients ages 16 through 40,[53] no FGAs were used, but patients were randomized to olanzapine, risperidone, or quetiapine and followed for one year. The fine print, however, revealed that patients could be ill for as long as five years and could have been treated with APs for as long as 16 cumulative weeks! For reasons not stated, a project officer allowed enrollment of 32 patients who had exceeded the time limits! Obviously, the term "first episode" has to be taken with the proverbial grain of salt.

The primary outcome measure was the number of patients who withdrew from the study before 52 weeks. The goal was to demonstrate that quetiapine was non-inferior to the other agents. (Of note, funding was provided by AstraZeneca, makers of quetiapine, and a number of investigators were stockholders in and/or employees of various drug companies.) As with the study just reviewed, the response rates were not significantly different and ranged from 58% to 65%, but dropout rates were high. Almost 80% of those treated with olanzapine gained at least 7% of their body weight. Sadly, five patients attempted suicide, two died of suicide, and one was alleged to have committed a homicide.

In 2016, in a comprehensive review and network meta-analysis of seven APs used in the treatment of early-onset schizophrenia,[54] only molindone, olanzapine, and risperidone led to a significant reduction in positive symptoms, but *none led to a significant reduction in negative symptoms*, again demonstrating that the SGAs had failed to improve the core symptoms of schizophrenia. Overall response rates varied between 38% to 65%, leaving patients with about a 50–50 chance of responding . . . not good!

More SGAs: Any Better?

Paliperidone (Invega)

In December 2006, the FDA approved paliperidone for schizophrenia, both in the acute phase and for maintenance. In April 2011, paliperidone was approved for the treatment of schizophrenia in adolescents ages 12 through 17, and in 2014, it was approved as monotherapy for schizoaffective disorder or as an adjunct to mood stabilizers or antidepressants for the same condition. This agent is simply a metabolite of risperidone, continuing a tradition we outlined earlier. The manufacturer emphasized a packaging twist to separate it from risperidone, in that paliperdone has an osmotic drug-release technology, reputed to minimize fluctuations in plasma levels. This enables once-daily dosing—but this can be done with most SGAs!

Three published RCTs of this agent were released in 2007.[55–57] All studies were six weeks long, with a combined population of 1,692 patients. The mean ages hovered around 38; 52% to 74% were men. The primary outcome was a 30% reduction in the PANSS score. Each study compared paliperidone with only 10 mg of olanzapine or placebo. Completion rates varied from 34% to 46% if taking placebo, 46% to 78% with paliperidone, and 45% to 70% with olanzapine, so about half dropped out. Response rates with placebo varied from 18% to 34%, while response rates with olanzapine ranged from 46% to 52%. Depending on the dose of paliperidone, response rates varied from 40% to a maximum of 61%, figures similar to those cited earlier. About 20% had more than a 7% increase in body weight, but there were few metabolic changes.

One potential problem: This drug is largely eliminated by the kidney, so if renal function is impaired, lower doses will be necessary. Paliperidone is similar to risperidone in that parkinsonian side effects occur in about 7% of patients and are more likely with doses of 9 mg daily or more. *Prolactin levels increase, as they do with risperidone*, with 4% reporting problems with amenorrhea and lactation. Paliperidone palmitate, a long-acting injectable, was FDA approved in 2009.

Asenapine (Saphris)

In August 2009, the FDA approved asenapine for the treatment of schizophrenia and the acute treatment of mixed or manic episodes in bipolar disorder, where it can be prescribed either as monotherapy or as an adjunctive agent. The FDA also approved it for use in pediatric bipolar disorder in 2015. Like the other SGAs, it is a blocker of multiple DA and 5-HT receptors and potently blocks adrenergic and histamine receptors. However, it does not block muscarinic cholinergic receptors, so it theoretically should not cause significant problems with dry mouth, constipation, or tachycardia. Asenapine is noteworthy for its ability to alter glutamate receptors (NMDA and AMPA), especially in the caudate, the putamen, and the nucleus accumbens—at least in rats.[58] The starting dose of 5 mg bid is a therapeutic dose, but in mania, the dose is 10 mg bid. The tablet is designed to be used sublingually, so if the patient swallows it, very little is absorbed. This could be a major problem in patients unable to follow directions.

In September 2011, the FDA amended the warning label[59] *due to 52 cases of type I hypersensitivity reactions*, which include angioedema, anaphylaxis, tachycardia, hypertension, wheezing, swelling of the tongue, and rash. In some cases, symptoms developed after the first dose. In 19 cases, hospitalization or ER visits were needed. In 15 cases, the symptoms resolved after discontinuation, but the FDA recommended *immediate* medical consultation for any symptoms of hypersensitivity.

Three studies were used to obtain FDA approval. A six-week study[60] compared asenapine with placebo and risperidone in the treatment of various subtypes of schizophrenia in adult patients. The population was largely male and had responded to at least one AP in the past. *Notice that the current APs were stopped only three days prior to study entry, not enough time to clear the brain.* Mood stabilizers were stopped about five days before entry. Did these sudden withdrawals contaminate the study? The authors did not address the question. The overall dropout rate was close to 60%, and the response rate was 53%, but only 35% for risperidone! Parkinsonian motor problems were rare, but 17% gained weight, and 14% had a 20% increase in fasting blood glucose. In the second study,[61] asenapine at 5 mg bid or 10 mg bid was compared with haloperidol 4 mg bid and placebo, with the PANSS again used as the primary outcome measure in 448 patients. Response rates varied from 44% to 48%, but in a third study,[62] neither the 5 mg per day nor the 10 mg per day beat placebo.

Asenapine may be less effective than other SGAs, but it appears to have fewer metabolic and neurologic side effects; *nevertheless, the allergic reactions are worrisome.*

Iloperidone (Fanapt)

Yet another me-too SGA that was approved for the treatment of acute episodes of schizophrenia on May 6, 2009, iloperidone comes with several cautionary notes, including the possibility of orthostatic hypotension (which may be more common than found with other SGAs) and heart block. As with other SGAs, it blocks both D2 and 5-HT receptors. The three published trials were similar to those we've previously described, in that they lasted only six weeks and compared various doses of iloperidone to placebo and/or a comparator drug such as haloperidol or risperidone. Two of the three published trials[63, 64, 65] examining response rates in acute schizophrenia *found no advantage of iloperidone over placebo,* but the third trial found it superior to placebo. In a four-week trial, iloperidone 24 mg daily was compared with ziprasidone or placebo, with a 72% response rate vs 52% with placebo, a significant difference. The latter two trials were accepted by the FDA as proof of efficacy.[63]

The review by Leslie Citrome just cited[63] did not capture a fascinating aspect of the early trials of this agent, a story described in detail by Steven Potkin and associates.[64] The problem was that after two failed trials, Vanda Pharmaceuticals no doubt was eager to find some way of obtaining FDA approval. (In fact, the FDA had failed to approve it in 2007.) This was accomplished in several ways, including a post-hoc analysis of three trials, in which additional data was examined from all patients who had completed at least two weeks of treatment. This was *a marked difference from the original protocol,* which had employed an intent-to-treat analysis with a last-observation-carried-forward (LOCF) analysis. In other words, the original protocol used data from patients who had taken at least one dose of the drug and had undergone at least one rating session.

(The LOCF tactic refers to the highly questionable assumption that the clinical state after x number of doses would be unchanged at study end. The authors correctly noted that the LOCF has been subject to heavy criticism, for obvious reasons. They were also concerned about the slower titration schedule with iloperidone, so they adjusted the time to end point.)

After all these post-hoc adjustments, the results improved considerably, with iloperidone showing improvement similar to that of 15 mg daily of haloperidol. However, this sort of post-hoc methodology is highly questionable. Further, every author on the Potkin paper was heavily involved with Vanda Pharmaceuticals. The subsequent paper in the supplement even included the company CEO as one author.[65]

Three trials[66] were aimed at comparing the long-term efficacy of iloperidone with haloperidol, but since there was no placebo, the FDA did not take the results into account. In the initial 6-week trial period, the response rates were 37% with iloperidone vs 38% with haloperidol, an equivalent outcome. This group then participated in a 46-week maintenance phase trial, with time to relapse as the end point. Time to relapse did not differ, nor did the relapse rate of 42%.

Finally, in another review of this agent,[67] the authors failed to describe the protocol changes in the three acute phase trials, leaving the reader unaware of the efforts made at obtaining statistically significant results. However, the authors did point out that these studies were published in company-sponsored journal supplements, which have been criticized for not meeting the same standards regarding peer review. In the interest of being fair and balanced, I should say that with regard to the *Journal of Clinical Psychiatry* supplement, the *Journal* noted that an "independent" member of the editorial board reviewed the material for objectivity and evidenced-based data. *Still, this is not the same as the usual peer-review process, in which two or three reviewers blindly assess the study, methodology, and results.*

Lurasidone (Latuda)

This SGA was FDA approved in October 2010 for the treatment of schizophrenia and in 2013 as either monotherapy or as an adjunctive agent for bipolar depression. Lurasidone wanders a bit off the beaten path in that it blocks a rather unusual serotonin receptor ($5HT_7$) that seems to have a role in spatial and contextual fear memory. The blockade of $5HT_7$ in animals has been shown to improve memory in some animal studies. In addition, lurasidone blocks several other receptors with a possible role in cognition, including 5-HT1a, and α_{2c}. Whether these receptor blockades yield clinically significant effects remains to be seen. Not surprisingly, it also blocks D2 and 5-HT2a and 5-HT1a receptors, as does every other SGA.[68]

The company web site (http://latuda/press-releasel.html, 2010) states that 40 clinical trials have been done—with 4 of these being the "pivotal" RCTs that led to FDA approval—but I located only two published trials. As with virtually all such studies, the Nakamura et al. trial (funded by the manufacturer and loaded with company employees)[69] was a six-week double-blind trial of hospitalized acutely ill patients with schizophrenia. Only a three-to-seven-day washout period was employed. A fixed dose of 80 mg daily was used, *without a taper up*. The primary outcome measure was the BPRS, with a 20% scale reduction used to define responders. Rates of discontinuation were high: 47% dropped out of the placebo arm while 42% dropped out of the lurasidone arm. A statistically significant drop in symptoms compared with placebo was seen by day three and continued through study completion. *However, as in most studies, the response rate was only 44%, vs 27% with placebo.*

Mean levels of cholesterol and triglycerides fell, and parkinsonian side effects were no more than reported with placebo. Given this data, lurasidone might well be preferable to some SGAs, especially olanzapine and quetiapine. On the other hand, this drug is metabolized by a CYP3A4 isoenzyme, so it should be avoided with inhibitors such as ritonavir and even grapefruit juice.

The Meltzer et al. trial[70] cited only the Nakamura et al. trial in the introduction to their study, with no mention of the other "pivotal trials" submitted to the FDA. The Meltzer trial was also six weeks in length and took place in the U.S. and overseas, with a number of company employees involved. Two doses of lurasidone, 40 mg and 120 mg, were compared for efficacy against placebo or 15 mg of olanzapine. Both doses of lurasidone were superior to placebo on the primary measure of efficacy, but the effect size was higher for the 40 mg dose, and the side effects were fewer. However, *neither dose of lurasidone was superior to placebo with regard to the standard measure of response*, i.e., a 20% drop on the PANSS.

I find it striking that while the authors mentioned the failure to find a difference in the response rate in the abstract, they did not comment on this in two pages of discussion, but simply wrote that the drug is an "effective treatment of schizophrenia." In a review of lurasidone published in the same supplement of the *Journal of Clinical Psychiatry*, John Kane[71] described several other studies, one of which found that 80 mg of lurasidone daily was superior to placebo, but another trial failed to find lurasidone or haloperidol superior to placebo. Three additional trials did find lurasidone superior to placebo. The most frequent adverse events included sedation, anxiety, akathisia, and other signs of parkinsonism, including dystonias.

The number of failed trials should give pause to prescribers and potential patients.

Brexipiprazole (Rexulti)

FDA approved in 2015 for the treatment of schizophrenia and as an adjunctive treatment for major depression, this drug is characterized as a "serotonin-dopamine activity modulator," but the same could be said for the other SGAs. It differs from aripiprazole (Abilify) in that its activity at D2 receptors is lower. Brexipiprazole is a partial agonist at D2 and 5-HT1a receptors, has moderate affinity for H1 receptors, is a partial agonist at D3 receptors, and blocks 5-HT7 receptors.[72] We should note its *very long half-life of 91 hours*, which is clinically meaningful in that the time required for effects of dose adjustments is quite lengthy, and side effects can persist for some time after the drug is stopped. (The same can be said for fluoxetine [Prozac], with a half-life of two weeks).

Despite the interesting biochemical profile of this drug, the results remain similar to those noted earlier, with *pooled response rates across studies of 45%*, with an NNT of seven.[73] A one-year maintenance study found that the relapse rate for brexipiprazole was 13% vs 38% for placebo,[74] a substantial difference. Parkinsonian side effects appear to be low, at 5.5% for akathisia, but rates for tardive dyskinesia are not known. At this point, weight gain appears to be less than that found with olanzapine and some other SGAs, but longer-term studies are needed.

What Can We Conclude?

We began this chapter by asking whether the biological revolution has delivered on the promise of improving the lives of patients via psychopharmacology and, more specifically, whether the SGAs have made a significant difference in both the symptoms and quality of life in those suffering from schizophrenia and other psychotic disorders.

The answer is no. Indeed, the results of the CATIE study[47] were largely unexpected, given the successful marketing of SGAs. By the time the FDA and the batteries of attorneys handling multiple class-action lawsuits got around to exposing the extent to which Big Pharma had hidden the results of their own studies with regard to weight gain, new-onset diabetes, and hyperlipidemia, it was too late: standard community practice clearly favored SGAs as the first-line treatment for schizophrenia, backed by the older treatment guidelines.[75]

Nevertheless, the CATIE study[47] and others precipitated a furious debate, which has continued to this day. Witness a number of soul-searching essays, such as "Second-generation antipsychotics for schizophrenia: can we resolve the conflict?"[76] "The rise and fall of the atypical antipsychotics,"[77] and, "CATIE and CUtLASS: can we handle the truth?"[78] wherein the authors noted a 30-fold increase in the global market for APs during the years 1980 to 2008, in part due to the rapid expansion of off-label use.[5, 6, pp. 78–80]

I strongly recommend the three critiques just cited, but I have to confess struggling with how to use this rather discouraging data in the clinic. Obviously, patients are in need of treatment, and, as we have seen, some do respond to medications, but the response rates are less than impressive, and the metabolic side effects can be both severe and a health threat. Unfortunately, all of us have been misled, to one extent or another, by the very aggressive marketing campaigns accompanying the development of the SGAs, campaigns that have led to multiple lawsuits and fines, largely secondary to illegal marketing practices.

For example, in 2009, Pfizer was accused of misbranding drugs, including ziprasidone, resulting in a $2.9 billion settlement. In 2011, GlaxoSmithKline paid $3 billion for illegal marketing of bupropion and paroxetine, antidepressants we shall discuss later, as well as several other drugs. In 2010, AstraZeneca paid $520 million for illegally marketing quetiapine to children, inmates, and the elderly. In 2012, Johnson & Johnson was fined some $1.1 billion for downplaying the risks of risperidone. The company had sent a letter to doctors claiming the drug did not increase the risk of DM and so was forced to retract it.[31, pp. 26–30]

Clinical Notes

I must insist that despite the hoopla and the remarkable dominance of SGAs in clinical practice, the scientific literature supports the following:

1. The response rates in schizophrenia are no better than those found with FGAs and in a few instances are worse. Response rates hover around 50%. The newest SGAs appear to have no advantages over the older SGAs, except for lower rates of the metabolic syndrome, but are much more expensive, pending the release of generic formulations.
2. We are now seeing a change in the stance of some clinical guidelines, given CATIE and CUtLASS, such that the American Psychiatric Association,[81] in its updated Practice Guideline for the Treatment of Patients with Schizophrenia, finally recognized that *"the distinction between first- and second-generation antipsychotics appears to have limited clinical utility"* (Emphasis mine). Similarly, the well-known Schizophrenia Patient Outcomes Research Team[82] emphasizes that simply recommending SGAs as first-line agents is not warranted. Nevertheless, the first-line use of SGAs remains the standard of practice in most communities.
3. A 2019 network meta-analysis[83] of 32 oral antipsychotics in 402 studies does find that clozapine, amisulpride (old FGA), zotepine (old FGA), olanzapine, and risperidone reduce overall symptoms to a greater extent than "many other drugs." *However, eight of the top 14 are FGAs, and the bottom ten included four of the newer APs*: lurasidone, cariprazine, iloperidone, and brexipiprazole. While clozapine, olanzapine, and risperidone may have "modest" advantages over FGAs, the serious metabolic effects—especially with clozapine and olanzapine—may well outweigh the small gains in symptom suppression. However, this study did not assess long-acting injectables, combinations of APs, or combinations of APs and other drugs.
4. In view of the less-than-ideal outcomes with APs, combinations are often used. A 2019 study[84] found that beginning an antidepressant with an AP resulted in a reduced risk of hospitalization, *but initiating a benzodiazepine resulted in a higher risk*. An earlier study[85] had found an increased risk of mortality when a benzodiazepine was used with an AP.
5. Data on social functioning has been limited,[83] but, remarkably enough, thioridazine, the second-oldest SGA, was at the top, followed by olanzapine, paliperidone, and seven others. Risperidone was ranked lower than placebo!
6. The negative symptoms of schizophrenia (poverty of speech, mood, and motivation) are *not* preferentially improved by SGAs, with the possible exception of clozapine, olanzapine, and asenapine, ranked in the top five in the network meta-analysis.[83]
7. There is some evidence that SGAs result in a better quality of life than do FGAs, but only ten studies assessed this issue in the network meta-analysis,[83] making the top choice of aripiprazole questionable.

8. Some—but not all—studies indicate a modest advantage of SGAs over FGAs in regard to parkinsonian side effects and tardive dyskinesia. However, this apparent advantage has done little to stem the flood of patients fleeing the studies. In a number of studies, there were no differences in the dropout rates of those taking either class of drug. Clearly, *patients are experiencing levels of discomfort not being captured* by the raters or rating scales. We shall say much more about the neurologic "side effects" of APs later in this volume.

9. None of the studies done in recent years have been of sufficient duration to fully capture the potential for the metabolic threats posed by the chronic use of SGAs, especially clozapine, olanzapine, and quetiapine. Nevertheless, we must emphasize that *metabolic changes have occurred even in short-term studies.* These observations were reinforced by an MRI study of abdominal fat in 46 patients with a first psychotic episode treated with either risperidone or chlorpromazine for ten weeks; none had been treated with APs previously.[86] Not only did the treated patients have a significant gain in abdominal and subcutaneous fat, but there was a three-fold increase in leptin, a hormone important in keeping body mass in equilibrium. (Interestingly, deficits in leptin usually result in weight gain, so this was unexpected and not easily explained.) Not surprisingly, increased levels of lipids and non-fasting blood glucose were also found. Similarly, inpatients treated with olanapine for six weeks had significant increases in visceral and subcutaneous fat, a change that has been associated with insulin resistance and diabetes mellitus.[87] As we shall see, *these changes may occur more rapidly in children and adolescents.*

10. With regard to long-term or maintenance treatment of schizophrenia, guidelines have recommended contrary approaches, with the American Psychiatric Association[81] recommending the lowest effective dose, while the Expert Consensus Guidelines have urged that we continue the dose used during the acute phase. A meta-analysis of this problem[88] found little difference between standard-dose and low-dose treatment and no differences in dropout rates between the two approaches. However, we still have insufficient trial data with regard to dosing,[89] and much of what is recommended is "not necessarily based on evidence."

11. There are still questions regarding the long-term use of APs for the maintenance treatment of schizophrenia, despite textbook[90] recommendations that AP be continued indefinitely and that continuous dosing is preferable, given the high rates of relapse. However, Moncrieff[91] has pointed to other studies showing that continuous treatment may worsen relapse compared with intermittent treatment. In addition, patients randomized to intermittent treatment had better social adjustment and higher rates of recovery. Adding to the debate is evidence showing that higher cumulative exposure over time is associated with loss of gray matter volume, this being more evident in patients using

higher doses of SGAs,[92] but one has to note that evidence also shows loss of gray matter volume with illness progression, even in the absence of medication.[93, 94] However, in 2015, a study of first-episode patients[95] found thinning of the prefrontal, parietal, temporal, and occipital cortices in those taking APs, but no thinning in the unmedicated group.

12. Yet the evidence continues to vary, with a review published in 2017 finding little data to support any negative or long-term effects of APs on outcomes.[96] However, I must note that five of the eight authors had received speaking or consultant fees from drug companies, as well as grant support or travel support, raising concerns over bias. In addition, this was a narrative review, not a systematic review or meta-analysis. In support of their conclusions, a prospective study[18] in Finland of 21,000 people with schizophrenia found a *reduction in mortality in those treated with reasonably dosed APs and ADs*, although the study was criticized on methodological grounds by Moncrieff and Steingard.[97] The variability of these studies led me to question whether the data permitted any definitive conclusions regarding brain changes and outcome in schizophrenia.[98]

13. About half of patients with schizophrenia do not respond well to what appears to be adequate treatment. In those instances, clozapine is often recommended, with its efficacy demonstrated in several meta-analytic studies, including the 2019 study,[83] but contradicted by others. Since the evidence was controversial, Samara and colleagues did an additional study[99] in 2016 that compared any AP with another AP or placebo and found *"little evidence" for the superiority of clozapine in treatment-resistant cases*. There was a small indicator of efficacy for olanzapine, risperidone, and clozapine when secondary outcomes were measured. In addition, a meta-analysis[100] of non-blinded ("cohort") studies in 2019 found that clozapine was associated with fewer hospitalizations, fewer risks of discontinuation, and better symptom improvement but increases in body mass index and type II diabetes mellitus.

14. Contrary to expectations, SGAs have not resulted in a significant increase in medication compliance. In Finland, for example, 54% of patients did not obtain a prescription for their AP within 30 days of discharge; many were taking an SGA.[101] The cost of drugs was not a factor, since patients were fully reimbursed.

15. Not surprisingly, those taking a long-acting depot drug (fluphenazine decanaoate and others) had a significantly lower risk of rehospitalization in a 2011study by Tiihonen and associates,[101] although others found no significant differences and more adverse events.[102] Yet long-acting formulations of risperidone and perphenazine have had substantially better outcomes than oral agents[103] while in another study in 2018 of patients with first-episode schizophrenia who were followed for 16 years, the risk of *rehospitalization and death was lowest for those with continuous AP treatment*,[104] whether with oral or injectable treatment! Indeed, a 30-year

follow-up study of schizophrenia[105] found that the standardized mortality ratio was stable, but the rate of suicide fell significantly. On the other hand, mortality from cancer and cardiovascular disease trended upward. Does this reflect the popularity of SGAs?

16. Despite the well-documented concerns over the AP-induced metabolic syndrome and neurologic side effects, 55% of office-based prescriptions for AP are written for adults not suffering from FDA-approved indications (schizophrenia, bipolar disorder, Tourette's syndrome, and treatment-resistant depression).[106] For those ages 65 and older, the rate is 75%! These data are consistent with the trend[5, 6] toward off-label prescribing during the years 1995 through 2008 and subsequently. This appears to reflect a *serious disregard on the part of practitioners to the black-box warnings and other obvious risks associated with APs, whether FGAs or SGAs. We shall see later that this is a serious problem in dementia, where a dose-response increase in mortality has been found with SGAs.*[107]

17. These data clearly underline the importance of thoroughly gauging the risk-benefit ratio in every patient. More independent research needs to be done on subgroups of patients, particularly older patients. Indeed, a study of patients over age 40 found no significant improvement after a trial of four SGAs, but 36% developed the metabolic syndrome, and 23% had serious adverse events.[108]

18. Psychosocial treatment must not be overlooked. A variety of well-investigated treatments are helpful, including assertive community treatment, cognitive behavioral therapy, family education, social skills training, cognitive remediation, and others.

Finally, the lack of substantial progress in developing more effective antipsychotics is based, at least in part, on the absence of new models that can serve Pharma with a different approach to screening compounds for efficacy. Obviously, as one examines the newer agents, they are characterized by their interactions with dopamine, serotonin, and NMDA receptors, the same set of interactions used for decades. This is true of cariprazine (Vraylar), FDA approved in 2015 for the treatment of schizophrenia and acute bipolar disorder. Here we have a relatively new SGA, with the pitch being its relatively selective effect on D3 receptors (vs D2 receptors), where it acts as a partial agonist. However, the response rate in the Kane et al. study[109] was 34.7% at the 6 to 9 mg dose, vs a placebo response rate of 24.8%. Remarkably, *the most serious AEs involved worsening of schizophrenia*, not an encouraging finding. Nevertheless, in an attempt to move past the standard model involving dopamine receptor antagonism, an elegant meta-analysis by Leucht et al.[110] in 2017 of 60 years of controlled trials of APs gives us some hope, in that APs improved functioning and quality of life, but the effect size was small. However, as we noted earlier, 51% had at least minimal improvement, but only 23% had a "good" response. Adding to this brighter outlook was a meta-analysis of FGAs vs SGAs with regard to relapse in schizophrenia,[111] where SGAs *collectively* were superior in preventing relapse at 3, 6, and 12 months; however the NNT was 17, exceeding the standard NNT of 10 for a clinically meaningful effect size, and the long-range effects of the metabolic syndrome were not investigated.

In the next chapter, we shall explore some additional factors important to this equation, including additional data on the metabolic risks, overall mortality rates, and movement disorders (tardive dyskinesia and parkinsonism).

References

1. Hobson JA, Leonard JA. *Out of Its Mind. Psychiatry in Crisis.* Perseus Publishing, Cambridge MA, 2001.
2. Carlat DB. *Unhinged: The Trouble with Psychiatry—A Doctor's Revelations About a Profession in Crisis.* Free Press, New York, 2010.
3. Andreasen NC. *The Broken Brain: The Biological Revolution in Psychiatry.* Harper and Row, New York, 1984.
4. Verdoux H, Tournier M, Bégaud B. Antipsychotic prescribing trends: a review of pharmacoepidemiological trends. *Acta Psychiatrica Scandinavica* 2010;121:4–10.
5. Alexander GC, Gallagher SA, Mascola A, et al. Increasing off-label use of antipsychotic medications in the United States, 1995–2008. *Pharmacoepidemiology Drug Safety* 2010;20:177–184.
6. Dean CE. The death of specificity: cheers or tears? *Perspectives in Biology and Medicine* 2012;55:443–460.
7. Saha S, Chant D, McGrath J. A systematic review of mortality in schizophrenia: is the differential mortality gap worsening with time? *Archives of General Psychiatry* 2007;64:1123–1131.
8. Hoang U, Stewart R, Goldacre MJ. Mortality gap between people with schizophrenia or bipolar disorders and the general population persists in England. *EBMH* 2012;15:14–15.
9. Olfson M, Gerhard T, Huang C, et al. Premature mortality among adults with schizophrenia in the United States. *JAMA Psychiatry* 2015. Doi:10.1001/jamapsychiatry.2015.1737.
10. Crump C, Winkleby MA, Sundquist K, et al. Comorbidities and mortality in persons with schizophrenia: a Swedish national cohort study. *American Journal of Psychiatry* 2013;170:324–333.
11. Dutta R, Murray RM, Allardyce J, et al. Mortality in first-contact psychosis patients in the UK: a cohort study. *Psychological Medicine* 2012;42:1649–1661.
12. Walker ER, McGee RE, Druss BG. Mortality in mental disorders and global disease burden implications. A systematic review and meta-analysis. *JAMA Psychiatry* 2015;72:344–341.
13. Ma J, Ward EM, Siegal RL, et al. Temporal trends in mortality in the United States, 1969–2013. *Journal of the American Medical Association* 2015;314:1731–1739.
14. Chetty R, Stepner J, Abraham S, et al. The association between income and life expectancy in the United States, 2001–2014. *Journal of the American Medical Association* 2016;315:1750–1766.
15. Walter F, Carr MJ, Mok PLH, et al. Premature mortality among patients recently discharged from their first inpatient psychiatric treatment. *JAMA Psychiatry* 2017. Doi:10.1001/jamapsychiatry.2017.0071.

16. Stewart R. Mental disorders and mortality: so many publications, so little change. *Acta Psychiatrica Scandinavica* 2015. Doi:10.1111/acps.12476.152:1694.

17. Sweeny J. The long-term effect of schizophrenia on the brain: dementia praecox? *American Journal of Psychiatry* 2013;170:571–573.

18. Tiihonen J, Mittendorfer-Rutz E, Torniainen M, et al. Mortality and cumulative exposure to antipsychotics, antidepressants, and benzodiazepines in patients with schizophrenia: an observational follow-up study. *American Journal of Psychiatry* 2016;173:600–606.

19. Hegarty JD, Baldessarini RJ, Tohen M, et al. One hundred years of schizophrenia: a meta- analysis of the outcome literature. *Archives of General Psychiatry* 1994;151:1409–1416.

20. American Psychiatric Association. *Diagnostic and Statistical Manual of Mental Disorders*, Third Edition. American Psychiatric Association, Washington DC, 1980.

21. American Psychiatric Association. *Diagnostic and Statistical Manual of Mental Disorders*, Fifth Edition. American Psychiatric Association, Arlington VA, 2013.

22. Baldessarini RJ, Cohen B, Teicher MH. Significance of neuroleptic dose and plasma levels in the pharmacological treatment of psychosis. *Archives of General Psychiatry* 1988;45:79–91.

23. Dean CE. Schizophrenia: a 100-year retrospective. *American Journal of Psychiatry* 1995;152:1694.

24. Piketty T. *Capital in the Twenty-First Century*. Translated from the French by Arthur Goldhammer. Belknap Press, Harvard University Press, Boston, MA. For a short version, see Piketty T, Sachs E. Inequality in the long run. *Science* 2014;344:838–842.

25. Engel GL. The need for a new medical model: a challenge for biomedicine. *Science* 1977;196:129–136.

26. Wilkinson R, Pickett K. *The Spirit Level: Why Greater Equality Makes Societies Stronger*. Bloomsbury Press, New York, 2009.

27. Talbott JA. Deinstitutionalization: avoiding the disasters of the past. *Hospital and Community Psychiatry* 1979;30:621–624.

28. Healy D, Harris R, Tranter P, et al. Lifetime suicide rates in treated schizophrenia: 1875–1924 and 1994–1998 cohorts compared. *British Journal of Psychiatry* 2006;188:223–228.

29. Fisher S, Greenberg R. Editors. *From Placebo to Panacea: Putting Psychiatric Drugs to the Test*. John Wiley & Sons, New York, 1997.

30. Valenstein ES. *Blaming the Brain. The Truth About Drugs and Mental Health*. The Free Press, New York, 1998.

31. Gøtzsche PC. *Deadly Medicines and Organized crime: How Big pharma Has Corrupted Health Care*. Radcliffe Publishing, London and New York, 2013.

32. Winkleman, NW Jr. An appraisal of chlorpromazine: general principles for administration of chlorpromazine, based on experience with 1,090 patients. *The American Journal of Psychiatry* 1957;113:961–971.

33. Kurland AA, Hanlon TE, Tatom MH, et al. The comparative effectiveness of six phenothiazine compounds, phenobarbital, and inert placebo in the treatment of acutely ill patients: global measures of severity. *Journal of Nervous and Mental Disease* 1961;133:1–8.

34. Cole JO. Phenothiazine treatment in acute schizophrenia. The national institute of mental health psychopharmacology service center collaborative study group. *Archives of General Psychiatry* 1964;344:246–261.

35. Leucht S, Komossa K, Rummel-Kluge C, et al. A meta-analysis of head-to-head comparisons of second-generation antipsychotics in the treatment of schizophrenia. *American Journal of Psychiatry* 2009;166:152–163.

36. Leucht S, Arbter D, Engel RR, et al. How effective are second-generation antipsychotic drugs? A meta-analysis of placebo-controlled trials. *Molecular Psychiatry* 2009;14:429–447.

37. Cohen J. *Statistical Power Analysis for the Behavioral Sciences*, Revised Edition. Academic Press, New York, 1977.

38. Ghaemi SN. The alchemy of meta-analysis. In: *A Clinician's Guide to Statistics and Epidemiology in Mental Health*. Cambridge University Press, New York, 2009.

39. Button KS, Ioannidis JPA, Mokrysz C, et al. Power failure: why small sample size undermines the reliability of neuroscience. *Nature Reviews | Neuroscience* 2013;14:365–376.

40. Ioannidis JPA. The mass production of redundant, misleading, and conflicted systematic reviews and meta-analyses. *The Milbank Quarterly* 2016;94:485–514.

41. de Vrieze J. The metawars. *Science* 2018;361:1185–1188.

42. Geddes J, Freemantle N, Harrison P, et al. Atypical antipsychotics in the treatment of schizophrenia: systematic overview and meta-regression analysis. *British Medical Journal* 2000;321:1371–1376.

43. Davis J, Chen N, Glick ID. A meta-analysis of the efficacy of second-generation antipsychotics. *Archives of General Psychiatry* 2003;60:533–564.

44. Leucht S, Wahlbeck K, Hamann J, et al. New generation antipsychotics versus low potency conventional antipsychotics: a systematic review and meta-analysis. *The Lancet* 2003;361:1581–1589.

45. Leucht S, Barnes TRE, Kissling W, et al. Relapse prevention in schizophrenia with new-generation antipsychotics: a systematic review and exploratory meta-analysis of randomized, controlled trials. *American Journal of Psychiatry* 2003;160:1209–1222.

46. Leucht S, Corves C, Arbter D, et al. Second-generation versus first-generation antipsychotic drugs for schizophrenia: a meta-analysis. *The Lancet* 2009;373:31–41.

47. Lieberman JA, Stroup TS, McEvoy JP, et al. Effectiveness of antipsychotic drugs in patients with chronic schizophrenia. *New England Journal of Medicine* 2005;353:1209–1223.

48. Swartz MS, Perkins DO, Stroup TS, et al. Effects of antipsychotic medications on psychosocial functioning in patients with chronic schizophrenia: findings from the NIMH CATIE study. *American Journal of Psychiatry* 2007;164:428–436.

49. Jones PB, Barnes TRE, Davies L, et al. Randomized controlled trial of the effect on quality of life of second-vs first-generation antipsychotic drugs in schizophrenia. Cost utility of the latest antipsychotics drugs in schizophrenia study (CUtLASS 1). *Archives of General Psychiatry* 2006;63:1079–1087.

50. Rosenheck R, Perlick D, Bingham S, et al. Effectiveness and cost of olanzapine and haloperidol in the treatment of schizophrenia: a randomized controlled trial. *Journal of the American Medical Association* 2003;290:2693–2702.

51. Lieberman JA, Tollefson G, Tohen M, et al. Comparative efficacy and safety of atypical and conventional antipsychotic drugs in first-episode psychosis: a randomized, double-blind trial of olanzapine versus haloperidol. *American Journal of Psychiatry* 2003;160:1396–1404.

52. Sikich L, Frazier JA, McClellan J, et al. Double-blind comparison of first- and second-generation antipsychotics in early-onset schizophrenia and schizoaffective

disorder: findings from the treatment of early-onset schizophrenia spectrum disorders (TEOSS) study. *American Journal of Psychiatry* 2008;165:1420–1431.

53. McEvoy JP, Lieberman JA, Perkins DO, et al. Efficacy and tolerability of olanzapine, quetiapine, and risperidone in the treatment of early psychosis: a randomized, double-blind 52-week comparison. *American Journal of Psychiatry* 2007;164:1050–1060.

54. Harvey RC, James AC, Shields GE. A systematic review and network meta-analysis to assess the relative efficacy of antipsychotics for the treatment of positive and negative symptoms in schizophrenia. *CNS Drugs* 2016. Doi:10.1007/s40263-015-0308-1.

55. Kane JM, Canas F, Kramer M, et al. Treatment of schizophrenia with paliperidone extended-release tablets: a 6-week placebo-controlled trial. *Schizophrenia Research* 2007;90:147–161.

56. Davidson M, Emsley R, Kramer M, et al. Efficacy, safety and early response of paliperidone extended-release tablets (Paliperidone ER): results of a 6-week, randomized, placebo-controlled study. *Schizophrenia Research* 2007;93:117–130.

57. Marder SR, Kramer M, Ford L, et al. Efficacy and safety of paliperidone extended-release tablets: results of a 6-week, randomized-controlled study. *Biological Psychiatry* Doi:10.1016/j.biosych.01.017.

58. Tarazi FLL, Choi YK, Gardner M, et al. Asenapine exerts distinctive regional effects on ionotropic glutamate receptor subtypes in rat brain. *Synapse* 2009;63:413–420.

59. FDA Drug safety communication: serious allergic reactions reported with the use of Saphris (asenapine maleate). http://fda.gov/Drugs/DrugSafety/ucm270243.htm. 09/01/2011.

60. Potkin SG, Cohen M, Panagides J. Efficacy and tolerability of asenapine in acute schizophrenia: a placebo-and risperidone-controlled trial. *Journal of Clinical Psychiatry* 2007;68:1492–1500.

61. Kane JM, Cohen M, Zhao J, et al. Efficacy and safety of asenapine in a placebo-and haloperidol-controlled trial in patients with acute exacerbation of schizophrenia. *Journal of Clinical Psychopharmacology* 2010;30:106–115.

62. Szegedi A, Verweij P, Duijnhoven W. Efficacy of asenapine for schizophrenia: comparison with placebo and comprehensive efficacy of all antipsychotics using all available head-to-head randomized trials using meta-analytical techniques. *Presented at the American College of Neuropsychopharmacology* December 2010, Miami, Florida. This data can be found in Szegedi A, Verweij P, van Duijnhoven W, et al. Meta-analysis of the efficacy of asenapine for acute schizophrenia: comparisons with placebo and other antipsychotics. *Journal of Clinical Psychiatry* 2012;73:1533–1540.

63. Citrome L. Iloperidone, a critical review. *Journal of Clinical Psychiatry* 2011;11(suppl 1):72, 19–23.

64. Potkin SG, Litman RE, Torres R, et al. Efficacy of iloperidone in the treatment of schizophrenia: initial phase 3 studies. *Journal of Clinical Psychopharmacology* 2008;28(suppl 1):S4–S11.

65. Weiden PJ, Cutler AJ, Polymeropoulos MH, et al. Safety profile of iloperidone: a pooled analysis of 6-week acute-phase pivotal trials. *Journal of Clinical Psychopharmacology* 2008;28(suppl 1):S12–S19.

66. Kane JM, Lauriello J, Laska E, et al. Long-term efficacy and safety of iloperidone. *Journal of Clinical Psychopharmacology* 2008;28(suppl 1):S29–S28.

67. Marino J, Caballero J. Iloperidone for the treatment of schizophrenia. *The Annals of Pharmacotherapy* 2010;44:863–870.

68. Ishibashi T, Horisawa T, Tokuda K, et al. Pharmacological profile of lurasidone, a novel antipsychotic agent with potent 5-hydroxytrptamine 7 (5-HT$_7$) and

5-HT1a receptor activity. *The Journal of Pharmacology and Experimental Therapeutics* 2010;334:171–181.

69. Nakamura M, Ogasa M, Guarino J, et al. Lurasidone in the treatment of acute schizophrenia: a double-blind, placebo-controlled trial. *Journal of Clinical Psychiatry* 2009;70:829–836.

70. Melzter HY, Cucchiaro J, Silva R, et al. Lurasidone in the treatment of acute schizophrenia: a randomized, double-blind, placebo-and olanzapine-controlled study. *American Journal of Psychiatry* 2011;168:957–967.

71. Kane JM. Lurasidone, a clinical review. *Journal of Clinical Psychiatry* 2011;72(suppl 1):24–28.

72. Maeda K, Sugino H, Akazawa H, et al. Brexpiprazole I: in vitro and in vivo characterization of a novel serotonins-dopamine activity modulator. *The Journal of Pharmacology and Experimental Therapeutics* 2014;350:589–604.

73. Citrome L. Brexipiprazole for schizophrenia and as adjunct for major depressive disorders. *Current Psychiatry* 2015;14:73–78.

74. Hobart M, Ouyang J, Forbes A, et al. Efficacy and safety of brexipiprazole (OPC-34712) as maintenance treatment in adults with schizophrenia: a randomized, double-blind, placebo-controlled study. *Poster presented at the American Society of Clinical Psychopharmacology Annual Meeting*, June 22–15, 2015. Miami, FL.

75. American Psychiatric Association. *Practice Guideline for the Treatment of Patients with Schizophrenia*, Second Edition. *American Journal of Psychiatry* 2004;161(suppl 2):1–114.

76. Leucht S, Kissling W, Davis JM. Second-generation antipsychotics for schizophrenia: can we resolve the conflict? *Psychological Medicine* 2009;39:1591–1602.

77. Kendall T. The rise and fall of the atypical antipsychotics. *The British Journal of Psychiatry* 2011;199:266–268.

78. Lewis S, Lieberman J. CATIE and CUtLASS: can we handle the truth? *The British Journal of Psychiatry* 2008;192:161–163. (The authors note a *30-fold increase* in the global market for APs from the late 1980s to 2008.)

79. Comer JS, Mojtabai R, Olfson M. National trends in the antipsychotic treatment of psychiatric outpatients with anxiety disorders. *American Journal of Psychiatry* 2011;168:1057–1065.

80. Leslie DL, Mohamed S, Rosenheck R. Off-label uses of antipsychotic medications in the Department of Veterans Affairs Health Care System. *Psychiatric Services* 2009;60:1175–1181.

81. Dixon L, Perkins D, Calmes C. Guideline watch (September 2009): practice guideline for the treatment of patients with schizophrenia. *PsychiatryOnline*. http://psychiatryonline.org.content.aspx?bookid=28&sectionid=16822'3:501001.

82. Buchanan RW, Kreyenbuhl J, Kelly DL, et al. The 2009 schizophrenia PORT psychopharmacological treatment recommendations and summary statements. *Schizophrenia Bulletin* 2010;36:71–93.

83. Huhn M, Nikolakopoulou A, Schneider J, et al. Comparative efficacy and tolerability of 32 oral antipsychotics for the acute treatment of adults with multiepisode schizophrenia: a systematic review and network meta-analysis. *The Lancet* 2019;394:939–951.

84. Stroup TS, Gerhardt T, Crystal S, et al. Comparative effectiveness of adjunctive psychotropic medications in patients with schizophrenia. *JAMA Psychiatry* 2019;76:508–505.

85. Tiihonen J, Suokas JT, Svissaari JM, et al. Polypharmacy with antipsychotics, antidepressants or benzodiazepines and mortality in schizophrenia. *Archives General Psychiatry* 2012;69:476–483.

86. Zhang Z-J, Yao Z-H, Liu W, et al. Effects of antipsychotics on fat deposition and changes in leptin and insulin levels. *British Journal of Psychiatry* 2004;184:58–62.

87. Gilles M, Hentschel F, Paslakis G, et al. Visceral and subcutaneous fat in patients treated with olanzapine: a case series. *Clinical Neuropharmacology* 2010;33:248–249.

88. Uchida H, Suzuki T, Takeuchi H, et al. Low dose vs standard dose of antipsychotics for relapse prevention in schizophrenia: meta-analysis. *Schizophrenia Bulletin* 2011;37:788–799.

89. Remington G. Antipsychotic dosing: still a work in progress. *American Journal of Psychiatry* 2010;167:623–625.

90. Minzenberg MJ, Yoon JH, Carter CS. Schizophrenia. In: *The American Psychiatric Publishing Textbook of Psychiatry*, Fifth Edition. Editors: Hales RE, Yudofsky SC, Gabbard G. American Psychiatric Publishing, Washington DC and London, 2008, p. 442.

91. Moncrieff J. Antipsychotic maintenance treatment: time to rethink? *Public Library of Science Medicine* 12(3):e1001861. Doi:10.1371/journal.pmed.1001861.

92. Fusar-Poli P, Smieskova R, Kempton MJ, et al. Progressive brain changes in schizophrenia related to antipsychotic treatment? A meta-analysis of longitudinal MRI studies. *Neuroscience and Biobehavioral Reviews* 2013;37:1680–1691.

93. Andreasen NC, Nopoulos P, Magnotta V, et al. Progressive brain changes in schizophrenia: a prospective longitudinal study of first-episode schizophrenia. *Biological Psychiatry* 2011;70:672–679.

94. Olabi B, Ellison I, McIntosh AM, et al. Are there progressive brain changes in schizophrenia: a meta-analysis of structural magnetic resonance imaging studies. *Biological Psychiatry* 2011;70:88–96.

95. Lesh TA, Tanase C, Geib BR, et al. A multi-modal analysis of antipsychotic effects on brain structure and function in first-episode schizophrenia. *JAMA Psychiatry* 2015;72:226–234.

96. Goff DC, Falkai P, Fleischhacker WW, et al. The long-term effect of antipsychotic medication on clinical course in schizophrenia. *AJP in Advance.* Doi:10.1176/appi.ajp.2017.160910161.

97. Moncrieff J, Steinberg S. A critical analysis of recent data on the long-term outcome of antipsychotic treatment. *Psychological Medicine* 2018;49:750–753.

98. Dean CE. Antipsychotic-associated neuronal changes in the brain: toxic, therapeutic, or irrelevant to the long-term outcome in schizophrenia? *Progress in Neuropsychopharmacology & Biological Psychiatry* 2006;30:174–189.

99. Smara MT, Dold M, Gianatsi M, et al. Efficacy, acceptability, and tolerability of antipsychotics in treatment-resistant schizophrenia. A network meta-analysis. *JAMA Psychiatry.* Doi:10.1001/jamapsychiatry.2015.2955. Published online February 3, 2016.

100. Masuda T, Misawa F, Takase M, et al. Association with hospitalization and all-cause discontinuation among patients with schizophrenia on clozapine vs other oral second-generation antipsychotics. A systematic review and meta-analysis of cohort studies. *JAMA Psychiatry* 2019;76:1052–1062.

101. Tiihonen J, Haukka J, Taylor M, et al. A nationwide cohort study of oral and depot antipsychotics after first hospitalization for schizophrenia. *American Journal of Psychiatry* 2011;168:603–609.

102. Kishi T, Oya K, Iwata N. Long-acting injectable antipsychotics for the prevention of relapse in patients with recent-onset psychotic disorders: a systematic review and meta-analysis of controlled trials. *Psychiatry Research* 2016;246:750–755.

103. Lähteenvuo M, Tanskanen A, Taipale H, et al. Real-world effectiveness of pharmacologic treatments for the prevention of rehospitalization in a Finnish nationwide cohort of patients with bipolar disorders. *JAMA Psychiatry*, published online 2018. Doi:10.1001/jamapsychiatry.2017.4711.

104. Tiihonen J, Tanskanen A, Taipale H. 20-year follow-up study on discontinuation of antipsychotic treatment in first-episode schizophrenia. *American Journal of Psychiatry* 2018;175:765–773.

105. Taskenen A, Tiihonen J, Taipale J. Mortality in schizophrenia: 30-year nationwide follow-up study. *Acta Psychiatrica Scandinavica* 2018;138:492–499.

106. Olfson M, King M, Schoenbaum M. Antipsychotic treatment of adults in the United States. *Journal of Clinical Psychiatry* 2015;76:1346–1353.

107. Maust DT, Kim HM, Seyfried LS, et al. Antipsychotics, other psychotropics and the risk of death in patients with dementia. *JAMA Psychiatry* 2015;72:438–445.

108. Jin H, Peian B, Golshan S, et al. Comparison of long-term safety and effectiveness of 4 atypical antipsychotics in patients over 40: a trial using equipoise-stratified randomization. *Journal of Clinical Psychiatry* 2013;74:10–18.

109. Kane JM, Zukin S, Wang Y, et al. Efficacy and safety of cariprazine in acute exacerbation of schizophrenia. Results from an international, phase III clinical trial. *Journal of Clinical Psychopharmacology* 2015;35:367–373.

110. Leucht S, Leucht C, Huhn M, et al. Sixty years of placebo-controlled antipsychotic drug trials in acute schizophrenia: a systematic review, Bayesian meta-analysis, and meta-regression of efficacy predictors. *American Journal of Psychiatry* 2017;174:927–942.

111. Kishimoto T, Agarwal V, Kishi T, et al. Relapse prevention in schizophrenia: a systematic review and meta-analysis of second-generation antipsychotics versus first-generation antipsychotics. *Molecular Psychiatry* 2013;18:53–66.

4   Antipsychotics and the Metabolic Syndrome, Cardiovascular Disease, and Mortality

Introduction

In previous chapters, we have discussed the development of APs and their putative of modes of action but also noted our failure to substantially improve their efficacy, which is similar in FGAs and SGAs. In contrast, we have seen a shifting set of side effects as drug development continued. As discussed in the previous chapters, the early FGAs (chlorpromazine, mesoridizine) were marked by significant anticholinergic side effects, such as constipation, dry mouth, urinary retention, and decreased sweating and also produced sedation, dizziness, postural hypotension and fainting, secondary to their blockade of alpha-adrenergic receptors. The blockade of dopamine receptors resulted in parkinsonism and, if chronic, tardive dyskinesia (TD). With the move to high-potency APs (haloperidol, thiothixene, fluphenazine), the anticholinergic and anti-alpha-adrenergic side effects diminished, but parkinsonism increased. Whether the higher-potency drugs led to more TD was questionable. With the introduction of SGAs (clozapine, olanzapine, risperidone), rates of parkinsonism appeared to decrease, although some blinded studies found similar rates. The incidence of TD, however, declined. Unfortunately, it soon became obvious that patients treated with SGAs were gaining significant amounts of weight and developing new-onset diabetes mellitus. Many went on to develop the full metabolic syndrome, a clear threat to their health and well-being.

The Metabolic Syndrome

The metabolic syndrome is characterized not only by weight gain but also hypertension, high levels of cholesterol and triglycerides, and insulin resistance, which, in turn, give rise to elevated levels of blood glucose and the eventual onset of type 2 diabetes mellitus (DM). This is very alarming, since it is well known that any component of the metabolic syndrome elevates the risk for cardiovascular disease, including strokes and myocardial infarction. In response, the American Diabetes Association, in conjunction with the American Psychiatric Association, the American Association of Clinical

Endocrinologists, and the North American Association for the Study of Obesity, held a consensus development conference in 2003[1] and concluded that clozapine and olanzapine were associated with the greatest risk of weight gain, hyperlipidemia, and DM, whereas risperidone and quetiapine had an intermediate risk, and aripiprazole and ziprasidone had little or no effect. The panel further noted that some patients might present with an *acute* onset of diabetic ketoacidosis, a clear-cut medical emergency.

The panel concluded that the serious health risks posed by the SGAs require "appropriate baseline screening and ongoing monitoring," which meant asking about the family history of cardiovascular disease, DM, hypertension, and hyperlipidemia. In addition, physicians should record data on weight and height in order to calculate the body mass index (BMI) and measure waist circumference, blood pressure, fasting blood glucose, and a fasting lipid panel.[1, p. 600] Dietary counseling might be appropriate, and the family should be educated with regard to the warning signs of DM and diabetic ketoacidosis. Weight should be assessed at four, eight, and twelve weeks after starting an SGA. Should the patient gain 5% or more of body weight, the physician should consider switching to a lower risk drug. At three months, one should measure fasting blood glucose and lipid levels, as well as blood pressure. Obviously, the onset of DM or significant increases in lipids should trigger a consultation with the appropriate specialist. These conclusions and recommendations were especially striking, since financial support for the conference was provided in part by the manufacturers of SGAs, and a number of participants had received financial support from the industry[1, p. 601]

While the conference recommendations were commendable, there is little doubt that Pharma fought tooth and nail against acknowledging the metabolic side effects of their drugs. Eli Lilly was especially blatant in its efforts to downplay the metabolic consequences of olanzapine by hiding or minimizing weight gain in publications and instructing their sales reps to avoid even mentioning the metabolic side effects.[2, 3, p. 142] On a personal note, one of the leading investigators from Eli Lilly met with the medical staff at the Minneapolis VA Medical Center on June 13, 2003, but refused twice to answer my questions regarding olanzapine-induced DM. Indeed, DM, weight gain, and other metabolic complications were seldom if ever mentioned in the four primary trials of olanzapine—trials that wound up spawning 234 publications.[3, p. 142]

The use of SGAs quickly spread to children and adolescents, prompting a *New York Times* editorialist[4] to cite evidence showing that olanzapine and risperidone were no more effective in youth than older agents but induced significant weight gain. Indeed, the metabolic effects of SGAs occur earlier and to a greater extent in youth, as shown by Correll et al.[5] Nevertheless, prescriptions for SGAs in youth increased from about 250 per 100,000 office visits in 1994 to almost 2,500 per 100,000 office visits in 2004.[5] By 2002, 92.3% of office-based prescriptions were written for SGAs.[6]

In October 2008, Eli Lilly paid $62 million to 32 states for illegally marketing olanzapine for off-label use, and in January 2009, the company agreed to a $1.4 billion payment to settle federal charges involving illegal marketing.[7] However, 2007 sales had reached $4.7 billion,[7] based in part on the widespread use of this drug for off-label conditions While off-label use is legal, a 2006 study of national trends in AP use in youth found a striking imbalance, with only 14% of AP prescriptions aimed at psychotic disorders, compared with 38% for disruptive behaviors, 32% for mood disorders, and 17% for developmental disorders.[6]

Other companies have had similar records, including AstraZeneca, which was fined $520 million in 2010 for illegal marketing of quetiapine and downplaying the risk of quetiapine-induced diabetes mellitus.[8] By 2011, the company had paid an additional $647 million to settle all but 250 of some 28,000 cases. As with the fines paid by Lilly, these fines did not significantly affect the bottom line since sales of quetiapine reached $ 4.9 billion in 2009 and grew to $5.3 billion worldwide by 2010. In 2012, Johnson & Johnson was fined $1.2 billion by an Arkansas Circuit Court judge as a result of 240,000 violations of that state's deceptive practices act, the accusation being that J&J had minimized or concealed the risks of risperidone.[9]

How Did Clinicians Respond?

In December 2003, the FDA finally ordered that a class warning be added to the labeling of SGAs, noting an increased risk of hyperglycemia, DM, and ketoacidosis. The FDA also sent letters to mental health professionals recommending monitoring of plasma glucose and careful attention to any symptoms of DM.[10, 11]

What effect did the ADA/APA Consensus Conference and the FDA-mandated labeling have on clinical practice? Not much. A study of three state Medicaid programs[12] found that testing of blood glucose did *not* increase from the baseline rate of 27% after the warnings were issued, while testing of blood lipids increased by only 1.7% from a baseline of 10%. The good news: Prescriptions of olanzapine dropped by 19.9% while those for aripiprazole (less likely to result in metabolic changes) rose by 12%. A meta-analysis of 48 studies with 290,000 patients[13] found somewhat better figures, in that rates of glucose testing rose from 33% to 48% post guidelines, but the changes in lipid monitoring were so minimal they could not be analyzed. In studies that examined monitoring *in the absence of guidelines*, 70% of patients had their blood pressure checked, but rates of monitoring for blood glucose and cholesterol fell to less than 50%.[13]

But what happens if clinicians find evidence of the metabolic syndrome? Are patients being adequately treated? In the CATIE study, rates of treatment for DM, lipid abnormalities, and hypertension were 70%, 12%, and 38%, respectively![14] This is unacceptable. While there is room for debate[15] over the difficulties in parsing the precise role of APs in the development of

DM and other metabolic changes, the bulk of the evidence clearly points to a significant metabolic risk with many of the SGAs. Nevertheless, we have to be mindful of obesity in the general population, as noted by de Leon.[15] Indeed, worldwide evidence in 2017[16] showed that age-standardized prevalence of obesity increased from 0.7% in 1975 to 5.6% in 2016 in girls and from 0.9% to 7.8% in boys. Prevalence of obesity is about 20% in a number of countries, including the United States.

Why do psychiatrists neglect these problems? Part of the answer lies in Pharma's fight to downplay or ignore the metabolic changes. Another ploy has been to emphasize the epidemics of obesity and diabetes in the general population, and another is to stress the well-known fact that people with many psychiatric disorders have an increased incidence of diabetes, obesity, and cardiovascular disease[15, 17] prior to the use of APs. While both these assertions are correct, the company line has been to stress the difficulties in clarifying cause and effect, rather than admitting that some APs make these metabolic problems worse. Such tactics are not new. Years ago, a number of prominent psychiatrists attempted to minimize the neurologic side effects of APs, especially tardive dyskinesia (TD), by pointing to its reversibility[18] and casually mentioning that it occurs in only a "few" patients.[19, p. 212]

For all the debate about cause and effect, the evidence of AP-induced weight gain continues to grow. For example, one group[20] reviewed 11 studies of AP-naïve patients not taking medications known to increase weight who then began an AP. The authors focused on weight gain and changes in the BMI (the ratio of weight in kilograms to height in meters squared, or kg/m^2) and found a *rapid and continuous gain in weight which was evident four weeks after starting APs*. The mean increase in weight was 4.85 kg, with a mean increase of 1.08 on the BMI. When they limited the analysis to hospitalized patients, the mean weight gain dropped to 3.8 kg; nevertheless, the results were highly significant. We should note, too, that the BMI *continued to increase* by 3.8 points in a few longer-term studies of 24 to 48 weeks. These data argue against the common belief that weight gain will plateau over time.

Unfortunately, the number of studies involving AP-naïve patients was too small to analyze the effect of individual APs. The authors noted that the rapid onset of weight gain was in contrast to data from an earlier and widely cited study by Allison et al.,[21] who found a significant gain in weight at ten weeks on average. However, that group did not take into account other risk factors and did not report on BMI.

While we have focused on schizophrenia, AP-induced metabolic changes can also occur in bipolar disorder, as shown in a meta-analysis[22] in which the risk of the metabolic syndrome significantly exceeded the risk in the general population. Unfortunately, those with bipolar disorder and schizophrenia had lower rates of glucose testing than adults in a state Medicaid program. Overall, *only* 41% had been tested for hyperlipidemia.[23]

Mortality and Morbidity in Excessive Weight Gain

While most people are aware of the serious consequences of diabetes and high cholesterol, we need to stress the devastating consequences of excessive weight gain. Perhaps the largest study to address this problem was published in 2009.[24] The authors examined the association between BMI and mortality in 57 prospective studies involving 900,000 adults after five years of follow-up. (Data for the first five years was excluded in order to limit the effects of pre-existing illness.)

The mean BMI at study entry was 24.8. (For reference, a BMI of 30 kg/m2 or greater is defined as obesity; a BMI from 25 to 29 is defined as being overweight.) The average age was 46, and 61% were men. After a mean follow-up of eight years, 72,749 deaths had occurred. For each 5 kg/m2 increase in BMI, overall mortality increased by 30%!

- At a BMI of 30 to 35, median life expectancy was reduced by two to four years.
- At a BMI of 40 to 45, median life expectancy was reduced by eight to ten years, similar to that found in smokers. No doubt these figures would have been even worse had it not been for the exclusion of participants with initial BMIs over 50, as well as those with a baseline history of heart disease or stroke.
- In all ages and both sexes, all-cause mortality was lowest at a BMI of 22.5 to 25. This isn't the only study with such findings. Guh and associates in Vancouver[25] did a meta-analysis of 89 studies that examined the rate co-morbid illnesses associated with obesity or excessive weight in Europe, North America, Australia, and New Zealand. They used both BMI and waist circumference as anchor points since increased waist circumference (WC) in some studies was a better predictor of cardiac disease and DM. (WC equal to or greater than 94 cm in males or 80 cm in females is defined as overweight; a WC of 88 cm or greater in females or 102 cm in males indicates obesity.)

Being overweight was *significantly* associated with DM, all cancers (except esophageal, pancreatic, and prostate), asthma, gallbladder disease, osteoarthritis, and back pain. Women who were overweight had a relative risk of 3.92 for type II DM: that is, almost four times the risk of those not overweight. With regard to obesity, the findings were almost identical, but the relative risk of type II DM in women increased to 12.41.

Additional Risks of Obesity and the Metabolic Syndrome

A number of studies have also found that the metabolic syndrome is a risk factor for cognitive decline in older adults.[26] These investigators set out to assess the association of the metabolic syndrome with cognitive impairment and markers of inflammation such as interleukin 6 and C-reactive protein in 2,600 people studied for five years. *Those with the metabolic syndrome had a 20% increase in risk of cognitive impairment.* A high level of inflammation yielded a 66% increase in risk.

In 2010, a meta-analytic study found a significant association between obesity and depressive disorder among adults aged 20 to 59 years and in those ages 60 and over.[27] Patients with baseline depression had an 18% increase in the risk of becoming obese, but the association was stronger in women. The authors confirmed that the association is bidirectional: *depression increases the risk of obesity by 58% while being overweight leads to a 27% increase in the risk of clinical depression. Obesity ups the risk to 55%!* Interestingly, the association between the risk of obesity-associated depressive disorder was stronger among Americans than Europeans, perhaps in part due to the fact that the average BMI in Americans was higher—no surprise here!

Well, if depression is increased by obesity, what about suicide? Mukamal et al. did a prospective study[28] of cause-specific mortality in 1.1 million adults followed from 1982 to 2004 as part of the American Cancer Society Cancer Prevention Study II. Consistent with several early studies, the authors found an *inverse relationship* between BMI and suicide in adults middle aged and older, despite the fact that increasing BMI was associated with DM. Interestingly, this inverse relationship held true across geographic regions (although the suicide rate differs dramatically across regions) and in both women and men but was "limited to married individuals." However, the authors cited other work showing an increased risk of suicide attempts in women having higher BMIs.[29]

Antipsychotics, Obesity, and Suicide in Adolescents and Children

None of the studies just reviewed addressed the risks of APs in children and adolescents. This is a matter of considerable importance, since AP prescriptions aimed at youth in the United States rose six-fold between 1993 and 2002.[6] In 2000 through 2002, SGAs had a 92% share of the AP market, but only 14% of the prescriptions for SGAs were being written for schizophrenia or other psychotic disorders. Instead, 38% were aimed at disruptive behavior, 31% for mood disorders, and 17% for developmental disorders. Similar increases have been found in the United Kingdom, with a three-fold increase for youth ages seven to twelve years[30] and in the Netherlands, where use of APs doubled between 1997 and 2005.[31]

Interestingly, the evidence suggests that APs may have efficacy for these non-psychotic conditions, with a number needed to treat (NNT) of only two to five, which is lower than in schizophrenia.[32] However, the risk-benefit ratio remains in question, especially when treatment is prolonged, due to the metabolic and neurologic side effects. Additional questions left largely unaddressed by these authors are the long-term effects of APs on brain structure and function, neuroendocrine function, and signaling pathways. (These results also underscore the lack of specificity found with use of APs, a topic we will explore later.)

This massive increase in the use of powerful APs was in part due to the hype surrounding SGAs, particularly the mistaken assumption that SGAs were more effective and had fewer neurologic side effects. While there may be some truth to the latter, the trade-off appears to be riskier than initially thought. Nevertheless, the increase in APs prescribed for youth is continuing, never mind the risks! I guarantee that the use of SGAs in youth will continue to rise, given three factors. (For additional details, see references 32–39).

First is the FDA decision in late 2009 to ramp up the approval rate for use of olanzapine and quetiapine in the treatment of schizophrenia and manic episodes in adolescents ages 13 to 17. Risperidone had been approved earlier for treatment of schizophrenia in adolescents ages 13 to 17 and for those as young as age 10 with bipolar disorder, a gift to Pharma, given the epidemic of bipolar illness. Risperidone has also been approved for the treatment of irritability in autism at *ages 5 to 16* years, as has aripiprazole, previously approved for schizophrenia in the those ages 13 to 17 and as an adjunct to lithium or valproate in bipolar mania in youth ages 10 to 17. Paliperidone is now approved for treatment of schizophrenia at ages 13 to 17.

It is truly mind boggling that the FDA has put its stamp of approval on the use of quetiapine and olanzapine in children, despite their well-known role in the development of the metabolic syndrome. It is even more inexplicable when one considers that the risks of the metabolic syndrome, neurologic side effects, and hyperprolactinemia are even higher in children than in adults, and the risk may persist for some time after the drug is stopped.[35–37] Indeed, the risk of DM increased by 51% in youths taking SGAs over a period of 17 months.[38]

Weight gain and adverse effects on health seem especially prevalent with olanzapine, which, according to Vitiello et al.,[39] *should not* be considered as a first-line drug in this age group. Indeed, others have noted[29] that in the first three months of treatment with SGAs, children ages 4 through 19 gain between 4.4 and 8.5 kg, compared with 0.2 kg in controls, as well as significant increases in cholesterol and triglycerides that are sometimes independent of weight gain. Vitiello et al.[39] also cite studies that have found elevated prolactin levels in almost 79% of children treated with SGAs for *less than a month*, with risperidone and olanzapine being at higher risk.

On the bright side—if there is one—aripiprazole tends to lower prolactin levels. On the dark side, there is growing evidence that no child, no matter how young, can escape the epidemic of medicating children. The FDA is playing into this, as we have seen earlier, with the FDA allowing children at age four to be medicated with APs. Over 20 years ago, Zito tracked the use of psychiatric drugs in *children ages two to four* in two state Medicaid programs and an HMO during the years 1991 through 1995.[40] These very young children experienced a 2.2-fold increase in the use of ADs, a 3-fold increase in the use of stimulants, and a 28-fold increase in the use of clonidine for attentional deficits, although there was little solid data to support the use of clonidine. They also cited evidence showing an increase in clonidine poisoning, not surprisingly.

Second, while psychiatrists must bear some responsibility for this state of affairs, I must note that political pressure on the FDA to approve drugs more rapidly seems to have diminished its regulatory efforts. For example, the approval rate of new drugs had increased from 60% to 80% by 2001. In addition, the number of warning letters to physicians fell by 50% in the late 1990s.[7, p. 14]

Third is the dramatic and very odd increase in the diagnosis of bipolar disorder in children and adolescents. A national survey of office-based physicians[41] found that in 1994 and 1995, the diagnosis of bipolar disorder in youth was made in 25 visits per 100,000 people. *Only ten years later, the diagnosis was being made in 1,003 visits per 100,000 people, a 40-fold increase, compared with a 2-fold increase in adults!* We shall explore this phenomenon later, but we have to insist that the biology of bipolar disorder, including its genetic roots and pathophysiology, can't be invoked as causal factors; rather, marketing and the growing acceptability of drug treatment are the likely explanations. As we have noted, the FDA has cooperated in this mass hysteria, approving increasing numbers of APs for the treatment of bipolar disorder, whether in children, adolescents, or adults.

Animal and Human Studies of Antipsychotic-Induced Metabolic Side Effects

While a review by Heidi Boyda and her colleagues[42] emphasized that weight gain is associated with an elevated risk of DM, others[43] have found that *15% of those with new-onset DM did not develop substantial weight gain, nor did 25% of cases with acute-onset diabetic ketoacidosis*, leaving the patient and provider without an early warning sign. Nevertheless, we need to closely monitor patients for unusual gains in weight. The liability of APs with regard to weight gain and DM is generally consistent across studies.[43, 44]

A meta-analytic study[45] of SGAs in 48 studies involving head-to-head comparisons produced additional data on both weight gain and differences among the SGAs with regard to their effects on cholesterol and blood glucose. Here are the rankings:

- Clozapine: more weight gain than olanzapine.
- Olanzapine: more weight gain than all other SGAs and greater increases in blood glucose than risperidone, quetiapine, aripiprazole, and ziprasidone, but not different from clozapine!
- Quetiapine: more increases in cholesterol than with risperidone and ziprasidone.

Numerous factors have been posited to explain the alarming increase in AP-induced weight gain, including blockade of the H1, muscarinic M3, and 5-HT2c receptors. Boyda et al.[42] also have noted multiple other possibilities, some of which we've already mentioned, including lifestyle, biological effects of the illness, and a direct effect on lipids, which, in turn, can lead to weight gain and insulin resistance. More specifically, there are *five key risk factors* for the eventual development of the metabolic syndrome: insulin resistance, glucose dysfunction, lipid and hormone changes, hypertension, and, of course, weight gain itself.

As one might imagine, we have seen a tremendous amount of research on risk factors, both in humans and in animals. Preclinical research using rodents has been especially important. The Boyda et al. review[42] cites 110 published in recent years. Her group concludes that these studies have had strong predictive validity; that is, APs that result in severe metabolic side effects in humans also have the strongest effects in rodents, with a few exceptions. The most consistent effects of APs have been on glucose regulation and insulin resistance, but rodent models of weight gain have been less consistent. For example, olanzapine induces weight gain only in female rats, a finding *not* replicated in humans, while the effects of clozapine are negative in rodents, in marked contrast to what we find in humans.

Human studies on weight gain have focused on clinical predictors, including a low baseline BMI, younger age, being female, non-white ethnicity, higher BMIs in parents,[46] and antipsychotic polypharmacy,[47] a key finding given the growing prevalence of polypharmacy, a topic we will explore in the Chapter 6. A number of genetic studies[48] have focused on various candidate genes, but the results have not been clinically useful due to the lack of specificity. A candidate gene analysis[49] of 756 schizophrenia patients in the CATIE study identified one polymorphism associated with discontinuation of quetiapine and another associated with improvement of verbal memory, but these results were "equivocal" and obviously in need of replication in a much larger sample size. Unfortunately, another GWAS[50] in a Han Chinese sample involved fewer than 1,100 subjects, a very small sample. A 2019 study[51] provided a review of twin and candidate gene studies that appeared to influence AP-induced weight gain, including variants in the serotonin 2c receptor, neuropeptide Y, the melanocortin 4 receptor, and several others, but *none of these have been sufficiently replicated* such that they can be used in the clinic.

Clinical Notes

1. *I never prescribe olanzapine or quetiapine to a new adult patient and would be even more reluctant to do so in children and adolescents.* I continue them only with reluctance in adult patients who are doing well clinically, have avoided the metabolic complications, and choose to continue them after a detailed discussion of their side effects. I am baffled by colleagues who

make olanzapine or quetiapine a first-line choice, given the large and ever-increasing number of alternatives, not to mention the well-known epidemics of obesity and DM in the general population—problems that are even worse in schizophrenia and bipolar disorder. It is particularly puzzling why many physicians use these agents for non–FDA approved conditions. This is especially disturbing when one considers the rampant use of quetiapine for insomnia, a condition for which multiple alternatives exist.

2. Clozapine is another matter, given its niche for use in highly treatment-resistant patients and the vetting that is done by the National Clozapine Coordinating Center before the drug can be given in the VA system. The VA actually requires that treatment-resistant patients be offered a trial of clozapine, although there are exceptions if contraindications exist and/or the patient cannot cooperate with the monitoring procedures. *Nonetheless, as with other SGAs, the VA requires yearly monitoring of blood glucose, lipids, and BMI.*

3. Finally, there is a desperate need for long-term (five to ten years) monitoring of SGAs, particularly in children. However, since the odds of a drug company sponsoring such as study are close to zero, any such work will need to be funded by the NIMH or NIH.

Antipsychotics and Cardiovascular Mortality

Do APs increase the risk of death from cardiovascular disease? This seems an obvious question in view of the metabolic effects of these drugs, especially SGAs. But does the risk actually differ among those taking FGAs and SGAs? Is the risk due to a direct cardiotoxic effect of the drugs and/or a consequence of the metabolic changes we've just described? Complicating matters are studies dating to the 19th century demonstrating that patients with schizophrenia have a mortality rate approximately twice that of the general population.[52]

However, excess mortality is not limited to schizophrenia but is substantially increased in substance abuse, depression, bipolar illness, eating disorders, and obsessive-compulsive disorder,[53–55] many of which are co-morbid with schizophrenia. This was confirmed in a 2012 study[56] of more than one million men in Sweden who were followed for 22 years after being drafted into the military. *The excess in mortality was not confined to those with psychotic disorders or those needing hospitalization.* Moreover, suicide was not the primary problem in this study, although suicide has accounted for a significant number of deaths in other studies, with a mortality rate at least 10 times higher in men and 18 times higher in women than in the general population.[57] However, we should stress that the *absolute number of deaths from suicide is low compared with deaths from natural causes*, with the highest rates secondary to cardiovascular disease.

Indeed, in subsequent study in Sweden[58] of first-admission patients with schizophrenia in 1976 through 1991 and followed through 1995 found that the rate of cardiovascular disease had increased to 4.7 in men and 2.7 in women, considerably above the all-cause mortality rate of 1.7 and 1.3, respectively. The authors stated that the "most probable explanation"[58, p. 484] was a 64% reduction in hospital bed days, similar to findings in other studies.[59, 60] I find it striking that not a word was written about the possible effects of APs, especially the shift toward high-dose FGAs, followed by the shift toward SGAs. In a more recent review, however, the authors acknowledged the use of SGAs as a contributory factor.[55, p. 756] They also pointed out that while many studies assess the role of unhealthy lifestyle, *all-cause mortality is still excessive, even when such risk factors are statistically controlled.*

Another—albeit smaller—study of cardiovascular events and all-cause mortality in schizophrenia[61] compared a control group with members of United Healthcare who were given an AP between 1995 and 1999. They also established whether patients had been diagnosed and treated for DM and whether they were being treated with cardiac and or antihypertensive drugs. Despite a small study sample, the results were similar to those of much larger studies, in that the mortality rate among patients with schizophrenia who were taking APs was four times that of the general population, although this was halved when suicides were excluded. *The risk of myocardial infarction in patients treated with FGAs* was five times higher than the control subjects, and the risk of new-onset DM was 75% higher, although the comparatively small study population has to be taken into account. In addition, note the following:

- The risk of myocardial infarction *decreased* with higher levels of AP exposure, although the risk of DM increased. This led the authors to speculate that lifestyle factors may have been more important than AP-induced cardiotoxicity. However, the authors were unable to assess possible complicating factors such as smoking, alcohol use, exercise, obesity, or a family history of heart disease.
- There was no difference in mortality rates between men and women, despite the well-established higher rate of cardiovascular disease in men. Despite my concern about polypharmacy, all-cause mortality was actually non-significantly lower among patients dispensed both SGAs and FGAs, although the data did not indicate the length of time during which agents were used simultaneously.
- Finally, it seems reasonable to assume that these patients had greater access to health care and a healthier lifestyle than do many patients with schizophrenia yet the authors still found a significantly higher mortality rate compared with controls.

A later study[62] of 46,000 patients with severe mental illness (SMI) in the United Kingdom found that people with SMI, when compared with a control population of 300,000 people, had a three-fold increase in cardio-vascular disease at a relatively young age (18–49), although this dropped to a two-fold increase between ages 50 and 75. With regard to cancer, the only significant increase was in respiratory tumors in the older age group, but this was not significant after adjustment for smoking and social deprivation. The authors also examined the influence of APs on mortality and found that patients never given an AP were still at an increased risk of cardiac disease and stroke, but the *risk was higher still in those taking the drugs and highest in those using higher doses. The use of SGAs, however, was not associated with increased risk.*

Given the debate over the possibility of an increase in mortality with SGAs, Tiihonen and colleagues published[63] an eleven-year study of all-cause mortality in Finnish patients with schizophrenia who were admitted between 1973 to 2004 and followed until 1996 through 2006. This yielded over 66,000 patients with a mean age of 51 at the start of the follow-up period. The study drugs included perphenazine, thioridazine, and haloperidol, as well as four SGAs. Drug companies were not involved in the study.

In marked contrast to other work, the authors found that *the long-term use of any AP was associated with a lower mortality rate than no use* and that the life expectancy of patients with schizophrenia did *not* decrease with the increased use of SGAs. However, the gap between the life expectancy of patients and the population was still present and was quite high at 25 years in 1995 and 2006. (We should also note that people in Finland have much better access to inexpensive medical care that we have in the U.S.) With regard to specific drugs, clozapine had a substantially lower mortality rate than did other agents, as well as a lower rate of suicide. On the other hand, *haloperidol, risperidone,* and *quetiapine increased* mortality by 37%, 34%, and 41%, *respectively, when compared with perphenazine.* The current use of polypharmacy was associated with a moderate degree of risk secondary to ischemic heart disease but did not affect overall mortality.

The authors found it striking that clozapine, despite the long-standing concerns over its safety, was associated with the lowest mortality rate. They also noted that restrictions on clozapine and thioridazine were never based on the overall risk-benefit ratio and went on to suggest that restricting the use of clozapine (and even thioridazine) may have "caused thousands of premature deaths" in patients prescribed other drugs. *Indeed, they suggested that clozapine be considered as a first-line agent,* although many patients refuse the drug due to the perceived risks and the need for weekly blood draws during the first six months. This study appeared to be quite powerful and, indeed, stimulated a detailed critique[64] that raised a number of questions about the methodology, including the lack of information on variables such as substance abuse, cardiovascular history, marital status, and socioeconomic status. Moreover, the risk of death with drugs other than clozapine seemed inflated and in marked contrast to research in which mortality rates with clozapine were higher. In contrast, another Swedish study in 2013[65] noted that all-cause mortality was lower in patients taking aripiprazole or olanzapine, but the results were mixed with regard to quetiapine.

Others have raised similar questions about mortality study methodologies,[66] particularly the lack of high-risk subjects in some samples, presumably due to concerns over safety. Nevertheless, such patients are given APs in clinical practice and therefore should be included in studies. The authors also called for more clinically relevant information, especially the number needed to harm.

Finally, in July 2011, the FDA added a warning to the labeling of quetiapine, noting that both short-acting quetiapine and its long-acting form, quetiapine XR, should be avoided in combination with 12 other drugs that can induce cardiac arrhthymias.[67] These included quinidine, amiodarone, pentamidine, and synthetic opioids including methadone (for a complete list, see the FDA website). *It appears that higher than recommended doses of quetiapine carry a greater risk.*

Antipsychotics and Venous Thrombo-Embolism

As reviewed by Parker et al.,[68] multiple studies have demonstrated an increased risk of deep vein thrombosis and pulmonary embolism with APs. However, the results were not consistent, in that some found an association with FGAs while others found an increased risk with SGAs, and still others found no association at all! In addition, the samples were often small and narrowly based with regard to age and residence. The authors therefore did a case-control study of the general practice database (11 million patients) in the United Kingdom.[68] The study population targeted all patients ages 16 to 100 who had suffered a first episode of venous thrombo-embolism between January 1996 and July 2007. They were divided into current users of APs, recent users (had a prescription between 4 and 12 months before the event), past users (13 to 24 months), or not exposed in the previous 24 months. The investigators gathered detailed historical and medical data on the 25,000 eligible patients and 89,000 controls. Fewer than 1% had major psychiatric diagnoses, while 1% had dementia.

Users of APs had an adjusted 32% increased risk of thrombotic episodes compared with non-users, but the risk jumped to 56% among current users, compared with 36% among recent users. Interestingly, 51% of users had received only one prescription in the previous 24 months! SGAs were associated with a higher risk: 73% vs 28% for FGAs. The adjusted risk was also increased in those given two or more APs, but there was no association between dose and risk. Other factors such as age, gender, BMI, and socioeconomic status did not affect the risk.

Despite these worrisome figures, the authors pointed out that the *absolute risk was small*, in that the number of excess cases of thrombotic disease per 10,000 treated patients ages 65 and over was (a) 10 among those using any AP in the past 24 months, (b) 29 for new users, and (c) 9 for continuing users.

Nevertheless, the authors concluded that APs themselves were responsible for the increased risk, rather than characteristics of the patients. In addition, they noted that APs were being used in almost all cases to treat nausea, vertigo, and agitation, rather than psychosis, Not surprisingly, they urged that more caution be used, especially where the patient has risk factors for thrombotic events. This is yet another instance of exposure to APs despite alternative choices. (Note that ADs also carry a risk for vascular events; see Chapter 10.)

Sudden Cardiac Death

In 2009, *The New England Journal of Medicine* published an outstanding study of over 93,000 Medicaid enrollees who were new or former users of SGAs and FGAs and compared their rates of sudden cardiac death with 186,600 non-user matched controls.[69] (Medicaid enrollees with a high risk of non-cardiac death were excluded.) The mean age was 45; 65% were women, and 70% were Caucasian. The authors found that the rate of sudden cardiac death in both groups was twice that of non-users, with *no* statistically significant difference between those taking SGAs vs FGAs, although the absolute rate with SGAs was increased (incidence rate-ratio of 2.26 vs 1.99). The authors took considerable pains to control for cardiovascular and behavioral risk factors and found that the risks remained elevated. Smoking, for example, had only a "minor effect" on risk estimates. (Controlling for such risk factors is called propensity scoring.)

With regard to my concerns about the earlier shift toward excessive dosing, *the risk of sudden cardiac death increased with higher doses of both SGAs and FGAs.* In an earlier study of 481,000 Tennessee Medicaid patients followed from 1988 to 1993, Ray and colleagues found similar results,[70] in that patients given a moderate dose of APs had twice the risk of sudden cardiac death than those taking a low dose, non-users, or those previously exposed within the year prior to death. Only FGAs were studied. A moderate dose was defined as greater than 100 mg daily of thioridazine or its equivalent (2 mg of haloperidol, 2 mg of fluphenazine, 5 mg of thiothixene, 100 mg of chlorpromazine, etc.). *Please note that these dose ranges of FGAs are much lower than those used in clinical practice.*

Given the results of the 2009 study, *The New England Journal of Medicine* published a lengthy editorial[71] in which the authors strongly recommended *that the use of APs be "sharply reduced" in children and the elderly with dementia.* They also noted that the rate of 2.9 sudden deaths per 1,000 patient years increases to 3.3 with higher doses and that this rate is much higher than the risk of death from agranulocytosis secondary to use of clozapine (0.2/1000 patient years) yet we do not routinely obtain EKGs or have in place a monitoring program remotely comparable to that found with clozapine. The authors recommended ordering an EKG before and after starting an AP, especially when higher doses are prescribed, but I've not seen any impact of this on clinical practice.

I am befuddled by the lack of attention given to these well-done and well-known studies. For example, the Schizophrenia Patient Outcomes Research Team (PORT) has repeatedly issued treatment recommendations for the acute and chronic phases of this disorder, but in 2010,[72] the report did not even mention AP-associated cardiovascular mortality, much less recommend pretreatment assessment of cardiac functioning—although it stressed the metabolic risks of SGAs. On the other hand, two popular textbooks[73, 74] have not only emphasized the metabolic syndrome and obesity, but have also stressed the risks of a prolonged QTc syndrome and arrthymias, especially with exposure to ziprasidone, mesoridazine, and thioridazine. Indeed, they recommend pretreatment EKGs in patients with cardiac risk factors, but not on a routine basis.

Finally, with regard to short-term mortality rates, a comprehensive analysis[75] in 2013 of the FDA Summary Basis of Approval for New Drug Applications (1990–2011) reinforced earlier data showing a 3.8-fold increase in mortality among patients with schizophrenia, a 3.1-fold increase in depression, and a 3-fold increase in bipolar disorder. However, the increased risk in mortality was *not* associated with exposure to newer psychotropic drugs (SGAs, SSRIs, or SNRIs) but rather with assignment to the older TCAs or tetracyclic ADs. Note that suicide was responsible for 41% of the 265 deaths registered among the 92,000 patients with diagnoses of schizophrenia, bipolar disorder, depression, anxiety disorders, and ADHD.

I should emphasize these studies were short-term: three to four months. Note, too, that patients with serious medical illnesses, significant suicidality, and active substance abuse were excluded, as required by the FDA. The authors also point out that the data did not permit evaluation of other key issues, including premorbid history, family history, course of illness, and findings at autopsy, nor were the FDA reports specifically designed to evaluate mortality risk. Obviously, we are still in need of *very long-term prospective studies* to more fully assess the impact of psychotropic drugs on mortality in everyday clinical practice, where many patients taking APs—or other psychotropics—are struggling with medical problems that would exclude them from almost all clinical research. Are there alternatives to APs?

Exercise

Let's further explore the exercise option. Multiple controlled trials have found exercise effective in improving symptoms in many chronic conditions, including arthritis, respiratory disease, cancer, and cardiovascular disease.[76] Not surprisingly, exercise improves memory,[77, 78] increases neurogenesis,[78, 79] and improves depression[80] as well as schizophrenia,[81] although one RCT of older patients in care homes noted that exercise failed to improve depression.[82]

A meta-epidemiological study[76] comparing the effectiveness of exercise and medications in the prevention of mortality found no differences between the two conditions in patients with coronary heart disease and prediabetes mellitus, but exercise was more effective than anticoagulants or antiplatelet drugs among patients with stroke. However, diuretics were more effective than exercise in heart failure. When head-to-head comparisons were done in patients with coronary artery disease, statins, ACE inhibitors, beta-blockers, antiplatelet drugs, and exercise *were not different* in their effects on mortality!

Unfortunately, the authors did not include psychiatric conditions in the study, but these results are very impressive, despite the fact that drug studies far outnumbered studies on exercise, leading the authors to view the results with some degree of uncertainty. However, they concluded that bias toward drug treatments in current research may hinder the development of the most effective treatment for a given condition.[76, pp. 4–5]

Fortunately, more investigators have taken an interest in the question of drugs vs other approaches and in the question of combination approaches. For example, a 2014 "meta-review" of 61 meta-analytic studies[83] of 21 psychiatric disorders involving over 137,000 participants compared drugs or psychotherapy to controls, head-to head comparisons of drugs to therapy, and combinations to monotherapy. This was a difficult and complex study due to methodological issues, variations in sample size, possible publication bias, and failure in some studies to blindly assess outcomes. What were the results?

- Drugs or therapy vs placebo or no treatment: mean effect size of 0.50, suggesting medium efficacy, with the effect sizes in drug studies being 0.58 vs 0.40 for therapy. However, differences in sample sizes and other methodological problems appeared to affect the outcome.
- Head-to-head comparisons of drugs and psychotherapy: an overall trend favoring psychotherapy, but the trend was significant only when treating bulimia and for the prevention of relapse in depression. Drugs were significantly more effective for treatment of schizophrenia (compared with psychodynamic therapy) and chronic depression (dysthymia, no longer in DSM-5).
- Combinations of drugs and psychotherapy: a *trend* favored combinations, with combinations reaching statistical significance in only 7 of 12 meta-analyses.
- There were no significant differences in the quality of meta-analytic studies of drugs or psychotherapies.
- The results were not specific to individual drugs, and there were *no large differences between drug classes.*

It seems clear that in many disorders, some form of psychotherapeutic intervention may be as effective as medication and should be considered, especially if the patient is burdened with medical risk factors, has difficulty in tolerating drugs, or is older. However, we should note the continuing debate over the efficacy of exercise, with studies in 2014 finding either no change in symptoms or BMI[84] or a reduction in symptoms of depression and schizophrenia.[85] Some thought should be given to alternatives to APs in pregnancy, although the largest study to date found no significant increase in the rate of birth defects following AP exposure, with the exception of risperidone.[86] Use of risperidone was associated with a 26% increase in the rate of cardiac events and the overall risk of malformations, although the reasons were not clear.

In the next chapter, we shall examine the role of APs in the treatment of dementia, in which many patients develop psychotic symptoms and/or behavioral disturbances.

Additional Clinical Notes

In this chapter, we have stressed the many health problems associated with psychiatric disorders and their treatment, especially the development of diabetes mellitus, weight gain, and cardiovascular disease. The primary prevention of these complications is difficult, especially given the increasingly widespread use of Aps and ADs and, as we shall see later, the legal and illegal use of stimulants, as well as prescription and non-prescription drug abuse. Making matters more difficult is the emphasis on relapse prevention, medication adherence, and very brief hospital stays, the latter ruling out lengthy inpatient efforts aimed at adjusting medications in a safe environment, a common practice years ago.

Yet common sense and the literature give patients, families, and clinicians several ways to minimize the risks of antipsychotic drugs. For example:

1. Avoid the use of antipsychotic drugs in non–psychotic conditions, particularly in the absence of randomized controlled trials.
2. What is the reasoning behind prescribing an AP? What are the goals? What are the side effects and risks? Are there any reasonable alternatives? In 2020, Correll and Kane[87] summarized meta-analytic studies noting that differences among APs were often gradual and non-significant, but that clozapine, olanzapine, and risperidone yielded better overall outcomes. However, each has significant adverse effects, so "do no harm" might be the best first approach.
3. Before starting an AP, baseline measurements of weight, blood glucose, lipids, BMI, and waist circumference should be done and repeated at three months, then yearly.
4. If dementia is present, APs should be avoided. (See the next chapter.)
5. Careful attention is needed in case of significant weight gain and/or elevations in blood glucose and lipids. Consultation with an internist is advised, and one should consider changing to an AP with a lower risk, perhaps aripiprazole. Yet remember that metabolic changes can occur with *any* of the APs.

6. DM can develop in the absence of weight gain and might present with diabetic ketoacidosis, an acute, *life-threatening event*. In that case, emergency medical consultation is necessary. Fortunately, I have never seen this in the clinic.

7. Avoid olanzapine and quetiapine as first-line agents. There many other options.

8. Patients and families should be educated regarding symptoms of stroke, heart attack, and thrombotic events and seek emergency help if any of these develop. Needless to say, the psychiatrist or other mental health professional should be able to recognize the symptoms and be prepared to take action. One patient walked into my office several years ago with his brother, who was concerned about the development of memory problems over the previous three days. One glance told me the patient was suffering from a stroke, prompting all of us to head for the emergency room. Sadly, the development of a facial droop and speech difficulties had gone unnoticed.

9. Avoid combinations of APs and higher doses: both carry clear-cut risks, although we shall discuss polypharmacy in more detail later.

10. Consider non-drug approaches, including cognitive behavioral therapy and exercise programs, either alone, if the clinical condition permits, or in combination with medications.

11. For all these cautions, keep in mind research that shows a *decrease* in mortality with APs and ADs. For example, a nationwide cohort of almost 30,000 patients with schizophrenia followed for 5.7 years[88] found that the use of long-acting injectables resulted in nearly a 30% lower risk of death compared with oral agents. The lowest rates were found with SGA long-acting injectables and oral aripiprazole. The authors noted that the *lack* of AP therapy is more likely to be associated with excess mortality than is AP treatment. However, this study was funded by Janssen Cilag, and several authors were company employees who provided critical revision of the manuscript for intellectual content.

12. Whether the adverse effects of psychotropic drugs would be increased by the presence of the COVID-19 virus is unknown. However, their sedative effects might put those with significant respiratory distress at additional risk. There is growing concern regarding obesity as a risk factor for COVID-19.

References

1. American Diabetes Association. Consensus development conference on antipsychotic drugs and obesity and diabetes. *Diabetes Care* 2004;27:596–601.

2. Berenson A. Eli Lilly said to play down risk of top pill. *The New York Times*, December 17, 2006, p. 1.

3. Healy D. *Pharmageddon*. University of California Press, Berkeley and Los Angeles CA, 2012, p. 142.

4. Editorial. Two more blockbusters fall short. *The New York Times*, September 18, 2008, p. A32.

5. Correll CU, Manu P, Olshanskiy V, et al. Cardiometabolic risk of second-generation antipsychotics used in the treatment of children and adolescents. *JAMA* 2009;302:1765–1773.

6. Olfson M, Blanco C, Liu L, et al. National trends in the outpatient treatment of children and adolescents with antipsychotic drugs. *Archives of General Psychiatry* 2006;63:679–685.

7. Wallace-Wells B. Bitter pill. www.rollingstone.com/politics/story/25569107_pill.

8. Wilson D. AstraZeneca has settled most of its Seroquel suits. *The New York Times*, July 29, 2011.

9. Thomas K. J&J fined $1.2 billion in drug case. *The New York Times*, April 12, 2012, p. B1.

10. Show 28: warning about hyperglycemia and atypical antipsychotic drugs [webcast]. *FDA Safety News*. June 2004. www.acccessdata.fda.gov/scripts/cdrh/cfdocs/psn/transcript.cfm?show=28.

11. Pfizer. Geodon (ziprasidone): dear healthcare provider letter, August 2004. www.fda.gov/Safety/MedWatch/Safety   Information//SafetyAlertsforHumanMedical-Products/ucm154977.htm.

12. Morrato EH, Druss B, Hartung DM, et al. Metabolic testing rates in 3 state Medicaid programs after FDA warnings and ADA/APA recommendations for second-generation antipsychotic drugs. *Archives of General Psychiatry* 2010;67:17–24.

13. Mitchell AJ, Delaffon V, Vancampfort D, et al. Guideline concordant monitoring of metabolic risk in people treated with antipsychotic medication: systematic review and meta-analysis of screening practices. *Psychological Medicine* 2012;42:125–147.

14. Nasrallah HA, Meyer JM, Goff DC, et al. Low rates of treatment for hypertension, dyslipidemia and diabetes in schizophrenia: data from the CATIE schizophrenia trial sample at baseline. *Schizophrenia Research* 2006;86:15–22.

15. de Leon J. Beyond the "hype" on the association between metabolic syndrome and atypical antipsychotics: the confounding effects of cohort, typical antipsychotics, severe mental illness, comedications, and comorbid substance use. *Journal of Clinical Psychopharmacology* 2008;28:125–131.

16. NCD Risk Factor Collaboration (NCD-RisC). World-wide trends in body-mass index, underweight, and obesity from 1975–2016: a pooled analysis of 2416 population-based measurement studies in 128.9 million children, adolescents, and adults. *Lancet* 2017;390:2627–2642.

17. Curkendall SM, Mo J, Glasser DB, et al. Cardiovascular disease in patients with schizophrenia in Saskatchewan, Canada. *Journal of Clinical Psychiatry* 2004;65:715–720.

18. Kline NS. On the rarity of "irreversible" oral dyskinesia following phenothiazines. *American Journal of Psychiatry* 1968;124(suppl):40–48.

19. Andreasen N. *The Broken Brain. The Biological Revolution in Psychiatry*. Harper & Row, New York, 1984.

20. Tarricone I, Ferrari B, Gozzi A, et al. Weight gain in antipsychotic-naïve patients: a review and meta-analysis. *Psychological Medicine* 2010;40:187–200.

21. Allison DB, Mentore JL, Heo M, et al. Antipsychotic-induced weight gain: a comprehensive research synthesis. *American Journal of Psychiatry* 1999;156:1686–1696.

22. Vancampfort D, Vansteelandt K, Correll CU, et al. Metabolic syndrome and metabolic abnormalities in bipolar disorder: a meta-analysis of prevalence rates and moderators. *American Journal of Psychiatry* 2013;170:265–274.

23. Morata EH, Campagna EJ, Brewer SE, et al. Metabolic testing for adults in a state Medicaid program receiving antipsychotics. Remaining barriers to achieving

population health prevention goals. *JAMA Psychiatry.* Published online May 11, 2016. Doi:10.1001/jamapsychiatry.2016.0538.

24. Prospective Studies Collaboration. Body-mass index and cause-specific mortality in 900 000 adults: collaborative analysis of 57 prospective studies. *The Lancet* 2009;373:1083–1096.

25. Guh DP, Zhang W, Bans back N, et al. The incidence of co-morbidities related to obesity and overweight: a systematic review and meta-analysis. *BMC Public Health* 2009;9:88. Doi:10.1186/1471-25458-9-88.

26. Yaffe K, Kanaya A, Lindquist K, et al. The metabolic syndrome, inflammation, and risk of cognitive decline. *Journal of the American Medical Association* 2004;292:2237–2242.

27. Luppino FS, de Wit LM, Bouvy PF, et al. Overweight, obesity, and depression. *Archives of General Psychiatry* 2010;67:220–229.

28. Mukamal KJ, Rimm EB, Kawachi I, et al. Body mass index and risk of suicide among one million US adults. *Epidemiology* 2010;21:82–86.

29. Bjerkeset O, Romundstad P, Evans J, et al. Association of adult body mass index and height with anxiety, depression, and suicide in the general population. *American Journal of Epidemiology* 2008;167:193–202.

30. Rani F, Murray ML, Byrne PJ, et al. Epidemiologic features of antipsychotic prescribing to children and adolescents in primary care in the United Kingdom. *Pediatrics* 2008;121:1002–1009.

31. Kalverdijk JJ, Tobi H, Van Den Berg PB, et al. Use of antipsychotic drugs among Dutch youths between 1997 and 2005. *Psychiatric Services* 2008;59:554–560.

32. Zuddas A, Zanni R, Usala T. Second generation antipsychotics (SGAs) for non-psychotic disorders in children and adolescents: a review of the randomized controlled studies. *European Neuropsychopharmacology* 2011;21:600–620.

33. Loy JH, Merry JN, Stasiak K. Atypical antipsychotics for disruptive behavior disorders in children and youths. *Cochrane Database Systematic Review* September 12, 2012;9:CD008559. Doi:10.1002/1465.CD008559.pub2.

34. Pathak P, West D, Martin BC. Weighing the evidence for pediatric antipsychotic use. *Psychiatric Services* 2010;61:325.

35. Kuehn BM. Studies shed light on risks and trends in pediatric antipsychotic prescribing. *Journal of the American Medical Association* 2010;303:1901–1903.

36. Correll CU, Carlson HE. Endocrine and metabolic adverse effects of psychotropic medications in children and adolescents. *Journal of the American Academy of Child and Adolescent Psychiatry* 2006;45:771–791.

37. Bobo WV, Cooper WO, Stein CM, et al. Antipsychotics and the risk of type 2 diabetes mellitus in children and youth. *JAMA Psychiatry* 2013;70:1067–1075.

38. Rubin DM, Kreider AR, Matone M, et al. Risk for incident diabetes mellitus following initiation of second-generation antipsychotics among Medicaid-enrolled youths. *JAMA Pediatrics* 2015;169(4):e6. Doi:10.1001/jamapediatrics.2015.0285.

39. Vitiello B, Correll C, van Zwieten-Boot B, et al. Antipsychotics in children and adolescents: increasing use, evidence for efficacy and safety concerns. *European Neuropsychopharmacology* 2009;19:629–635.

40. Zito JM, Safer DJ, dosReis S, et al. Trends in the prescribing of psychotropic medications to preschoolers. *Journal of the American Medical Association* 2000;283:1025–1030.

41. Moreno C, Laje G, Blanco C, et al. National trends in the outpatient diagnosis and treatment of bipolar disorder in youth. *Archives of General Psychiatry* 2007;64:1032–1039.

42. Boyda HN, Tse L, Procyshan RM, et al. Preclinical models of antipsychotic drug-induced metabolic side effects. *Trends in Pharmacological Sciences* 2010;31:484–497.
43. Newcomer JW. Second-generation (atypical) antipsychotics and metabolic side-effects: a comprehensive literature review. *Central Nervous System Drugs* 19(suppl 1):1–93.
44. Allison DB, Casey DE. Antipsychotic induced weight gain: a review of the literature. *Journal of Clinical Psychiatry* 2001;62:272–276.
45. Rummel-Kluge C, Komossa K, Schwartz S, et al. Head-to-head comparisons of metabolic side-effects of second generation antipsychotics in the treatment of schizophrenia: a systematic review and meta-analysis *Schizophrenia Research* 2010;123:225–233.
46. Gebhardt S, Haberhausen M, Heinzel-Gutenbrunner M, et al. Antipsychotic-induced body weight gain: predictors and a systematic categorization of the long-term weight course. *Journal of Psychiatric Research* 2009;43:620–636.
47. Maayan L, Correll CU. Weight gain and metabolic risks associated with antipsychotic medications in children and adolescents. *Journal of Child and Adolescent Psychiatry* 2011;21:517–535.
48. Adkins DE, Åberg K, McClay JL, et al. Genome-wide pharmacogenomic study of metabolic side effects to antipsychotic drugs. *Molecular Psychiatry* 2011;16:321–332.
49. Need AC, Keefe RSE, Dongliang Ge, et al. Pharmacogenetics of antipsychotic response in the CATIE trial: a candidate gene analysis. *European Journal of Human Genetics* 2009;17:946–957.
50. Yu H, Wang L, Lv L, et al. Genome-wide Association Study suggesting the PTPRD polymorphisms were associated with weight gain effects of atypical antipsychotic medications. *Schizophrenia Bulletin* 2016;42:814–823.
51. Malgorzata M, Gorbovskaya I, Tiwari AK, et al. Genetic validation study of protein tyrosine receptor type D (PTPRD) gene variants and the risk for antipsychotic-induced weight gain. *Journal of Neural Transmission* 2019;126:27–33.
52. Brown S. Excess mortality of schizophrenia: a meta-analysis. *British Journal of Psychiatry* 1997;171:502–508.
53. Harris EC, Barraclough B. Excess mortality of mental disorder. *British Journal of Psychiatry* 1998;173:11–53.
54. Meier SM, Matthiesen M, Mors O, et al. Mortality among people with obsessive-compulsive disorder in Denmark. *JAMA Psychiatry* 2016;73:268–274.
55. Lawrence D, Kisely S, Pais S. The epidemiology of excess mortality in people with mental illness. *Canadian Journal of Psychiatry* 2010;55:752–760.
56. Gale CR, Batty D, Osborn DPJ, et al. Association of mental disorders in early adulthood and later psychiatric hospital admissions and mortality in a cohort study of more than one million men. *Archives of General Psychiatry* 2012;69:823–831.
57. Allebeck P, Wisted B. Mortality in schizophrenia: a ten-year follow-up based on the Stockholm county inpatient register. *Archives of General Psychiatry* 1986;43:650–653.
58. Österg U, Correia N, Brandt L, et al. Time trends in schizophrenia mortality in Stockholm county Sweden: cohort study. *British Medical Journal* 2000;321:483–484.
59. Nordentoft M, Laursen TM, Agerbo E, et al. Change in suicide rates for patients with schizophrenia in Denmark, 1981–1997: nested case-control study. *British Medical Journal* 2004;229(7470):261–266.
60. Hamer M, Stamatakis E, Stephoe A. Psychiatric hospital admissions, behavioral risk factors, and all-cause mortality in the Scottish Health Survey. *Archives of Internal Medicine*, 2008;168:2474–2479.

61. Enger C, Weatherby L; Reynolds RF, et al. Serious cardiovascular events and mortality among patients with schizophrenia. *The Journal of Nervous and Mental Disease* 2004;192:19–27.

62. Osborn DJP, Levy G, Nazareth I, et al. Relative risk of cardiovascular and cancer mortality in people with severe mental illness from the United Kingdom's general practice research database. *Archives of General Psychiatry* 2007;64:242–249.

63. Tiihonen T, Lonnqvist J, Wahlbeck K, et al. 11year follow-up of mortality in schizophrenia: a population-based cohort study (FIN11 study). *The Lancet* 2009;374:620–627.

64. de Hert M, Correll CU, Cohen D. Do antipsychotic medications reduce or increase mortality in schizophrenia? A critical appraisal of the FIN-11 study. *Schizophrenia Research* 2010;117:68–74.

65. Crump C, Winkleby MA, Sundquist K, et al. Comorbidities and mortality in persons with schizophrenia: a Swedish national cohort study. *American Journal of Psychiatry* 2013;170:324–333.

66. Correll CU, Nielsen J. Antipsychotic-associated all-cause mortality: what should we worry about and how should the risk be assessed? *Acta Psychiatrica Scandinavica* 2010;122:341–344.

67. Wilson D. Heart warning added to label on popular antipsychotic drug. *The New York Times*, July 18, 2011.

68. Parker C, Coupland C, Hippisley-Cox J. Antipsychotic drugs and risk of venous thromboembolism: nested case-control study. *British Medical Journal* 2010;341:c4245. Doi10:1136/bmj.c4245.

69. Ray WA, Chung CP, Murray KT, et al. Atypical antipsychotic drugs and the risk of sudden cardiac death. *New England Journal of Medicine* 2009;360:225–235.

70. Ray WA, Meredith S, Thapa PB. Antipsychotics and the risk of sudden cardiac death. *The New England Journal of Medicine* 2001;58:1161–1167.

71. Schneeweis S, Avorn J. Antipsychotic agents and sudden cardiac death—how should we manage the risk? *The New England Journal of Medicine* 2009;360:294–296.

72. Buchanan RW, Kreyenbuhl J, Kelly DL, et al. The 2009 schizophrenia PORT psychopharmacological treatment recommendations and summary statements. *Schizophrenia Bulletin* 2010;36:71–93.

73. Tasman A, Kay J, Lieberman JA, First MB, Maj M. Editors. *Psychiatry*, Third Edition. Wiley-Blackwell, Chichester, West Sussex, 2008.

74. Roberts LW. Editor. *The American Psychiatric Association Publishing Textbook Psychiatry*, Seventh Edition. American Psychiatric Association Publishing, Washington DC, 2019.

75. Khan A, Faucett J, Morrison S, et al. Comparative mortality risk in adult patients with schizophrenia, depression, bipolar disorders, anxiety disorders, and attention-deficit/hyperactivity disorder participating in psychopharmacology clinical trials. *JAMA Psychiatry* 2013;70:1091–1099.

76. Naci H, Ioannidis JPA. Comparative effectiveness of exercise and drug interventions on mortality outcomes: meta-epidemiological study. *British Medical Journal* 2013;347:15577. Doi:10.1136/bmj.15577 Published October 1, 2013.

77. Erickson KI. Exercise training increases size of hippocampus and improves memory. *Proceedings of the National Academy of Sciences of the United States of America* 2011;108:3017–3022.

78. Morroni F, Kitazawa M, Drago D, et al. Repeated physical training and environmental enrichment induce neurogenesis and synaptogenesis following neuronal injury in an inducible mouse model. *Journal of Behavioral and Brain Science* 2011;1:199–209.

79. Kim S-E, Ko I-G, Kim B-K, et al. Treadmill exercise prevents age-induced failure of memory through an increase in neurogenesis and suppression of apoptosis in rat hippocampus. *Experimental Gerontology* 2010;45:357–365.
80. Bridle C, Spanjers K, Patel S, et al. Effect of exercise on depression severity in older people: systematic review and meta-analysis of randomized controlled trials. *British Journal of Psychiatry* 2012;201:180–185.
81. Scheewe TW, Backx FJG, Takken T, et al. Exercise therapy improves mental and physical health in schizophrenia: a randomised controlled trial. *Acta Psychiatrica Scandinavica* 2013;127:464–473.
82. Underwood M, Lamb SE, Eldridge S, et al. Exercise for depression in elderly residents of care homes: a cluster randomised controlled trial. *The Lancet* 2013. Doi:10.1016/S0140-6736(13)606492-2.
83. Huhn M, Tardy M, Spinelli LM, et al. Efficacy of pharmacotherapy and psychotherapy for adult psychiatric disorders. A systematic overview of meta-analyses. *JAMA Psychiatry* 2014;71:707–715.
84. Pearsall R, Smith DJ, Pelosi A, et al. Exercise therapy in adults with serious mental illness: a systematic review and meta-analysis. *BMC Psychiatry* 2014. Doi:10.1186/1471-244X-14-117.
85. Rosenbaum S, Tiedemann A, Sherrington C, et al. Physical activity interventions for people with mental illness: a systematic review and meta-analysis *Journal of Clinical Psychiatry* 2014;75:964–974.
86. Huybrechts KF, Hernandez-Diaz S, Patorno E, et al. Antipsychotic use in pregnancy and the risk for congenital malformations. *JAMA Psychiatry*. Doi:10.1001/jamapsychiatry.2016.1520.
87. Correll CU, Kane JM. Ranking antipsychotics for efficacy and safety in schizophrenia. *JAMA Psychiatry* 2020;77:225–226.
88. Taipale H, Mittendorfer-Rutz E, Alexanderson K, et al. Antipsychotics and mortality in a nationwide cohort of 29,83 patients with schizophrenia. *Schizophrenia Research* 2018;197:274–280.

5   Antipsychotics and Mortality in the Elderly With Dementia

Introduction

On April 11, 2005, the FDA issued a health advisory,[1] warning that the use of second-generation antipsychotics (SGAs) in older patients with dementia doubled the risk of death compared with placebo. This is not insignificant since at least 70% of patients with dementia develop behavioral problems and psychotic symptoms, with Jeste et al. noting a *lifetime* risk of 100%.[2] At least 25% of patients in nursing homes are treated with antipsychotics (APs),[3] often for non-psychotic conditions. The FDA has not approved any antipsychotics for the treatment of agitation or psychosis in dementia. However, risperidone has been approved by Health Canada for management of aggression or psychosis in severe Alzheimer's disease (AD).[4] Risperidone is also licensed in the United Kingdom for treatment of aggression in AD, with a six-week limit; it has also been licensed in Finland. After additional studies, the FDA in June 2008 expanded the black-box warning to include first-generation antipsychotics (FGAs).[5]

The FDA Health Advisory was issued in the context of a rapidly aging population, such that some 14 million people in the U.S. will be suffering from Alzheimer's disease (AD) by 2050.[6] About 47 million people worldwide have Alzheimer's disease, according to the World Health Organization.[7] We are therefore facing an enormous public health problem, from the standpoint of both overall costs for dementias, which in 2019 were around $290 billion,[6] and deaths secondary to AD, which increased by 145% between 2000 and 2017, compared with a 9% drop in heart disease.[6] On a county-wide level in the U.S., Dwyer-Lindgren et al. found an 18% increase in deaths from neurological disorders during the years 1980 through 2014.[8]

Antipsychotics and the Risk-Benefit Ratio

No doubt Pharma has been embracing the opportunity to expand the use of APs, despite the long-standing reports of SGA-induced strokes, transient ischemic episodes (TIAs), and increased mortality rates,[9, 10] data we reviewed in Chapters 3 and 4. As early as 2002, Health Canada[4] warned physicians that the risk-benefit ratio of APs should be reassessed, and caregivers should quickly assess any symptoms suggestive of a stroke so physicians could rapidly begin treatment. Did these warnings have any substantial effect on the use of APs in dementia? History suggests they didn't, given the lack of significant changes following recommendations for the assessment of metabolic parameters before and after prescriptions for APs. On a positive note, the FDA warnings about APs and mortality did result in a significant decline in the use of SGAs in 2003, at least in the Department of Veteran's Affairs.[11]

The growing concerns regarding AP-associated increases in mortality in dementia patients were reinforced by a meta-analytic study of 15 published trials of SGAs in 3,353 patients treated over an 8-to-12-week period with SGAs.[9] Of these patients, 87% had been diagnosed with Alzheimer's disease. Patients taking SGAs had a *54% increase in mortality vs placebo, with a significant risk for cerebrovascular events, especially if taking risperidone.* (The authors noted that some of the data on mortality and adverse events was obtained from other studies, including a 2005 meta-analysis by the same authors.[10]) Please note that the *increase in mortality was found after no more than three months of treatment!* The number needed to harm (NNH) with drug treatment was 100, although the confidence interval was very broad. The number needed to treat (NNT) ranged from 4 to 12.

These figures indicated that there would be one death for every 9 to 25 patients who had received some benefit.[10] There was *no* evidence that any individual drug was at greater risk, with the possible exception of risperidone. However, the *absolute number of events was small*: 3.5% with drugs vs 2.3% with placebo. I must say that a mortality rate approaching 4% may be small technically, but whether families would have the same view is doubtful. Another issue to consider in this study is dropout rates, which exceeded those we reviewed previously. With olanzapine, 80% discontinued the drug; with quetiapine, 82%; and with risperidone, 77%! *The response rates varied from 21% to 32%, but what can one make of these figures, given the dropout rates?* Clearly, patients found the drugs difficult to tolerate.

Making matters worse, a case-control study[12] in 2015 of 90,786 patients in the Veteran's Health Administration found that the effects of APs on mortality were higher than previously reported, with an NNH of 27 to 50 for those taking SGAs, quite the contrast to the NNH of 100 reported by Schneider and associates.[10] Once again, *risperidone had the highest risk—* despite the recommendation by Health Canada and approval in Finland and elsewhere—compared with olanzapine and quetiapine, but haloperidol took first place when compared with the SGAs, valproic acid, and ADs. While quetiapine had the lowest risk among the SGAs, with a NNH of 50, other work has shown that quetiapine has fewer benefits.[9]

Another key finding: *the mortality risk with SGAs increased with higher doses*,[11] a common finding, as we shall see. Still, the question of FGAs vs SGAs lingered. In an earlier study, Wang and colleagues[13] had examined the six-month mortality rate in 23,000 patients ages 65 and over who had started either FGAs or SGAs during the years 1994 through 2003. They found a significantly higher adjusted mortality rate of 37% in patients taking FGAs than in those taking SGAs. An elevated risk was found at all time intervals, regardless of the presence or absence of dementia. The greatest risk was found *early* in the course of treatment and with *higher doses.*

The primary lesson: *FGAs are not safer* than SGAs in dementia and in the elderly. The discerning reader will no doubt point out that the high risk of death within the first weeks and months of treatment might indicate that this group of patients was sicker and had additional risk factors which biased the results—a good point, but not so. The investigators used *propensity scoring* to control for risk factors such as DM, cardiovascular disease, cancer, psychiatric disorders, hospitalizations, nursing home residence, and the use of other medications, including other psychiatric drugs. Nevertheless, the difference in mortality remained, but with time, the SGA and FGA mortality rates began to converge.[13]

The short-term risk has been confirmed by other studies, including a population-based study in Ontario, Canada, of over 20,000 older adults with dementia and 20,000 matched controls.[14] *Within 30 days of starting an AP, those taking an SGA were three times more likely to have a serious adverse event* including death, hospitalization for fractures, cerebrovascular events, and movement disorders. More bad news for FGAs, which had almost four times the risk. Propensity scoring indicated that the patients taking APs differed from the controls only in the use of APs.

Poor Results: Why?

One problem might be differences in the health care systems and safety nets across countries. However, several studies have found alarming increases in mortality even in countries with better access to health care. For example, a study[15] in British Columbia examined mortality rates in 37,000 patients ages 65 and over who were given SGAs or FGAs from 1996 through 2004. Patients with cancer were excluded, since FGAs are sometimes used to treat vomiting. The sample was also restricted to new users of APs in order to avoid any effects from prior treatment. Although this study was not intended as a comparative study of health care systems, the results were similar to those found in the U.S., in that patients given FGAs had an adjusted risk of death 32% higher than those given SGAs. As in the Wang et al. study,[13] the *mortality rate was higher in those treated with higher doses and during the first 40 days.* Prescriptions for FGAs resulted in four additional deaths in every 100 patients. Compared with risperidone, haloperidol doubled the mortality rate!

Another Canadian study[16] examined the six-month all-cause mortality rate in demented patients ages 66 and over who were new users of APs and who were living either in the community or in long-term care residential settings. Propensity scoring was used to examine the influence of a host of risk factors. Risk of death was examined at 30, 60, 120, and 180 days after starting an AP. The most commonly prescribed SGA was risperidone (75%), whereas haloperidol was the most commonly used FGA (60%), whether patients were living in the community or in long-term care. As we have seen in other studies, the *mortality risk was significantly elevated at 30 days* compared with non-users. The risk varied from 31% with SGAs to 55% with FGAs, albeit with small differences between the community-dwelling and residential-dwelling groups. Unfortunately, the investigators were not able to study dose-response relationships, nor did they have data on the causes of death. The authors concluded that the risk with SGAs is a class effect and that switching between individual agents is not recommended. They also concluded, as have other authors, that FGAs may carry even greater risks than do SGAs.

It appears that faulty prescribing and deviation from guidelines play significant roles[5] in the significant risks associated with APs. Indeed, despite this research, and despite the FDA-mandated black-box warning, an audit of the Medicare program in 2007 revealed that 83% of prescriptions for elderly residents of nursing homes were for non-approved conditions, which in 88% of the cases meant dementia.[17] Even where APs were prescribed for approved conditions, *22% did not meet standards set for reasonable dosing and length of use.* The erroneous use of APs resulted in wrongful payment of $116 million in a six-month period. The inspector general of the Department of Health and Human Services stated that all of us, whether patients, families, or caregivers, should be outraged by the results.[17]

Similar and very worrisome results were found in another study that examined the quality of AP drug prescribing, using a database of 2.5 million Medicare beneficiaries in the years 2000 and 2001.[18] Only 42% of AP use was consistent with nursing home guidelines, and 25% had no appropriate indication. *Worse, 17% were given excessive doses, while 18% had no approved indication.*

Ongoing Mortality Rates

Data from 2012 continued to demonstrate serious increases in mortality, as shown by another study[19] of Medicaid and Medicare data on 75,000 new users of APs in nursing homes who were given haloperidol, risperidone, aripiprazole, ziprasidone, or quetiapine. Six months later, those taking haloperidol had double the risk of dying than those using risperidone, while users of quetiapine had a decreased risk. The other APs carried no increase in risk, and there were no differences in causes of death. The authors recommended, as have many others, that *APs not be used unless there is clear need,* but it appears that prescribers have a very generous idea of what constitutes need.

Few studies have examined mortality in longer-term use of APs or with regard to polypharmacy. In 2017, these risks were evaluated in a sample of

70,718 community-dwelling patients with AD in Finland.[20] Users of APs in this population suffered a 61% increase in mortality risk, and, as in other studies, the increased risk was noticeable shortly after use began, *but the risk continued after two years of use*, although adjusted hazard ration dropped to 30%. AP polypharmacy almost *tripled* the risk (adjusted hazard ratio of 2.88)! Once again, quetiapine had a lower risk than risperidone, despite the fact that risperidone has been licensed in Canada, the UK, Europe, and Australia! Note, too, that risperidone increased the risk for cerebrovascular events in the study reported by Schneider et al.,[9] leaving the clinician and families with sets of inconsistent data.

Additional Risks of Antipsychotics in Dementia

Hip fractures have been shown to increase disability, mortality, and institutionalization across multiple studies,[21, 22, 23] with twice to three times the rate of hip fractures in AD.[24] In a 2017 study of community-dwelling persons with AD,[25] use of APs was associated with a 54% increase in the risk of hip fracture, with the increase in risk starting within the first days of use. The risk was similar for those taking risperidone or quetiapine during the first 2.7 years of use, but from 2.7 years to 4.1 years, the risk was lower with quetiapine. *Note that a higher dose risperidone (over 0.5 mg/day) led to a 72% increase in risk.* Fortunately, the doses were quite low, with a median dose of 0.7 mg/day for risperidone and 31 mg/day for quetiapine, indicating sensitivity to the risks of high doses.

Falls, Injuries, Hospitalizations

A nationwide study in Denmark[26] of 1.2 million persons over age 65 found that injuries from falls were strongly associated with use of antidepressants, while mortality and hospitalizations were strongly related to use of APs. In this era of polypharmacy, we should stress a relationship between the number of psychotropics and the risks of falls, hospitalizations, and death. Indeed, among persons with dementia, those taking *four psychotropics* had a 99% increased risk of death!

APs, Cognition, and Metabolic Changes

Earlier, we discussed the CATIE trial,[27] which compared SGAs with perphenazine, an old SGA, and noted that the outcomes were similar. The NIMH then funded a subsection of CATIE (CATIE-AD), designed to compare the effectiveness of olanzapine, risperidone, and quetiapine vs placebo in Alzheimer's disease. CATIE-AD was designed to take place in usual-care settings and took into account changes in medications and dosages based on the clinician's judgment. For a full description of the design, testing, and other details, see Schneider et al.[28] In a subsequent paper on CATIE-AD, the specific results of the extensive neuropsychological test battery were described by Vigen et al.,[29] who noted that the 421 participants showed a steady decline in cognition during the 36-week trial period—regardless of the drug or placebo and regardless of the initial level of impairment. Although patients were enrolled due to their agitated and aggressive behaviors, only 47 patients had no follow-up cognitive data available.

Unfortunately, patients randomized to APs demonstrated a significantly greater rate of decline, as shown by a 2.46 greater decrease on the Mini-Mental Status Examination. Differences between the SGAs could not be determined due to the sample size. The authors did cite several earlier studies that had found greater cognitive decline with olanzapine and quetiapine vs placebo, although another study had failed to find any significant decline in those treated with olanzapine, risperidone, or quetiapine. However, that study was done in younger patients.

I also note the results of the first phase of the CATIE-AD study published in 2008, where results were assessed at a median of 7 weeks, rather than 36 weeks.[30] (The first phase ended when the clinician felt that treatment was not optimal.). At week 12, there were *no differences between drug and placebo on the cognitive subscale* of the Alzheimer's Disease Assessment Scale or on quality of life, as reflected in ratings by caregivers. (This was not addressed in the Vigen et al. study.[29]) Interestingly, olanzapine, at the last observation in phase I, demonstrated worse functional status and worsening symptoms on withdrawal/depression vs quetiapine and risperidone, although it was superior on ratings of hostility/suspiciousness.

A number of post-hoc analyses of CATIE-AD have been carried out. Among them was a study by Nagata et al.[31] in 2018, which found that preservation of neurocognitive functioning was associated with greater improvement in neuropsychiatric symptoms over the 36-week trial. On the other hand, a study[32] of baseline predictors of treatment continuation and response at 8 weeks noted that only 48% continued the initial treatment, in an echo of Schneider et al.[9] In Caucasian patients, *baseline predictors of clinical response included poorer cognition and psychotic symptoms,* while DM and global physical status predicted more improvement. No doubt this was a function of the scales, wherein those with worse scores often show more improvement, assuming the intervention is effective.

In an editorial[33] examining the Vigen et al. study,[29] Devanand et al. reminded us that in addition to antipsychotics and antidepressants, anticonvulsants and anxiolytics have been shown to impair cognitive functioning. They also noted that cognition may be adversely affected during a crossover from one drug to another. The editorialists also cited several large-scale studies carried out after the FDA black-box warning was issued, none of which found an increase in mortality or hospital admissions secondary to the use of either FGAs or SGAs. In an updated editorial published in 2017, Devanand[34] observed that predicting response to antipsychotics in persons with dementia "remains a conundrum." I would add that we should not forget the metabolic complications of SGAs, which seem neglected in these studies. However, another analysis[35] of CATIE-AD did find significant weight gain among women, but not men, which became worse over time. At 24 weeks and beyond, the odds of experiencing a 7% increase in weight tripled *among women!* In addition, HDL levels decreased. Olanzapine and quetiapine were the principal culprits. Given our earlier review of the consequences of significant weight gain, patients with dementia should be carefully monitored for changes in weight.

A Focus on Individual Antipsychotics

As these studies indicate, there appears to be inconsistency regarding the efficacy and safety of the individual APs. This leaves the clinician unsure as to the initial choice of drug. Of course, one must take into account the history of cardiovascular disease, obesity, DM, and hyperlipidemia, as well as any information regarding prior experience with APs and ADs. Whether pharmacogenetic testing might be helpful is not clear, except where the patient has a history of inability to tolerate psychotropic drugs, in which case we might suspect that he or she is a poor metabolizer. Might this be a factor in the high dropout rates just cited?

One of the largest studies examining mortality rates with individual APs was published in 2012 by Kales et al.[36] The study sample included 33,604 veterans with dementia age 65 and older who were treated during 1999 through 2008. The focus was on risperidone, olanzapine, quetiapine, haloperidol, and valproic acid derivatives (Depakote) and their impact on mortality within 180 days. Only patients taking a single drug (monotherapy) were included.

Across a variety of analyses, haloperidol carried the greatest risk for morality in the first 30 days of use, but the risk then fell significantly, in part due to the shorter exposure period. Interestingly, 78% of patients taking haloperidol were seen in non-psychiatric visits, perhaps secondary to its use in delirium. These patients were also older and sicker. *After haloperidol, the risks were highest in risperidone, olanzapine, and divalproex. Quetiapine had the lowest risk.* Among these four drugs, the risks were most significant in the first 120 days of treatment, then fell in the next 60 days. After 120 days of treatment, there were *no differences* in mortality risks with any individual AP.

Although risperidone has been licensed or approved in a number of different countries for the treatment of behavioral problems in dementia, the studies just reviewed have shown that risperidone carries a greater risk for cardiovascular disease,[9] a greater risk for mortality,[12] and a greater risk for hip fractures at higher doses.[25] While these are only a few of the extant studies, the data appears to undercut the approval of risperidone as a top-line agent.

Nevertheless, Davies et al.,[37] in an effort to develop a drug treatment algorithm for use in agitation and aggression in Alzheimer's disease, recommended risperidone as the first-step AP, followed by quetiapine, aripiprazole, and then non–APs, including carbamazepine, citalopram, gabapentin, and prazosin. However, the evidence for carbamazepine is very weak, and the risks are considerable. The evidence for gabapentin and prazosin is quite weak and, indeed, based on clinical reports and one RCT. *Note that olanzapine was excluded due to its metabolic risks.* More evidence for aripiprazole can be found in a 2014 meta-analysis,[38] in which aripiprazole showed no difference vs placebo for almost all adverse events other than sedation and a significantly lower risk for time to discontinuation. This study of 16 RCTs found no differences in mortality for any single AP, in contrast to studies just cited in the previous paragraph. *With certainty, we can say that higher cumulative doses of APs are associated with increased mortality rates.*[39]

Alternatives to Antipsychotics

Antidepressants

While antidepressants (ADs) have been proposed for treatment of depression in dementia, a multi-center RCT of mirtazapine and sertraline found no benefits.[40] However, a double-blind comparison of citalopram and risperidone in the treatment of behavioral and psychotic symptoms found, rather surprisingly, no significant differences between the two drugs, but the burden of side effects was less with citalopram.[41] Interestingly, citalopram was equivalent to risperidone with regard to parkinsonism. (In Chapter 10, we will discuss the neurological side effects of SSRIs).

A CitAD study[42] examined the effectiveness of citalopram in 186 patients with Alzheimer's disease, with patients randomized to psychosocial intervention plus either citalopram or placebo. Any ongoing psychotropic medications had to be discontinued, but lorazepam and trazodone were allowed as rescue medications. Memantine and cholinesterase inhibitors were allowed if dosing had been stable for one month prior to study entry. Patients with a QTc of > 450 ms for men and 475 ms for women were excluded due to safety concerns. An EKG was obtained at week three and after the dose reached 30 mg daily. Citalopram was started at 10 mg daily, with a target dose of 30 mg daily.

Citalopram was superior to placebo on multiple rating scales and reduced caregiver distress scores. Agitation was significantly reduced, with a response rate of 40% vs 26% on placebo, but there was no improvement in quality of life or in lesser use of rescue lorazepam, which seems odd. Unfortunately, *citalopram also resulted in worsening cognition, but the decrease was only one point on the MMSE. Citalopram also led to QT interval prolongation.* The latter two findings prompted the authors to state that citalopram *cannot be generally recommended* at a dose of 30 mg. However, the data were insufficient to judge its efficacy at lower doses.

Psychosocial Interventions

A systematic review[43] of psychological approaches found over 1,600 studies, of which only 162 met preset criteria for inclusion. The authors used evidence-based guidelines for recommendations, but only nine studies were rated as having top-level evidence! The overall quality of research was poor. *Only behavioral management, some specific types of caregiver and residential staff education, and possibly cognitive stimulation had any lasting effect.* Indeed, in a 2015 review of interventions,[44] the best evidence was found for involvement of family caregivers.

Yet in 2017, Hane et al.[45] cited evidence for the efficacy of physical activity, building on work that found an association between high levels of walking and an increased volume of gray matter and a lower risk of cognitive impairment. Resistance training and cognitive training were also effective in reducing the decline found with mild cognitive impairment. Whether these efforts will be significantly effective in more severe cases of dementia is not clear. Other strategies[46] have included training of caregivers; provision of more recreational activities, including preferred music; aromatherapy; pet therapy; reminiscence therapy; and bright light therapy, although the last three have low levels of confidence.

In a fascinating study[47] of health-related quality of life in people living in care homes, each care home was randomized to at least one of three interventions, including antipsychotic review, social intervention, and personalized exercise. All homes received person-centered care training for nine months prior to randomization. Trained therapists provided training and education, while the reviewers of antipsychotic therapy followed guidelines from several sources.

The results of the antipsychotic review carried out in eight homes was mixed, with a significant 50% reduction in the use of APs and a 30% drop in mortality, also significant. However, this resulted in a *significant worsening* on health-related quality of life scores, a drop that approached statistical significance, while statistically significant worsening was found on negative emotions and appearance. On the other hand, homes randomized to a combination of antipsychotic review and social interaction found *no* decline in quality of life. *Social interaction alone significantly benefitted quality of life.* In contrast to studies noted earlier, exercise had no effect on quality of life measures but did increase positive emotions.

The primary problems with watchful waiting and psychosocial interventions are the time required, the likelihood of higher costs, and allotting time for the staff training. Let's face it: Giving APs is much less expensive, at least in the short term, and may yield rapid but very short-term benefits—but one has to balance these benefits with the long-term costs of diagnosing and treating the metabolic syndrome, cardiovascular events, and neurological side effects, all of which place additional stress on the family and other caregivers.

Finally, I must stress that this chapter has addressed our efforts at treating the behavioral consequences of dementia but not the underlying pathology. For a review of these issues, please see Hane et al.,[45] who describe the many efforts aimed at reducing and preventing toxic amyloid aggregates found in the brains of people with Alzheimer's disease. At least a dozen of these drugs have failed, as have other disease-modifying therapies.[48] Other approaches have included immunotherapy,[49] stem cell therapy,[50] and targeting the GABAergic system,[51] but the results of these studies will not be known for some time. In the meantime, we struggle to treat symptoms and support caregivers in their difficult tasks, The advent of COVID-19 has made these problems dramatically worse. However, it is not yet clear how many of the deaths in nursing home and care centers have occurred in the context of AD.

Clinical Notes

1. The demand for treatment of behavioral difficulties and psychotic symptoms that occur in almost all patients with Alzheimer's disease presents clinicians, families, and patients with a series of difficult choices. How do we balance the immediate therapeutic needs with the fact that APs increase the mortality rate in dementias?
2. In a 23-page summary of these issues,[2] Jeste and colleagues stressed the "modest efficacy" of APs in the treatment of agitation and aggression associated with dementia, and pointed out that the NNT (the number of patients needed to treat in order to see an effect greater than placebo) ranged from 9 to 14, depending on the outcome measure. An NNT of 10 is usually regarded as a benchmark, so this figure, if accurate, would seem to provide some reassurance.
3. *Perhaps the most positive advice in this admittedly complex and difficult field would be to stop the increasingly widespread use of APs for non-psychotic conditions.* The risks do not justify using APs for simple irritability, insomnia, and anxiety. Other therapeutic approaches are available, including various forms of therapy that clearly have fewer risks. Even non-AP drug therapy has a considerably lower mortality rate, with the possible exception of anticonvulsants and benzodiazepines.
4. Families need to be fully informed of the risks vs benefits of APs when caring for a loved one with dementia and should know that *no psychotropic agents have been FDA approved in the United States for the behavioral problems associated with dementia.*
5. Another dimension to this debate can be found in another off-shoot of the CATIE-AD study, in which Rosenheck et al.[52] did a cost-benefit analysis of SGAs and placebo in the treatment of Alzheimer's disease and found that "watchful waiting," a term they substituted for placebo, did not differ from the effects of SGAs on multiple measures of quality

of life. *Indeed, placebo yielded greater net health benefits* at a lower cost! As a corollary, patients taking olanzapine did worse on activities of daily living than did those taking placebo.

6. While the evidence for psychosocial interventions is not top notch, behavioral management, caregiver and staff education aimed at dealing with behavioral problems, and cognitive stimulation techniques do have a better evidence base and need to be emphasized.

7. Here's a thought: If the patient isn't doing well, or perhaps is getting worse, consider tapering and stopping the AP and putting more emphasis on caregiving.

8. Physicians and caregivers should also note that the mortality rate of APs in dementia is linked to the cumulative dose, even after taking into account severity and co-morbid illnesses. Similarly, a dose-response relationship between mortality risk and the total number of psychotropic drugs taken in persons older than 65 found a significant increase in the risk of injuries from falls and the rate of readmissions. Families and caregivers should inquire about the risks and benefits of both the dose and the number of drugs being prescribed.

9. Families and physicians should keep in mind that federal regulations require that APs prescribed in nursing homes be stopped after three to four months unless documentation supports their continuance.

10. In addition, the staff should properly evaluate the patient for the presence of parkinsonian side effects, especially akathisia (motor restlessness), which is often mistaken for agitation/belligerence, in which case the antipsychotic dose is raised—precisely the wrong move! Similar efforts should be made to ensure that the patient is being appropriately treated for any subtle medical problems, including urinary retention, urinary tract infections, gait abnormalities, edema, constipation, anemia, and vitamin deficiencies.

11. Remarkably enough, our ability to predict response to APs in dementia remains murky at best.

12. We hope that more progress can be made soon in treating and preventing the underlying pathology of Alzheimer's disease and other dementing disorders. Without such progress, we are limited to treating symptoms.

References

1. Public Health Advisory. *Deaths with Antipsychotics in Elderly Patients with Behavioral Disturbances.* US Food and Drug Administration, Washington DC, April 11, 2005. www.fda.gov/cder/drug/advisory/antipsychotics.htm. Accessed October 15, 2015.
2. Jeste DV, Blazer D, Casey D, et al. ACNP White Paper: update on use of antipsychotic drugs in elderly persons with dementia. *Neuropsychopharmacology* 2008;33:957–970.
3. Rabins PV, Lyketsos CG. Antipsychotic drugs in dementia: what should be made of the risks? *Journal of the American Medical Association* 2005;294:1963–1965.

4. *Health Canada.* Risperidone. Restriction of the dementia indication. http://healthycanadians.gc.ca/recall-alert-rappel-avis/hc-sc/2015/43797a-eng.php. Accessed December 18, 2019.

5. *Transcript for FDA Media Briefing on Safety Labeling Changes for Antipsychotic Drugs*, June 16, 2008. http://fda.gov/downloads/NewsEvents/Newsroom/MediaTranscripts.UCM169331.pdf.

6. Alzheimer's Association. Alzheimer's Disease Facts and Figures, 2019.

7. *WHO Fact Sheet.* Dementia 2015. World Health Organization [online]. www.who.int/mediacentre/factsheets//fs.362/en/#. Accessed March 27, 2016.

8. Dwyer-Lindgren L, Bertozzi A, Stubbs RW, et al. US county-level trends in mortality rates for major causes of death, 1980–2014. *JAMA* 2016;316:2385–2401.

9. Schneider LS, Dagerman KS, Insel PS. Efficacy and adverse effects of atypical antipsychotics for dementia: meta-analysis of randomized, placebo-controlled trials. *American Journal of Geriatric Psychiatry* 2006;14:191–210.

10. Schneider LA, Dagerman KS, Insel P. Risk of death with atypical antipsychotic drug treatment for dementia: meta-analysis of randomized, controlled trials. *JAMA* 2005;294:1934–1943.

11. Kales HC, Zivin K, Kim HM, et al. Trends in antipsychotic use in dementia 1999–2007. *Archives of General Psychiatry* 2011;68:190–197.

12. Maust DT, Kim HM, Seyfried LS, et al. Antipsychotics, other psychotropics, and the risk of death in patients with dementia. Number needed to harm. *JAMA Psychiatry* 2015;72:438–445.

13. Wang PS, Schneeweiss S, Avorn J, et al. Risk of death in elderly users of conventional vs. atypical antipsychotic medications. *New England Journal of Medicine* 2005;353:2335–2341.

14. Rochon PA, Normand S-L, Gomes T, et al. Antipsychotic therapy and short-term serious events in older adults with dementia. *Archives of Internal Medicine* 2008;168:1090–1096.

15. Schneeweis S, Setoguchi S, Brookhart A, et al. Risk of death associated with the use of conventional versus atypical antipsychotic drugs among elderly patients. *Canadian Medical Association Journal* 2007;176:627–632.

16. Gill SS, Bronskill SE, Normand S-LT, et al. Antipsychotic drug use and mortality in older adults with dementia. *Annals of Internal Medicine* 2007;146:775–786.

17. *Office of the Inspector General, Department of Health and Human Services.* Medicare atypical antipsychotic drug claims for elderly nursing home residents. Department of Health and Human Services, 2011.

18. Briesacher BA, Limcango R, Simoni-Wastila L, et al. The quality of antipsychotic drug prescribing in nursing homes. *Archives of Internal Medicine* 2005;165:1280–1285.

19. Huybrechts KF, Gerhard T, Crystal S, et al. Differential risks of death in older residents in nursing homes prescribed specific antipsychotic drugs: population-based cohort study. *British Medical Journal* 2012;344:e977. Doi:10.1136/bmj.e977, published February 23, 2012.

20. Koponen M, Taipale H, Lavikainen P, et al. Risk of mortality associated with antipsychotic monotherapy and polypharmacy among community-dwelling persons with Alzheimer's disease. *Journal of Alzheimer's Disease* 2017;56:107–118.

21. Kirke PN, Sutton M, Burke H, et al. Outcome of hip fracture in older Irish women: a 2-year follow-up of subjects in a case-control study. *Injury* 2002;33:387–391.

22. Willig R, Kenänen-Kiukaaniemi S, Jalovarra P. Mortality and quality of life after trochanteric hip fracture. *Public Health* 2001;115:323–327.

23. Haentjens P, Magaziner J, Colón-Emeric CS, et al. Meta-analyis: excess mortality after hip fracture among older women and men. *Annals of Internal Medicine* 2010;152:380–390.

24. Baker NL, Cook MN, Aright HM, et al. Hip fracture risk and subsequent mortality among Alzheimer's disease patients in the United Kingdom, 1988–2007. *Age Ageing* 2011;40:49–54.

25. Kopenen J, Taipale H, Lavkainin P, et al. Antipsychotic use and hip fracture among community-dwelling persons with Alzheimer's disease. *Journal of Clinical Psychiatry* 2017;78:e257–e3263. https://doi.org/10.4088/JCP.15m10458.

26. Johnell K, Bergman GJ, Fastborn J, et al. Psychotropic drugs and the risk of fall injuries, hospitalisations and mortality among older adults. *International Journal of Geriatric Psychiatry* 2016;32:414–420.

27. Lieberman JA, Stroup TS, McEvoy JP, et al. Effectiveness of antipsychotic drugs in patients with chronic schizophrenia. *New England Journal of Medicine* 2005;353:1209–1223.

28. Schneider LS, Ismail MS, Dagerman K, et al. Clinical antipsychotic trials of intervention effectiveness (CATIE): Alzheimer's disease trial. *Schizophrenia Bulletin* 2003;29:57–72.

29. Vigen CLP, Mack WJ, Keefe RSE, et al. Cognitive effects of atypical antipsychotic medications in patients with Alzheimer's disease: outcomes from CATIE-AD. *American Journal of Psychiatry* 2011;168:831–839.

30. Sultzer DL, Davis SM, Tariot PN, et al. Clinical symptom responses to atypical antipsychotic medications in Alzheimer's disease: phase 1 outcomes from the CATIE-AD effectiveness trial. *American Journal of Psychiatry* 2008;165:844–854.

31. Nagata T, Shinagawa S, Nakajima S, et al. Association between neuropsychiatric improvement and neurocognitive change in Alzheimer's disease: analysis of the CATIE-AD study. *Journal of Alzheimer's Disease* 2018;66:139–148.

32. Nagata T, Nakajima S, Shinagawa S, et al. Baseline predictors of antipsychotic treatment continuation and response at 8 weeks in patients with Alzheimer's disease with psychosis or aggressive symptoms: an analysis of the CATIE-AD study. *Journal of Alzheimer's Disease* 2017;60:263–272.

33. Devanand DP, Schultz SK. Editorial. Consequences of antipsychotic medications for the dementia patient. *American Journal of Psychiatry* 2011;168:767–769.

34. Devanand DP. Prediction of response to antipsychotics in patients with dementia remains a conundrum. *American Journal of Geriatric Psychiatry* 2017. http://dx.doi.org/10.1016/j.jagp.2017.04.005.

35. Zheng L, Mack WJ, Dagerman KS, et al. Metabolic changes associated with second-generation antipsychotic use in Alzheimer's disease: the CATIE-AD study. *American Journal of Psychiatry* 2009;166:583–590.

36. Kales HC, Kim HM, Zivin K, et al. Risk of mortality among individual antipsychotics in patients with dementia. *American Journal of Psychiatry* 2012;169:71–79.

37. Davies SJC, Burhan AM, Kim D, et al. Sequential drug treatment algorithm for agitation and aggression in Alzheimer's and mixed dementia. *Journal of Psychopharmacology* 2018;32:509–523.

38. Ma H, Huang Y, Cong Z, et al. The efficacy and safety of atypical antipsychotics for the treatment of dementia: a meta-analysis of randomized, placebo-controlled trials. *Journal of Alzheimer's Disease* 2014;42:915–937.

39. Nielsen RE, Lolk A, Valentin JB, et al. Cumulative dosages of antipsychotic drugs are associated with increased mortality rate in patients with Alzheimer's dementia. *Acta Psychiatrica Scandinavaca* 2016;134:314–320.

40. Banerjee S, Hellier J, Dewey M, et al. Sertraline or mirtazapine for depression in dementia (HTA-SADD): a randomized, multicenter double-blind, placebo-controlled trial. *Lancet* 2011;378:403–411.

41. Pollock BG, Mulsant BH, Rosen J, et al. A double-blind comparison of citalopram and risperidone for the treatment of behavioral and psychotic symptoms associated with dementia. *American Journal of Geriatric Psychiatry* 2007;15:942–952.

42. Portsteinsson AP, Drye LT, Pollock BG, et al. Effect of citalopram on agitation in Alzheimer disease. The CitAD randomized clinical trial. *JAMA* 2014;311:682–691. Doi:10.1001/jama.2014.93.

43. Livingston G, Johnson K, Katona C, et al. Systematic review of psychological approaches to the management of neuropsychiatric symptoms of dementia. *American Journal of Psychiatry* 2005;162:1996–2021.

44. Kales HC, Gitlin LN, Lyketsos C. Assessment and management of behavioral and psychological symptoms of dementia. *British Medical Journal* 2015;350:h369. Doi:10.1136/bmj.h369.

45. Hane FT, Robinson M, Lee BY, et al. Recent progress in Alzheimer's disease research, part 3: diagnosis and treatment. *Journal of Alzheimer's Disease* 2017;57:645–665.

46. Loi SM, Eratne D, Kelso W, et al. Alzheimer disease: non-pharmacological and pharmacological management of cognition and neuropsychiatric symptoms. *Australasian Psychiatry* 2018;26:358–365.

47. Ballard C, Orrell M, Sun Y, et al. Impact of antipsychotic review and non-pharmacological intervention on health-related quality of life in people with dementia living in care homes: WHELD—a factorial cluster randomized controlled trial. *International Journal of Geriatric Psychiatry* 2016. Doi:10.1002/gps.4572.

48. Forester BP, Patrick RE, Harper DG. Setbacks and opportunities in disease-modifying therapies in Alzheimer disease. *JAMA Psychiatry* 2020;77(1). https://jamanetwork.com.

49. Schwartz M, Ramos JMP, Ben-Yehuda H. A 20-year journey from axonal injury to neurodegenerative diseases and the prospect of immunotherapy for combating Alzheimer's disease. *The Journal of Immunology* 2020;204:243–250.

50. Zhang F-Q, Jiang J-L, Zhang J-T, et al. Current status and future prospects of stem cell therapy in Alzheimer's disease. *Neural Regeneration Research* 2019. Doi:10.413/1673-5374,265544.

51. Guzmán BC-F, Vinnakota C, Govindpani K, et al. The GABAergic system as a therapeutic target for Alzheimer's disease. *Journal of Neurochemistry* 2018;146:649–669.

52. Rosenheck RA, Leslie DL, Sindelar JL, et al. Cost-benefit analysis of second-generation antipsychotics and placebo in a randomized trial of the treatment of psychosis and aggression in Alzheimer disease. *Archives of General Psychiatry* 2007;64:1259–1268.

6 Psychotropic and Antipsychotic Polypharmacy

Common Practice, Good Medicine?

Introduction

In previous chapters, we underscored the dramatic increase in the numbers of prescriptions for antipsychotics (APs) and antidepressants (ADs), which to some extent corresponded with the expansion of mental disorders listed in successive editions of the *Diagnostic and Statistical Manual*. However, the rates of schizophrenia itself had not increased, in marked contrast to the doubling of adult inpatients with bipolar disorder during the years 1996 through 2004. Even more strikingly, bipolar disorder increased four-fold in adolescents, and six-fold in children.[1] This fit nicely with data on the outpatient treatment of children and adolescents with APs in the years 1993 to 2002,[2] when office visits accompanied by prescriptions for APs rose from 201,000 to 1,224,000, a six-fold increase. SGAs were prescribed in 92% of the visits, regardless of concerns over the metabolic syndrome. In office-based visits, 39% of youth received prescriptions for APs, as did 32% of those with mood disorders, 17% of those with pervasive developmental disorders or mental retardation, but only 14% of those with a psychotic disorder.[2]

This phenomenon was not limited to youth. Zuvekas[3] in 2005 reported that prescription drug use in households rose rapidly starting in 1996, so that by 2001, another 5.5 million Americans were being treated for mental disorders, reflecting a 7.4% increase in the use of APs within each diagnostic category.[3] Much of this was stimulated by the release of SSRIs in the late 1990s and by the marketing of SGAs starting in 1993,[4] as well as the popularity of off-label use.[5]

In the meantime, *total drug costs* in the U.S. amounted to $17 billion in 1972, with $10 billion spent on prescription drugs.[6] Total drug costs had climbed to $234 billion by 2008, to $392 billion in 2013, and to $480 billion in 2016, of which $323 billion went to Pharma.[7, 8] Spending on personal health care ballooned to $30 trillion in the years 1996 to 2013, with $154 billion of that spent on five mental health disorders.[9]

We should note that these dramatic increases took place in the context of a drug-saturated society. Indeed, 12% of the U.S. population is dependent on alcohol and 3% on illicit drugs.[10] In youth ages 13 to 18, the combined rates of dependence and abuse are 6.5% for alcohol and 9% for illicit drugs. People in the U.S. account for almost 100% of the world's consumption of hydrocodone and 81% of the global consumption of oxycodone.[11] (Despite this epidemic, some in psychiatry are now proposing[12] the use of opioids for the treatment of depression; see Chapter 12.) In our never-ending search for new sources of comfort, some have turned to bath salts[13] and energy drinks,[14] often with serious consequences.

Psychotropic Polypharmacy

In the context of our drug-saturated society,[15, pp. 20–34] the remarkable increase in the use of ADs and APs for an expanding array of symptoms should not be surprising, nor should the increasing use of psychotropic polypharmacy.[16] Patients and providers seem to expect that drugs of whatever kind are the answer to life's problems, so if one drug is good, why not two, three, or more? This was corroborated in a national survey[17] of office-based psychiatrists in which the percentage of visits resulting in the use of two more psychotropics increased from 43% in 1996 and 1997 to almost 60% in 2000 through 2005. During that period, visits with prescriptions for three or more drugs increased from 17% to 33%. (These figures held up after controlling for background characteristics.)

There is a semblance of reasonable behavior in some of these results, since combinations of APs and ADs were given more frequently when the diagnosis was schizophrenia, bipolar disorder, or major depression. A combination of ADs and mood stabilizers was more common with diagnoses of bipolar or schizophrenia,[18] but note a possible increase in the number of manic episodes with the use of ADs. (We shall examine both these issues later.)

What about the simultaneous use of two or more antipsychotics (antipsychotic polypharmacy, or APP)? Mojtabai et al.[17] found an increase from 1.2% in 1995 to 5% in 2005. APP was used significantly more often in schizophrenia but less so in depression. In a study of patients with schizophrenia, rates of APP increased from 5.7% in 1995 to almost 25% in 1999,[18] with the low rate in the 1990s confirmed in another study[19] that found *no* AP polypharmacy in discharged psychiatric patients in 1995, but this increased to 16% in 2000. However, the rate *varies* with the population and setting, with rates of 30% to 40% on inpatient units and 11% to 30% in outpatient clinics.[20]

There is little doubt that the figures found by Clark et al.[18] have climbed considerably, with rates ranging from 57% in a study of naturalistic (uncontrolled) treatment of schizophrenia to over 90% in Japan.[21] In a European study of patients with schizophrenia who began a single atypical antipsychotic at baseline, 27% had switched to APP at 12 months.[22] In North America, the median prevalence of APP increased from 12.7% in the 1980s to 17% in the 2000s.[23]

Others have taken note of the wide variation in these rates, pointing to the aforementioned differences in settings, as well as the duration of APP and the exclusion of APs when used on an as-needed (prn) basis. Other factors include variations in the health care systems, prescription costs, socioeconomic factors, and the burden of other non-psychotropic drugs and concomitant non-psychiatric illnesses.[24, 25] Unfortunately, many studies fail to account for these factors.

Another major methodological problem lies in separating out patients for whom APP represents a therapeutic transition, in which one AP is substituted for another. In that case, APP is rational since the first drug should be tapered down while the new drug is tapered up. But if the study goal is to examine point prevalence, the tapering process will inflate the rate of APP. A related problem is the lack of consensus regarding the time needed for a cross-taper. It seems obvious that this could vary considerably, given the clinical situation, but a 60-day range seems reasonable, unless the patient is taking a long-acting injectable AP (LAI), for which the time needed may stretch to 70 days. Given these issues, better information can be gained by examining rates of APP over longer periods of time, thus minimizing the cross-taper problem.

Persistent APP

With regard to the interaction of time and APP, a VA study[26] of 61,000 patients with schizophrenia found considerably different rates of APP depending on the time period. The prevalence rate was 20% in a 30-day period, 13% at 60 days, and 9.5% at 90 days. The authors also reviewed previous cross-sectional studies and found that variations in definitions resulted in the failure to identify as many as 32% to 89% who received APP for 90 days or longer. I am gratified that persistent APP was found in only 10% of the VA population but not happy that 74% received a combination of an SGA and FGA, despite the alleged superiority of SGAs and the faults of FGAs—but, as we shall see, this is not uncommon.

In APP lasting at least 60 days, one group[27] found rates of 30% in schizophrenia, 17% in bipolar disorder, and, remarkably enough, 14% in major depression. Despite the potential for serious metabolic complications, *quetiapine was the most commonly prescribed SGA in APP* (44%), *with olanzapine a close second!* Even worse, these patients were given excessively high doses, and 50% were also treated with anticholinergic drugs, used to treat EPSE, compared with 36% of those taking monotherapy, a significant difference.

In a study[28] of 31,000 Medicaid patients with schizophrenia, the overall rates of APP rose from 32% in 1998 to 41% in 2000. Of the latter group, 23% were treated with APP for an average of almost eight months, far exceeding the time needed for a cross-taper. *Remarkably,* 29% of patients taking clozapine were given long-term APP, despite clozapine's reputation as the best drug for treatment-resistant schizophrenia, while 68% of all long-term cases were treated with a combination of an SGA and an FGA, similar to the results noted earlier. And, given the metabolic risks of quetiapine, it is inexplicable that this drug had the strongest association with APP, trailed by olanzapine, another high-risk drug, and risperidone.

At this point, we have described *persistent* APP in a VA population, a Medicaid population, and a community setting in Canada, so let's move on to Denmark, where a nationwide study[29] in 2015 of people with schizophrenia taking APP for at least four months found rates of 17% in 1996, 31% in 2006, and 25% in 2012. *Higher daily doses were three times more likely with APP and treatment with clozapine.* Those treated with APP had double the odds of receiving ADs, perhaps reflecting the severity of illness.

Adverse Events With APP

In Chapter 4, we explored the interactions of AP use, dosage, the metabolic syndrome, and mortality. With regard to the adverse effects of APP, we should note that where two non–clozapine SGAS were combined,[28] there was a 70% increase in the risk of COPD and a doubling of the risk for cardiac arrythmias, asthma, and complicated DM. With the combination of an SGA and an FGA, the risk of a myocardial infarction was tripled, while the combination of two FGAs increased the risk of a clotting disorder six-fold. These are very alarming figures, but the high confidence intervals (reflecting a lack of precision) led the authors to write that they *could not assign causal relationships*. Nevertheless, they recommended EKGs for those treated with APP, another recommendation often ignored.

It seems likely that adverse events in APP are tied, at least in part, to excessive dosing, despite the early optimism that APP could result in lower doses. However, there is strong evidence of excessive dosing with APP. That being the case, it shouldn't be surprising that a 2012 review[23] of APP found eight studies noting that the use of anticholinergic drugs (benztropine and others) occurred more often with APP. This is consistent with other work[30] demonstrating an increase in parkinsonian side effects with APP, as well as an increase in prolactin levels, with both reflecting the widespread use of an FGA combined with an SGA—a strategy that seems irrational, as discussed earlier. Indeed, the three most commonly used drugs were olanzapine, risperidone, and haloperidol. The combination of olanzapine and haloperidol strikes me as an odd couple indeed since the patient is exposed not only to a metabolically risky SGA, but also to a neurologically risky FGA! Nevertheless, in a global study[23] of APP, the combination of an FGA and SGA was found in 42% of patients. What is the rationale?

The use of anticholinergic agents in APP is not a minor issue since they have significant side effects,[31] including tachycardia, constipation, urinary retention, decreased sweating, vulnerability to heat-related illnesses, dry mouth, an increased frequency of caries, and blurred vision. Anticholinergics may worsen memory loss, especially in older patients; have been subject to abuse; and, at higher doses, can result in a toxic delirium. With regard to memory, in a study[32] of stable outpatients with schizophrenia (mean age of 43), higher blood levels of anticholinergics at baseline were correlated with greater impairment of verbal learning and working memory—areas that lie at the core of schizophrenia. After cognitive training, it was clear that higher anticholinergic levels were associated with less improvement in cognition, with an *impact greater* than age, IQ, or severity of symptoms. Clearly, efforts at cognitive rehabilitation in schizophrenia must be accompanied by efforts at minimizing the use of anticholinergic drugs, but we must stress that many of the older ADs and APs are inherently anticholinergic; that is, they block muscarinic cholinergic receptors.

In a naturalistic 2018 study of 1,087 patients in Norway,[33] the authors reported a significantly higher burden of adverse events with an increasing number of APs and a progressive increase in the defined daily dose. Patients using APs reported triple the risk of galactorrhea, four times the risk of motor slowing, triple the risk of sleepiness, and twice the risk of erectile dysfunction, weight gain, and restlessness. *The risk with three APs was surprisingly similar*, with almost triple the risk of motor slowing and more than triple the risk of akathisia. Only 5% reported that side effects constituted a severe burden, but this was greater than reported by investigators. Females reported a greater burden of side effects than males.

APP, Other Psychotropics, and Non-Psychiatric Drugs

In a 2012 review[23] of APP prevalence and correlates, psychiatrists in North America used ADs as co-medication in 19% of cases, antianxiety agents and hypnotics in 23%, mood stabilizers in 28%, lithium in 7%, and, in the case of anticholinergics, 33%. In a large VA study[30] of patients taking AP mono-therapy or APP, antianxiety agents were used more frequently with APP (42% vs 38%), as were mood stabilizers (38% vs 30%) and anticholinergics (50% vs 38%). However, there was no difference in the use of ADs, which is fortunate, since adding ADs to APs increases the risk of drug interactions secondary to the potent effects of ADs on the cytochrome P450 enzyme system, a system largely responsible for the metabolism of psychotropic drugs.

Yet, in another naturalistic study of 374 patients with schizophrenia published in 2012,[34] 16% were prescribed ADs with APs, while 11% received a combination of APs and mood stabilizers, 20% received APP, and *only 20% received AP monotherapy*. Drugs from three psychotropic classes were used in 16% of the cases, and anticholinergics were prescribed in 5% to 8%. We should note as well that about 50% of patients taking AP monotherapy are treated with antidepressants, mood stabilizers, or benzodiazepines,[22] which is not surprising, given the high rates of co-morbidity found in schizophrenia.

Making matters even more complicated, few of the studies cited in this chapter have investigated the rates, types, or doses of drugs used to treat co-existing medical disorders such as diabetes mellitus, hypertension, obesity, hyperlipidemia, or heart disease. Yet use of such agents is fairly common, as shown by Ganguly et al. in their study[28] of Medicaid-eligible patients with schizophrenia. The most common drugs were antihypertensives (24%), antiepileptics (47%), parkinsonian agents (71%), and drugs used for hyperlipidemia (7%). The use of parkinsonian agents and antiepileptic drugs was significantly more common in those on APP, no doubt reflecting the greater use of anticholinergics and mood stabilizers in APP.

The paucity of data on these "medical drugs" and the lack of recognition of their side effects are unfortunate and leave us with an incomplete picture. I recognize that including data on drugs aimed at non-psychiatric disorders complicates data analysis, but statisticians can work miracles. The use of anti-hyperlipidemic drugs, as well as antidiabetic drugs, is of particular importance, given the association between APs and the metabolic syndrome.

APP and the Metabolic Syndrome

In Chapter 4, we reviewed the extensive evidence documenting the association between use of APs and the development of the metabolic syndrome, with its potential for shortening the life span and increasing the risk of cardiovascular events. We noted concerns over this issue dating to 2003, when a Consensus Development Conference[35] warned of the metabolic risks posed by SGAs. The risks appeared greater with clozapine and olanzapine, followed by quetiapine and risperidone, while aripiprazole and ziprasidone seemed to have little or no effect. But, as we noted in Chapter 4, the FDA then proceeded to approve the use of olanzapine and quetiapine for the treatment of schizophrenia and manic episodes in adolescents and even for use in children as young as age ten who have a diagnosis of childhood bipolar disorder! Indeed, quetiapine has been commonly used in APP![28, 36]

In 2007, Correll and colleagues reviewed[37] these developments and posed the obvious question: Might APP further increase the risk of the metabolic syndrome? Given the absence of relevant studies, they decided to do a point-prevalence study of randomly selected inpatient admissions from August, 2004 to March 2005. All physicians had been instructed to follow the recommendations of the Consensus Development Conference with regard to monitoring of weight and the other components of the metabolic syndrome. What were the results?

Of the 364 patients, 19% were receiving APP, with a combination of two SGAs in 70%; quetiapine was used in 43% of the cases. In a logistic regression analysis, *the metabolic syndrome was found in 50% of those using APP vs 34% on monotherapy.* APP was accompanied by a higher BMI, an older age, a diagnosis of schizophrenia or bipolar disorder, and co-treatment with an FGA. However, when using a multivariate analysis that included demographic and clinical variables, the metabolic syndrome was *not* independently associated with APP, nor was there an association with a drug class (FGA vs SGA) or with combinations of clozapine/olanzapine vs aripiprazole/ziprasidone, which is surprising. The authors postulated an interaction between underlying risk factors (BMI, age, schizophrenia, bipolar disorder, gender, race) and AP treatment and concluded that APP should be reserved for patients with a mood or psychotic disorder resistant to clozapine, those who refuse clozapine, or those whose medical disorders argue against clozapine.[37]

This was a well-done study, but I must stress that the population was rather young (age 43 ± 15 years), largely male, and Caucasian. Some 50% to 58% were smokers. Note, too, that this was not a longitudinal study but simply a one-time cross-sectional view. It seems odd that Correll and Gallego, in their 2012 review[38] of APP, did not mention any concerns regarding APP and the metabolic syndrome.

Another cross-sectional study[39] of 334 outpatients with schizophrenia done in Japan found APP in 50% of the patients but failed to find a significant association with the full metabolic syndrome. However, unlike most studies, they divided metabolic factors into four classes, including a "pre-metabolic" syndrome, defined as visceral obesity combined with only one of the three other components (dyslipidemia, elevated blood glucose, elevated blood pressure). In this group, *the risk of the pre-metabolic syndrome was doubled, providing a warning sign* to clinicians, patients, and families!

Perhaps more relevant to the United States is a cross-sectional study[40] in Sweden, in which both clozapine and olanzapine were the most frequently used APs in a naturalistic study of 269 patients with schizophrenia. The overall prevalence of the metabolic syndrome was 34.6%, with the use of clozapine in 51%. APP was used in 20%, of whom 40% had the metabolic syndrome, but this was *not* significantly different from monotherapy. In another naturalistic study[41] of patients with a psychotic disorder in the Netherlands, 35% had the metabolic syndrome at baseline and 32% at a one-year follow-up evaluation. *This study was unique in tracking the course of the metabolic syndrome and found that 33% had a reversal over the course of a year* while it developed in 13%. This is quite striking and reflects the difficulties in establishing a consistent picture of the long-term metabolic effects of APs and APP. It did appear, however, that chronicity, smoking, a family history of cardiovascular disease, abdominal obesity, and dyslipidemia were associated with a higher risk. Unfortunately, active treatment for cardiovascular problems or DM did not increase the possibility of reversal.

Given the results of these studies and the lack of large, long-term, and well-controlled investigations, the evidence strongly suggests that APP is associated with a risk of the metabolic syndrome beyond that found with monotherapy.

APP in Bipolar Disorder

We have focused on schizophrenia, but the FDA approval of multiple SGAs for treatment of bipolar disorder will no doubt lead to many of the same problems and issues surrounding the use of APP in schizophrenia. Indeed, there was a nearly 7-fold increase in the use of SGAs for the treatment of bipolar disorder during the years 1995 to 2008,[42] despite concerns over their metabolic effects and the very high initial costs. This rapid increase was accompanied by the aforementioned 40-fold increase in the outpatient diagnosis of childhood bipolar disorder[43] and a 45-fold increase in the rate of publications on the subject, rates certainly not explained by any genetic factors or even social changes. Adding to the diagnostic and treatment problem in youth is a co-morbid diagnosis in 32% of ADHD, a condition with many similar symptoms.

With regard to the more general issue of polypharmacy in treatment-resistant mood disorders, a two-decade long study[44] of patients discharged from the National Institute of Mental Health, 3% of patients left the hospital with three or more psychotropic medications in the mid-1970s, 9% in the mid-1980s, 35% in the late 1980s, and 44% by the mid-1990s. This clearly reflects the growing emphasis on intensive pharmacotherapy and polypharmacy in the years following the introduction of SSRIs and SGAs. With regard to bipolar disorder, a survey[45] of five state Medicaid programs found that APP was found in 13% to 21% of patients with bipolar disorder. This is considerably fewer than those found in schizophrenia (64%–69%), but not an insignificant number and comparable to the 10% rate found in a multi-site NIMH study of bipolar illness published in 2011.[46]

In Chapters 8 and 9, we will focus on polypharmacy in depression.

Polypharmacy and APP in Youth: A Growing Problem

We should first note a 75% increase in the number of child and adolescent office-based visits that involved mention of a psychotropic drug from the mid-1990s to 2004 through 2007.[47] During that decade, the percentage of visits in which youth were treated with psychotropic polypharmacy rose from 14% to 20%, but, if a psychiatric illness had been diagnosed, the percentages rose from 22% to 32%. This era was remarkable for a six-fold increase in the co-prescription of APs and other medications for ADHD, accompanied by a five-fold rise in co-prescriptions for APs and ADs, although, as the authors admitted, "little is known about the safety and efficacy" of multi-class psychotropics for youth.[47]

Despite the newfound freedom to prescribe APs and ADs for children, there had been no significant increase in the diagnoses of co-morbid psychiatric disorders (including psychotic disorders) in the *very* young, except for a doubling of the diagnoses of autism spectrum disorders and mental retardation in *children ages two to five years*.[48] Indeed, non-psychotic disorders were the dominant diagnoses in youth, with pervasive developmental disorder/mental retardation leading the way with 28%, ADHD in 24%, no diagnosis in 17%, and disruptive behavior disorders in 13%. Yet Olfson et al.[48] found that the annual rate of prescriptions for APs in children ages two through five doubled from 1999–2000 to 2007. Despite the gravity of giving powerful APs to children this young, most had not been seen by a psychiatrist, nor had they had a mental health evaluation visit or psychotherapy in the year in which the drug was prescribed! Given these figures, it shouldn't be surprising to learn that children and adolescents with ADHD and behavioral disorders accounted for 45% and 30%, respectively, of all APP use in a Florida Medicaid program.[49]

In a 2014 review of 15 studies examining APP in youth,[50] Toteja and colleagues found a prevalence rate of 9.6% in children and 12% in adolescents, with the most common combination (70%) being an FGA and an SGA, despite the lack of logic in such a strategy. While the authors did not find a correlation between APP and individual diagnoses, there was a correlation between use of APP when a diagnosis of bipolar disorder was combined with schizophrenia spectrum disorders. Nevertheless, the authors strongly cautioned that the high prescribing rates of APs for youth with oppositional defiant disorder and ADHD are "clearly of concern." They also took note of a 2011 study[51] in which *youth in foster care had a 43% increase in the odds of receiving APP.* In contrast to the use of APP in adults, there was no correlation between APP and use of anticholinergics, long-acting injectables, male sex, or use of clozapine.

Unfortunately, a 2017 study[52] found that a combination of an AP with an SSRI or SNRI (selective norepinephrine reuptake inhibitor) increased the risk of type II DM by 80%, with higher doses and length of treatment associated with the increase in risk. Obviously, youth treated with this combination should be monitored *very* carefully Fortunately, the combination of an AP and a stimulant medication did not carry an increased risk.

Implications, Concerns Regarding Psychotropic Drugs in Youth

In Chapter 4, we reviewed and cited a number of studies on the metabolic consequences of APs in youth, but let's focus briefly on the risks of APP. McIntyre and Jerrill carried out a retrospective cohort study[53] of AP treatment in 4,140 youth and 4,500 controls in a South Carolina Medicaid program and found some very disturbing data. Compared to the non-exposed group, youth treated with APP had *double the risk for obesity/weight gain and new-onset type 2 DM, and five times the risk for dyslipidemia.* The risk for obesity was also doubled in a review[54] of 34 head-to-head studies of youth with psychotic and bipolar disorders, accompanied by a 72% increase in the risk of any cardiovascular, cerebrovascular, or hypotensive adverse event.

Parents should take note of a 2019 study[55] of risk factors for polypharmacy that included the presence of multiple prescribers; this was an independent risk factor and underscores the risks of a shifting set of prescribers. The involvement of a psychiatrist upped the risk considerably, but note that youths with bipolar disorder were more likely to be seen by a psychiatrist, so this raises the issue of case complexity. Polypharmacy was much more common in Caucasians and males but less common in Hispanics. The differences in ethnicity were not explained, but see Zito's work, which follows.

Psychotropics in the Very Young: Why?

Twenty years ago, Zito and colleagues[56] drew attention to the use of psychotropic agents in very young children, stressing a three-fold increase in children ages two to four during the years 1990 through 2005, an era already familiar to us. The paper seemed to have little impact, given the *five-fold rise in the use of APs in ages two to four.*[57] Zito went on to publish an essay[58] with a relevant title, "On the Medicalization of Emotional and Behavioral Problems in Youth," in which she emphasized data showing that race and ethnicity play a role in the prescription of psychotropics in youth, as does the widening gap in socioeconomic status, a subject we will stress in Chapter 14.

Nevertheless, prescribers continue to hand out APs and ADs to children as young as age two. This caught the attention of a writer for the *New York Times*, Alan Schwartz,[59] who examined data from IMS Health and noted that in 2014, some 20,000 prescriptions for risperidone and other APs were aimed at *children two years and younger.* This represented a 50% increase from 2013! Prescriptions for fluoxetine in the same age group rose by 23% to 83,000! In 2014, 10,000 children ages two to three were diagnosed with ADHD and treated with stimulants, despite the absence of guideline recommendations. Schwartz added that he had interviewed multiple experts in the field who said they had never heard of children younger than three being given these drugs—nor could they offer a rationale.

What can account for this disturbing trend, at least in part, is marketing. This seems especially true for risperidone, heavily marketed to pediatricians. This paid off, with 20% of the sales of risperidone coming from treatment aimed at youth.[60] Underscoring the success of this strategy, risperidone accounted for 66% of all AP prescriptions written for children ages six or under in a Kentucky Medicaid population.[61] However, only 32% were written by psychiatrists while general practitioners and pediatricians accounted for 34%. Almost one third of the children in this age group were prescribed risperidone for at least 12 months.

By 2004, sales of risperidone had reached $3 billion in the U.S. and some $30 billion globally, despite heavy fines for Johnson & Johnson, the manufacturer, which suppressed data showing that risperidone often led to breast development in boys.[62] Given the sales figures, no wonder that Pharma continues to push the FDA for the right to legally market drugs for off-label use.[62]

Yet we do have some positive news from a 2018 national study of prescription patterns for youth (n = 6,351,482), with the focus on antidepressants, stimulants, and antipsychotics[63] prescribed according to age groups and medication class. In general, percentages of young people ages 3 to 24 years prescribed psychotropics were consistent with the epidemiologic patterns of indications for ADHD, anxiety, and depression. For those ages 3 to 5, 0.8% were given one of the three classes; for ages 6 to 12, 5.4%; and for ages 19 to 24, 6.0%. The peak age for stimulant prescriptions was 11 (5.7%); for antidepressants, 16 (4.8%); and for antipsychotics, 16 (1.3%). Interestingly, the percentage of youth taking stimulants is lower than the 8.6% prevalence of ADHD while the percentage of youth taking ADs is lower than the prevalence of mood/anxiety disorders, leading to concerns regarding undertreatment, rather than overtreatment. Regarding APs, the estimated prevalence of psychotic disorders, including psychotic mood disorders, is about 3.6%.

These data are at least somewhat reassuring, but note the caveats described by the authors. First, the analysis was based on 2008 prescription data and, therefore, may have missèd the impact of SGAs on the treatment of bipolar disorder in youth. Second, there was no information regarding clinical diagnoses, severity of symptoms, or whether the recipients actually took the medication. I found no data on APP. I must note that while three of the authors reported no conflicts of interest, the second author has been heavily supported by Pharma and has testified for at least three drug companies.

In a 2019 study[64] on psychotropic medication use in Canadian children from 2012 through 2016, the news was mixed. First, prescriptions for APs fell by 10%, much in contrast to a 114% increase found between 2005 and 2009. While this seems to reflect more concern over the appropriateness of APs for children, the previous massive increase was not significantly affected. In addition, consistent with the off-label use of APs we described earlier, ADHD and conduct disorder were the primary diagnoses in prescribing APs. Similarly, AP prescriptions for autism rose by 34% and by 27% for ADs.

The authors stressed that several guidelines were published in 2012 and 2015 in Canada that strongly recommended psychosocial interventions for first-line treatment of maladaptive aggression in youth.[64] Should medication be necessary, the guidelines recommended stimulants, alpha agonists, and atomoxetine for first-line use, followed by risperidone if the earlier steps failed. In addition, risperidone should be limited to three months and tapered down and off if at all possible.

APP and Mortality

Does APP may increase mortality? The data is limited, but a study from Finland[65] found that over a 17-year follow-up, the relative risk of mortality increased by 2.50 with each AP added, even after controlling for multiple risk factors. These results were similar to those found in an earlier 10-year follow-up study,[66] in which APP was associated with a shortened survival time in schizophrenia. In an Australian study,[67] *APP among older veterans and war widows led to a five-fold increase in all-cause mortality.* However, we have to recognize that only *FGAs* were involved in these studies, which were also marked by small sample sizes.

With a much larger sample size, APP did *not* result in an increase in the rate of natural deaths when compared with monotherapy.[68] Interestingly enough, *APP was associated with* a *lower mortality rate* than was found in the absence of APs. However, the number of medications used to treat various physical diseases was associated with increasing mortality rates, reaching an adjusted odds ratio of almost 27 when ten or more drugs were prescribed. The use of an AP combined with a long-acting benzodiazepine increased the risk of death by 78%! Yet caution is indicated, since it was not clear if patients were using a benzodiazepine at the time of death.

The risk of benzodiazepines, almost always used as adjunctive therapy, was also highlighted by a Finnish study[69] of patients with schizophrenia, in which the authors found a *91% increase in mortality risk with benzodiazepine use*, whether used alone or in combination with 'ADs or APs, largely due to increases in suicide and non-suicide deaths. As with the Danish study, mortality risk was not increased by APP when compared with monotherapy. And, in marked contrast to data we cited previously, the *absence of an AP doubled the mortality risk.* On the other hand, a recent study[70] of monotherapy vs polypharmacy among community-dwelling persons with Alzheimer's disease found that use of AP monotherapy was associated with a 60% increase in the risk of mortality, *while APP almost tripled the risk.*

More bad news for youth: A retrospective cohort study of Medicaid enrollees[71] aged 5 through 24 years focused on those taking APs who had *no* diagnoses of schizophrenia or related psychoses, tic disorder, or Tourette syndrome (FDA approved for use of APs) and no history of severe medical illnesses. The control group was taking stimulants, ADs, or α-agonists. The AP-exposed group had an 81% increase in the risk of death, primarily due to 3.5-fold increase in the risk of unexpected death in the higher-dose group, defined as an initial dose of over 50 mg of chlorpromazine equivalents. This persisted for unexpected deaths not due to overdose, with a 4.3-fold increased risk of death secondary to metabolic or cardiovascular disease. The higher-dose group had a greater prevalence of mood disorders and more exposure to mood stabilizers and other psychotropics. We must note as well *that rates of polypharmacy were increased in the higher-dose group,* with 45% taking medications for ADHD and 42% taking ADs. These data prompted an editorial[72] in 2019 expressing additional concerns about off-label prescribing, an issue we have emphasized throughout this volume—but it continues.

Although the data on mortality is not consistent, the increasing use of polypharmacy in older patients is worrisome, since this is a vulnerable population. For example, an analysis[73] of prescription data in patients older than 70 found a significant increase in the use of two or more psychotropics during the period from 1990 to 1999. The heaviest use was concentrated in females and in those 85 years and older. Unfortunately, this increase was not confined to psychotropics. Inappropriate prescribing was common, with 92% receiving one or more inappropriate medications. Indeed, a 2015 review[74] of inappropriate polypharmacy cited 50 studies examining various aspects of this problem, including recommendations for taking corrective steps, or "deprescribing." However, psychotropics were generally not the focus of these efforts, nor was APP. This is surprising, given data showing the detrimental effects of APs in this population, especially in those with dementia, as we reviewed in Chapter 5. On the other hand, a 2014 study of medications with questionable benefit in dementia *did not list any psychotropic drug* as an offender.[75] Instead, cholinesterase inhibitors and memantine topped the list.

Nevertheless, it's clear that that more attention needs to be given to the effects of APP in the elderly, as well as in youth. But what are we to do with such inconsistent results? One always must take note of the study population, the specific drugs studied, dosing, study length, co-morbidity, sample size, the health care system, and any evidence of bias. Few of these studies take into account the socioeconomic status of the enrollees. There indeed must be huge gaps between the socioeconomic status of people in the U.S. Medicaid programs and the study populations in Denmark, Finland, and Sweden.

The Costs of APP

Ganguly et al.[28] compared the costs of polypharmacy and monotherapy in Georgia and California. Use of APP led to an annual cost to Medicaid of almost $500,000 in Georgia and over $6 million in California, although these estimates almost certainly are low since administrative and monitoring costs were not included. Had these states implemented a prior authorization rule, Georgia could have saved $419,000 per year and California $5 million per year, but this step would also have increased the burden on clinic staff.

The cost of APP was as much as 300% higher than monotherapy in a Medicaid outpatient study[76] while an investigation in New Hampshire found that the rising rates of APP increased the average monthly cost by $400 per patient.[77] A controlled trial[78] of over 300 patients with schizophrenia or schizoaffective disorder found that adding risperidone to a previous AP resulted in an additional monthly cost of $57, while the addition of quetiapine led to an additional monthly cost of $101. Additional cost studies can be found in a 2012 review by Correll and Gallego,[38] although many studies were done prior to the FDA approval of lower-cost generic SGAs.

I have been unable to locate any current investigations that have taken the lower costs of generic SGAs into account or, for that matter, any comparative cost-benefit analyses of APP across countries with markedly different drug costs and health care systems.

Does APP Result in Lower Doses of Individual Drugs?

One tenet of APP enthusiasts has been the idea that APP would result in lower doses and, presumably, a lower rate of side effects.[79] We have already debunked the latter, but what about dosing practices? (In Chapters 4 and 5, we documented well-done studies that found an association between higher doses and an increased risk of sudden cardiac death, cardiac disease, stroke, and all-cause mortality.)

Given these data, it seems obvious that we need to find a reasonable way of restraining the urge to order higher doses of APs, but APP hasn't helped, and in fact has made matters worse. Centorrino and associates[80] found a 46% increase in the dose experienced by inpatients from 1988 to 1999. The same lead author sampled another group of patients hospitalized at McLean in 2004 and 2009[81] and found that the final AP dose in 2009 had increased by 97%! Nevertheless, there was no increase in adverse events and "possibly superior clinical improvement." The trend toward excessive dosing is not limited to hospitalized patients or those enrolled in Medicaid programs. In a study of eight community health teams in Vancouver,[27] excessive dosing was found in all patients taking APP, regardless of diagnoses, and was significantly higher than with monotherapy. In a lengthy naturalistic study[46] of almost 1,700 bipolar patients taking SGAs, the mean olanzapine dose in monotherapy was 10 mg daily, compared with 12 to 16 mg daily in SGA polytherapy. In the case of quetiapine, the results were even more striking; the dose in polytherapy almost doubled to 469 mg daily. APP was *not* associated with improvement in clinical status or functioning, but instead was associated with more dry mouth, tremor, constipation, and sexual dysfunction. Symptom severity at baseline was not associated with APP, in contrast to claims made in other studies.[38]

Are There Benefits of APP?

Gören and associates[20] found only six controlled trials of APP in treatment-resistant schizophrenia. Five of the six examined AP augmentation of clozapine, with four of these using risperidone and the others using sulpiride, not available in the United States. The results were not impressive. Three of the studies found *no* significant differences in symptom outcome, while a fourth found that clozapine *alone* produced significantly better symptom outcome but no difference in the quality of life. Goren et al.[20] also cited three RCTs of APP in patients *without* documented resistance to monotherapy for schizophrenia or schizoaffective disorder. *None of these studies found an advantage for APP*, while sedation and constipation were worse. In uncontrolled studies of APP in non-treatment-resistant patients, five of six studies found no advantages with polypharmacy, nor did a study of polypharmacy in hospitalized patients,[81] even while controlling for age, gender, diagnoses, and initial ratings of psychotic symptoms.

Better support for APP can be found in a meta-analytic study[82] of 19 controlled trials of APP vs monotherapy in schizophrenia, involving 1,216 subjects. Interestingly, only SGA + FGA combinations were superior to monotherapy with regard to all-cause discontinuation and inefficacy. The greatest effects were seen in patients with an acute exacerbation of schizophrenia and in patients who were treated with two APs started simultaneously. However, the superiority of APP was found *only* in studies lasting longer than ten weeks. In contrast to the many studies reviewed earlier, a higher dose of APs was not found in those studies that found APP superior to monotherapy, nor was there an increase in use of anticholinergics, movement disorders, weight gain, or other metabolic abnormalities. The exception was an increase in prolactin levels when risperidone or sulpiride was added to clozapine.

This seemed reassuring, but the authors added that "the lack of conclusive adverse effect data that makes it difficult to weigh potential benefits against risks." In addition, the reviewed studies were highly heterogeneous, and there was evidence of publication bias, suggesting a tilt toward publication of positive studies.[82] In the same year, a Cochrane database review[83] of clozapine combined with different APs found no evidence of superiority for *any* type of APP compared with monotherapy.

I must conclude that despite the popularity of APP, the benefits are slim while the evidence for adverse events is substantial. The proposal that APP could result in lower dosing of individual APs and fewer adverse events has been debunked. In 2008, Goodwin et al.[79] stated that there is no biological or evidence-based rationale indicating that APP should be superior to monotherapy. In fact, a 2017 Swedish study[84] of AP treatment in schizophrenia found that the risk of rehospitalization was lowest with monotherapy with long-acting injectable APs (LAIs), including paliperidone, risperidone, perphenazine, and oral clozapine. All LAIs were superior to their oral equivalents. Please note that oral quetiapine and perphenazine were associated with the greatest risk of rehospitalization. In another study[85] of monotherapy vs APP, APP was superior to monotherapy only in open-label and low-quality trials.

Rather than prescribing APP, why not change to an LAI, or clozapine? Both, however, present their own problems from the standpoint of requiring accepting injections, tolerating the side effects of clozapine, and accepting the need for blood samples in order to monitor plasma levels and white cell counts. Both clozapine and LAIs lend more certainty regarding medication adherence, for obvious reasons.

From APP to Monotherapy: Is It Feasible?

We earlier noted instances where persistent APP was the result of the failure to complete the transition from one AP to another or reluctance on the part of the provider, patient, and family to "rock the boat" if improvement has occurred. Yet there is evidence suggesting that a switch to monotherapy is often successful. An investigation by Essock et al.[86] is worth describing in more detail, since it involved *randomly* assigning 127 outpatients with schizophrenia to continue APP or switch to monotherapy. Patients could not be enrolled if they were judged to be in need of a rapid medication change, whether due to side effects or an exacerbation of symptoms. APP was limited to two APs, the presence of which was confirmed by blood levels. Psychotropic drugs other than APs were permitted. Tapering to monotherapy had to be completed in 30 days. This was a six-month trial with a six-month naturalistic follow-up. The primary outcome was all-cause time to drug discontinuation. Secondary outcomes included symptom rating scales and others aimed at measuring subjective complaints. Considerable effort was put into maintaining blinded ratings. Results?

Time to discontinuation was significantly shorter for those switched to monotherapy, of whom 31% stopped the assigned medication. The survival curves began to differ at two months. Conversely, *67% successfully switched to monotherapy, with no differences on ratings of psychotic symptoms* compared with APP. There were no differences in ratings of parkinsonism or tardive dyskinesia, sexual side-effects, or hospitalizations. Body mass index (BMI), however, fell significantly with a switch to monotherapy, but the absolute change in BMI was quite small, translating into a weight loss of five pounds from a baseline average weight of 203 pounds. Unfortunately, no data was given on adjunctive medications, their doses, or prior use of other therapies.

This study was published in 2011 but was the *first* randomized trial to address the outcome of a switch to monotherapy, despite the lengthy history of APP. Several other studies[87–89] have had positive results, including educational efforts and feedback from pharmacists to providers. Of special interest is a Cochrane Database Review[90] of withdrawal of APs from patients with dementia. The trial was successful in 80% of the patients. Additional studies noting the success of "desprescribing" in different populations can be found in Scott et al.[74] who also include information on strategies.

Clinical Notes

1. There is little evidence to support the long-term use of two APs simultaneously but considerable evidence noting an increased risk of adverse events, including an increase in mortality, a higher cumulative dose, more use of anticholinergics, more adverse events, more metabolic problems, and an increase in costs.

2. Rather than APP, good evidence shows that use of a single long-acting injectable AP can forestall relapse and hospitalization in those with schizophrenia. Monotherapy with clozapine is also very effective, but the demands on the patients are more significant, given the side effects and need for ongoing laboratory studies.

3. The evidence in children and adolescents does not support APP, and the risk of adverse events is clear, including a higher likelihood of the metabolic syndrome and neurological side effects. These may have a rapid onset and can occur with low doses.

4. Youth are now being liberally treated with combinations of APs, ADs, and stimulants, some of which work at cross-purposes. Evidence suggests that in some instances, there has been no psychiatric consultation before starting such combinations, which is unacceptable. In other instances, there has not been a mental health assessment, again unacceptable! We know very little about the long-term effects of these combinations on the developing brain. Parents should be skeptical in the extreme about such drug combinations.

5. If APs are necessary, please advocate for the lowest possible dose, given the evidence for additional harm at higher doses, whether with monotherapy or APP.

6. I would never prescribe APs in children ages two through five. This borders on the bizarre and has no supporting data. Even in children ages 6 to 11, I would demand evidence of effectiveness balanced against the risks. Again, the longer-term effects on the developing brain are completely unknown but, given the effects of APs on the mature brain, one must suspect that the effects of central nervous system drugs on the brains of very young children must be significant. It is highly doubtful that a study aimed at assessing the risks will ever be done.

7. At the other end of the age scale, APP is being used in patients older than 70 and even past the age of 85, often in combination with other harmful medications. Families should insist on a detailed review of all APs and may wish to consider an independent review by another psychiatrist or a clinical pharmacist. Pharmacy staff can be extremely helpful.

8. There is no doubt that psychiatrists and other physicians are flouting guidelines for use of APP. Several studies have shown that APP has been the first step in treatment,[37, 50, 77] contrary to guidelines.

9. A 2017 study[91] found 29 meta-analyses of 42 combinations of APs and other drugs, including anti-inflammatories, various classes of ADs, lithium, oxytocin, anticonvulsants, and others. While 14 combinations were better than placebo, *the effect sizes were far less in high-quality studies,* leaving the authors to conclude that no single strategy deserves a recommendation.

10. Studies indicate that many patients can be successfully tapered off combinations of psychotropic drugs. This should always be explored, as should the availability of non-drug treatment, as noted in previous chapters. Indeed, exercise, cognitive training, and psychosocial rehabilitation may be quite helpful.

References

1. Blader JC, Carlson GA. Increased rates of bipolar diagnoses among U.S. child, adolescent, and adult in-patients, 1996–2004. *Biological Psychiatry* 2007;62:107–114.

2. Olfson M, Blanco C, Liu L, et al. National trends in the outpatient treatment of children and adolescents with antipsychotic drugs. *Archives of General Psychiatry* 2006;63:679–685.

3. Zuvekas SH. Prescription drugs and the changing patterns of treatment for mental disorders, 1996–2001. *Health Affairs* 2005;24. Doi:10.1377/hlthaff.24.1.195.

4. Crystal S, Olfson M, Huang C, et al. Broadened use of atypical antipsychotics: safety, effectiveness, and policy challenges. *Health Affairs* 2009. Doi 10.1377/hlthaff.28.5.w770.

5. Dean CE. The death of specificity in psychiatry: cheers or tears? *Perspectives in Biology and Medicine* 2012;55:443–460.

6. Silverman M, Lee PR. *Pills, Profits, & Politics*. Harper and Row, New York, 1984.

7. Thomas K. Prices soaring for specialty drugs, researchers find. *The New York Times*, April 14, 2014, p. B1.

8. Yu NL, Atteberry P, Bach PB. Spending on prescription drugs in the US: where does all the money go? *Health Affairs Blog* 2018. Doi:10.1377/hblog20180726,670593.

9. Dieleman JL, Baral J, Birger M, et al. US spending on personal health care and public health, 1996–2013. *JAMA* 2016;316:2677–2646.

10. Merikangas K, McClair VL. Epidemiology of substance abuse disorders. *Human Genetics* 2012;131:779–780.

11. Volkow ND. America's addiction to opioids: heroin and prescription drug abuse. *Presented to the Senate Caucus on International Narcotics Control*, May 14, 2014.

12. Kosten TR. An opioid for depression? *American Journal of Psychiatry* 2016;173:446–447.

13. Rasimas JJ. "Bath salts" and the return of the serotonin syndrome. *Journal of Clinical Psychiatry* 2012;73:1126–1127.

14. Meir B. Reports on energy drinks show gaps in safety policy. *The New York Times*, October 26, 2012.

15. Alcabes P. Medication nation. *The American Scholar* Winter 2016.

16. Kantor ED, Rehm CD, Haas JS, et al. Trends in prescription drug use among adults in the United States from 1999–2012. *Journal of the American Medical Association* 2015;314:1818–1834.

17. Mojtabai R, Olfson M. National trends in psychotropic medication polypharmacy in office-based psychiatry. *Archives of General Psychiatry* 2010;67:26–36.

18. Clark RE, Bartels SJ, Mellman TA, et al. Recent trends in antipsychotic combination therapy of schizophrenia and schizoaffective disorder: implications for state mental health policy. *Schizophrenia Bulletin* 2002;28:75–84.

19. McCue RE, Waheed R, Urcuyo L. Polypharmacy in patients with schizophrenia. *Journal of Clinical Psychiatry* 2003;64:984–989.

20. Gören JL, Parks JJ, Ghinassi FA, et al. When is antipsychotic polypharmacy supported by research evidence? Implications for QI. *The Joint Commission on Quality and Patient Safety* 2008;34:571–582.

21. Tranulis C, Skalli L, LaLonde P, et al. Benefits and risks of antipsychotic polypharmacy. An evidence-based review of the literature. *Drug Safety* 2008;31:7–20.

22. Novick D, Ascher-Svanum H, Brugnoli R, et al. Antipsychotic monotherapy and polypharmacy in the treatment of outpatients with schizophrenia in the European schizophrenia outpatients health outcomes study. *Journal of Nervous and Mental Disease* 2012;200:637–643.

23. Gallego JA, Bonetti J, Zhang JP, et al. Prevalence and correlates of antipsychotic polypharmacy from the 1970s to 2009. Prevalence and correlates of antipsychotic

polypharmacy: a systematic review and meta-regression of global and regional trends from the 1970s to 2009. *Schizophrenia Research* 2012;138:18–28.

24. Lochmann van Bennekom MWH, Gijsman Hj, Zitman FG. Antipsychotic polypharmacy in psychotic disorders: a critical review of neurobiology, tolerability, and cost effectiveness. *Journal of Psychopharmacology* 2013;27:327–336.

25. Sernyak MJ, Rosenhec R. Clinician's reasons for antipsychotic co-prescribing. *Journal of Clinical Psychiatry* 2004;65:1597–1600.

26. Kreyenbuhl J, Valenstein M, McCarthy JF, et al. Long-term combination antipsychotic treatment in VA patients with schizophrenia. *Schizophrenia Research* 2006;84:90–99.

27. Procyshyn RM, Honer WG, Wu TK, et al. Persistent antipsychotic polypharmacy and excessive dosing in the community psychiatric treatment setting: a review of medication profiles in 435 Canadian outpatients. *Journal of Clinical Psychiatry* 2010;71:566–573.

28. Ganguly R, Kotzan JA, Miller S, et al. Prevalence, trends, and factors associated with antipsychotic polypharmacy among Medicaid-eligible schizophrenia patients, 1998–2000. *Journal of Clinical Psychiatry* 2004;65:1377–1388.

29. Sneider B, Pristed SF, Correll CU, et al. Frequency and correlates of antipsychotic polypharmacy among patients with schizophrenia in Denmark: a nation-wide pharmacoepidemiological study. *European Neuropsychopharmacology* 2015;25:1669–1676.

30. Kreyenbuhl JA, Valenstein M, McCarthy JF, et al. Long-term antipsychotic polypharmacy in the VA health system: patient characteristics and treatment patterns. *Psychiatric Services* 2007;58:489–495.

31. Stanilla JK, Simpson GM. Drugs to treat extrapyramidal effects. In: *The American Psychiatric Press Textbook of Psychopharmacology*, Fourth Edition. Editors: Schatzberg AF, Nemeroff CB. American Psychiatric Publishing, Washington, DC and London, 2009, pp. 669–694.

32. Vinogradov S, Fisher M, Warm H, et al. The cognitive cost of anticholinergic burden: decreased response to cognitive training in schizophrenia. *American Journal of Psychiatry* 2009;166:1055–1062.

33. Iversen TSJ, Steen NE, Dieset I, et al. Side-effect burden of antipsychotic drugs in real life—Impact of gender and polypharmacy. *Progress in Neuropsychopharmacology & Biological Psychiatry* 2018;82:263–271.

34. Längle G, Steinert T, Weiser P, et al. Effects of polypharmacy on outcome in patients with schizophrenia in routine psychiatric treatment. *Acta Psychiatrica Scandanavica* 2012;125:372–381.

35. American Diabetes Association, American Psychiatric Association, American Association of Clinical Endocrinologists, et al. Consensus development conference on antipsychotic drugs and obesity and diabetes. *Journal of Clinical Psychiatry* 2004;65:267–272.

36. Jaffe AB, Levine J. Antipsychotic coprescribing in a large state hospital system. *Pharmacoepidemiology and Drug Safety* 2003;12:41–48.

37. Correll CU, Frederickson AM, Kane JM, et al. Does antipsychotic polypharmacy increase the risk for metabolic syndrome? *Schizophrenia Research* 2007;89:91–100.

38. Correll CU, Gallego JA. Antipsychotic polypharmacy. A comprehensive evaluation of relevant correlates of a long-standing clinical practice. *Psychiatric Clinics of North America* 2012;35:661–681.

39. Misawa F, Shimizu K, Fujii Y, et al. Is antipsychotic polypharmacy associated with metabolic syndrome even after adjustment for lifestyle effects? a cross-sectional study. *BMC Psychiatry* 2011;11:118.

40. Hägg S, Lindblom Y, Mjörndal T, et al. High prevalence of the metabolic syndrome among a Swedish cohort of patients with schizophrenia. *International Clinical Psychopharmacology* 2006;21:93–98.

41. Schorr SG, Slooff CJ, Bruggeman R, et al. The incidence of metabolic syndrome and its reversal in a cohort of schizophrenic patients followed for one year. *Journal of Psychiatric Research* 2009;43:1106–1111.

42. Lewis S, Lieberman J. CATIE and CUtLASS: can we handle the truth? *British Journal of Psychiatry* 2008;192:161–163.

43. Moreno C, Laje G, Blanco C, et al. National trends in the outpatient diagnosis and treatment of bipolar disorder in youth. *Archives of General Psychiatry* 2007;64:1032–1039.

44. Frye MA, Ketter TA, Leverich GS, et al. Increasing use of polypharmacy for refractory mood disorders:22 years of study. *Journal of Clinical Psychiatry* 2000;61:9–15.

45. Morrato EH, Dodd S, Oderda G, et al. Prevalence, utilization patterns, and predictors of antipsychotic polypharmacy: experience in a multistate Medicaid population, 1998–2008. *Clinical Therapeutics* 2007;29:183–195.

46. Brooks JO, Goldberg JF, Ketter TA, et al. Safety and tolerability associated with second-generation antipsychotic polytherapy in bipolar disorders: findings from the systematic treatment enhancement program for bipolar disorder. *Journal of Clinical Psychiatry* 2011;72:240–247.

47. Comer JS, Olfson M, Mojtabai R. National trends in child and adolescent psychotropic polypharmacy in office-based practice, 1996–2007. *Journal of the American Academy of Child and Adolescent Psychiatry* 2010;49:1001–1010.

48. Olfson M, Crystal S, Huang C, et al. Trends in antipsychotic drug use by very young, privately insured children. *Journal of the American Academy of Child and Adolescent Psychiatry* 2010;49:13–23.

49. Constantine RJ, Boaz T, Tandon R. Antipsychotic polypharmacy of children and adolescents in the fee-for-service component of a large state Medicaid program. *Clinical Therapeutics* 2010;32:942–959.

50. Toteja N, Gallego JA, Saito E, et al. Prevalence and correlates of antipsychotic polypharmacy in children and youth receiving antipsychotic treatment. *International Journal of Neuropsychopharmacology* 2014;17:1095–1105.

51. dosReis S, Yesel Y, Rubin DM, et al. Antipsychotic treatment among youth in foster care. *Pediatrics* 2011;128:1459–1466.

52. Burcu M, Zito J, Safer DJ, et al. Concomitant use of atypical antipsychotics with other psychotropic medication classes and the risk of type 2 diabetes mellitus. *Journal of the American Academy of Child and Adolescent Psychiatry* 2017;56:642–651.

53. McIntyre RS, Jerrell JM. Metabolic and cardiovascular adverse events associated with antipsychotic treatment in children and adolescents. *Archives of Pediatric and Adolescent Medicine* 2008;162:929–935.

54. Maayan L, Correll CU. Weight gain and metabolic risks associated with antipsychotic medications in children and adolescents *Journal of Child and Adolescent Psychopharmacology* 2011;21:517–535.

55. Medhekar R, Aparasu R, Bhatara V, et al. Risk factors of psychotropic polypharmacy in the treatment of children and adolescent with psychiatric disorders. *Research in Social and Administrative Pharmacy* 2019;15:395–403.

56. Zito JM, Daniel JS, dosReis S, et al. Trends in the prescribing of psychotropic medications to preschoolers. *Journal of the American Medical Association* 2000;283:1025–1030.

57. Zito JM, Safer DJ, Valluri S, et al. Psychotherapeutic medication prevalence in Medicaid insured preschoolers. *Journal of Child and Adolescent Psychopharmacology* 2007;17:195–204.

58. Zito JM. On the medicalization of emotional and behavioral disturbances in youth. *The Hedgehog Review* 2012;14:73–84.

59. Schwartz A. Still in a crib, yet being given antipsychotics. *The New York Times*, December 11, 2016, pp. A1, A27.

60. Kristoff N. Drug crime that paid billions. *The New York Times*, September 17, 2015, p. A31.

61. Lohr WD, Chowning RT, Stevenson MD, et al. Trends in atypical antipsychotics prescribed to children six years of age or less on Medicaid in Kentucky. *Journal of Child and Adolescent Psychopharmacology* 2015;25:440–443.

62. Kristoff N. Drugs, greed, and a dead boy. *The New York Times*, November 5, 2015, p. A25.

63. Sultan RS, Correll CU, Schoenbaum M, et al. National patterns of commonly prescribed psychotropic medications to young people. *Journal of Child and Adolescent Psychopharmacology* 2018;28:158–165.

64. Pringsheim T, Stewart DG, Chan P, et al. The pharmacoepidemiology of psychotropic medication use in Canadian children from 2012 to 2016. *Journal of Child and Adolescent Psychiatry* 2019;XX:1–6. Doi:10.1089/cap.2019.0018.

65. Joukamma M, Heliövaara M, Knekt P, et al. Schizophrenia, neuroleptic medication and mortality. *British Journal of Psychiatry* 2006;188:122–127.

66. Waddington JL, Youseff HA, Kinsella A. Mortality in schizophrenia. Antipsychotic polypharmacy and absence of anticholinergic agents over the course of a 10-year prospective study. *British Journal of Psychiatry* 1998;173:325–329.

67. Hollis J, Touyz S, Grayson D, et al. Antipsychotic medication dispensing and associated odds ratio of death in elderly veterans and war widows. *Australian and New Zealand Journal of Psychiatry* 2006;40:981–986.

68. Baandrup L, Gasse C, Jensen VD, et al. Antipsychotic polypharmacy and risk of death from natural causes in patients with schizophrenia: a population-based nested case-control study. *Journal of Clinical Psychiatry* 2010;71:103–108.

69. Tiihonen J, Suokas JT, Suvisaari JM, et al. Polypharmacy with antipsychotics, antidepressants, or benzodiazepines and mortality in schizophrenia. *Archives of General Psychiatry* 2012;69:476–483.

70. Koponen M, Taipale H, Lavikainen P, et al. Risk of mortality associated with antipsychotic monotherapy and polypharmacy among community-dwelling persons with Alzheimer's disease. *Journal of Alzheimer's Disease* 2017;56:107–118.

71. Ray WA, Stein M, Murray KT, et al. Association of antipsychotic treatment with risk of unexpected death among children and youths. *JAMA Psychiatry* 2019;76:162–171.

72. Geller B. Antipsychotics, excess deaths, and paradoxes of child psychiatry. *JAMA Psychiatry* 2019;76:111–112.

73. Hanlon JT, Artz MB, Pieper CF, et al. Inappropriate medication use among frail elderly inpatients. *Annals of Pharmacotherapy* 2004;38:9–14.

74. Scott IA, Hilmer SN, Reeve E, et al. Reducing inappropriate polypharmacy: the process of deprescribing. *JAMA Internal Medicine* 2015;175:827–834.

75. Tjia J, Briesacher BA, Peterson D, et al. Use of medications of questionable benefit in advanced dementia. *JAMA Internal Medicine* 2014;174:1763–1771.

76. Stahl SM, Grady MM. A critical review of atypical antipsychotic utilization: comparing monotherapy with polypharmacy and augmentation. *Current Medicinal Chemistry* 2004;11:313–327.

77. Clark RE, Bartels SJ, Mellman TA, et al. Recent trends in antipsychotic combination therapy of schizophrenia and schizoaffective disorder: implications for state mental health policy. *Schizophrenia Bulletin* 2002;28:75–84.

78. Rupnow MF, Greenspan A, Gharabawi GM, et al. Incidence and costs of polypharmacy: data from a randomized, double-blind, placebo-controlled study of risperidone and quetiapine in patients with schizophrenia or schizoaffective disorder. *Current Medical Research Opinion* 2007;23:2815–2822.

79. Goodwin G, Fleischhacker W, Arango C, et al. Advantages and disadvantages of combination treatment with antipsychotics. ECPN Consensus Meeting, March 2008, Nice. *European Neuropsychopharmacology* 2009;19:520–532.

80. Centorrino F, Eaken M, Bahk W-M, et al. Inpatient antipsychotic drug use in 1988, 1993, and 1989. *American Journal of Psychiatry* 2002;159:1932–1935.

81. Centorrino F, Ventriglio A, Vincenti A, et al. Changes in medication practices for hospitalized psychiatric patients; 2009 versus 2004. *Human Psychopharmacology* 2010;25:179–186.

82. Correll CU, Rummel-Kluge C, Corves C, et al. Antipsychotic combinations vs monotherapy in schizophrenia: a meta-analysis of randomized controlled trials. *Schizophrenia Bulletin* 2009;35:443–457.

83. Cipriani A, Boso M, Barbui C. Clozapine combined with different antipsychotic drugs for treatment-resistant schizophrenia. *Cochrane Database Systematic Review* 2009;8(3):CD00634.

84. Tiihonen J, Mittendofer-Rutz E, Majak M, et al. Real-world effectiveness of antipsychotic treatments in a nationwide cohort of 29 823 patients with schizophrenia. *JAMA Psychiatry* 2017;74:686–693.

85. Galling B, Roldan A, Hagi K, et al. Antipsychotic augmentation vs. monotherapy in schizophrenia: systematic review, meta-analysis and meta-regression analysis. *World Psychiatry* 2017;16:77–89.

86. Essock SM, Schooler NR, Stroup TS, et al. Effectiveness of switching from antipsychotic polypharmacy to monotherapy. *American Journal of Psychiatry* 2011;168:702–708.

87. Suzuki T, Uchida H, Tanaka KF, et al. Revising polypharmacy to a single antipsychotic agent for patients with chronic schizophrenia. *International Journal of Neuropsychopharmacology* 2004;7:133–142.

88. Hazra M, Uchida H, Sproule B, et al. Impact of feedback from pharmacists in reducing antipsychotic polypharmacy in schizophrenia. *Psychiatry Clinical Neuroscience* 2011;65:676–678.

89. Borlido C, Remington G, Graff-Guerrero A, Arenovich T, et al. Switching from 2 antipsychotics to 1 antipsychotic in schizophrenia.: a randomized, double-blind, placebo-controlled study. *Journal of Clinical Psychiatry* 2016;77:e14–e20. Doi:10.4088/JCP.14m09321.

90. Van Leeuwen E, Petroic M, van Driel, M, et al. Discontinuation of long-term antipsychotic drug use for behavioral and psychological symptoms in older adults aged 65 years and older with dementia. *Journal of the American Medical Directors Association* 2018;19:1004–1014.

91. Correll CU, Rubio JM, Inczedy-Farkas G, Birnbaum ML, et al. Efficacy of 42 pharmacologic cotreatment strategies added to antipsychotic monotherapy in schizophrenia. Systematic overview and quality appraisal of the meta-analytic evidence. *JAMA Psychiatry* 2017. Doi:10.1001/jamapsychiatry.2017.0624.

7 The Neurologic Consequences of Antipsychotics

From Parkinsonism to Tardive Dyskinesia

Introduction

In Chapter 2, we noted that the first clinicians who began prescribing chlorpromazine in 1954 noticed that many patients were developing signs of parkinsonism, including tremor, muscle stiffness, and a gait disturbance marked by short, rapid steps and loss of balance when changing directions.[1] Over time, this set of abnormal motor movements has been labeled neuroleptic-induced parkinsonism (NIP), antipsychotic-induced parkinsonism (AIP), or extrapyramidal side effects (EPSE), the term I will use. With regard to EPSE, the gait disturbance became infamous as the "Thorazine shuffle" and, some years later, as the "Haldol shuffle." Only a few years after the introduction of chlorpromazine, observers described a set of motor movements with abnormal blinking, jaw movements, tongue protrusions, lip smacking, and irregular movements in the arms and legs. Patients and families found them more disturbing than EPSE, since they were common in the face, lips, and tongue. Since these appeared later in the course of AP therapy, the term "tardive dyskinesia" was applied.[2] While both disorders are secondary to APs, their course, pathogenesis, and treatment differ markedly. Although the advent of second-generation antipsychotics (SGA) has resulted in fewer instances of TD, the manufacturers continue to emphasize the dangers of abnormal movements on television and in printed material, often noting that the movements associated with TD may be irreversible, although this is uncommon.

The Clinical Impact of TD

There is no question but that the appearance of TD marked the start of a long era of discontent on the part of patients, families, and clinicians. I distinctly recall my first haloperidol-treated patient, a young soldier seen at the Second General Hospital in Landstuhl, Germany, who developed severe facial grimacing, tongue protrusion, and jaw movements, prompting me to wonder if the treatment for his psychosis was worse than the illness! However, the pioneers of AP treatment in the 1950s were so alarmed by

EPSE that they predicted an epidemic of parkinsonism and encephalitis.[1] Lehmann and Hanrahan likened the effects of chlorpromazine to a lobotomy,[3] with patients becoming emotionally blunted and motorically slowed, a clinical state which *clearly was the goal* of these first prescribers. Suppression of psychotic symptoms was an afterthought. (For additional details, see Chapter 2.)

The descriptions of abnormal movements were in marked contrast to the first public accounts of chlorpromazine in the *New York Times*, *Time* magazine, and other news outlets, where chlorpromazine was hailed as a miraculous drug that brought peace of mind and freedom from anxiety and confusion. Indeed, the public presentation of APs was marked by an absence of detail about the EPSE and TD.[4, p. 152] It appears, too, that William Winkelman, who initially was concerned about EPSE, had a change of heart after being hired by Smith, Kline & French (SKF), the manufacturer, to lead the studies on chlorpromazine. By 1957, he claimed that only one patient had developed "full-blown" parkinsonism while only two developed gait disturbances and masked facies, out of 1,090 outpatients. He added that other side effects were mild and disappeared spontaneously after the dose was modified.[5, pp. 966–967]

The financial impact of chlorpromazine enormous. SKF took in $75 million in the drug's first year of sales[6, p. 97] and had a return of 33% on its invested capital by 1958. Revenues increased from $53 million in 1953 to $347 million by 1970,[4, p. 155] a harbinger of the massive returns achieved by Pharma in the years to come. Nevertheless, as one psychiatrist later wrote,[7] chlorpromazine "engulfed the whole treatment spectrum of psychiatric disorders" and ushered in the era of psychopharmacology.

Nevertheless, psychiatry and Pharma had a major problem, both clinically and from a public relations standpoint. The money had begun to roll in, and Pharma was not stingy with its assets. The popular media, as well as many in the medical community, had hailed APs as not just revolutionary but miraculous, and some even wrote of "curing" mental illness. Yet observations of patients told another story, a story not only of lethargy and lack of motivation, but of EPSE and TD.

Psychiatry's Response to Tardive Dyskinesia: The Early Years

How did psychiatry respond to this sometimes devastating neurologic syndrome? Two words come to mind: *massive ambivalence!* In the course of a literature review of TD, an associate and I found clearly opposing points of view on TD.[8] Some investigators had written that most cases of TD were irreversible while others pointed to a largely reversible course. In 1968, for example, Nathan Kline[9] wrote that only 54 patients of several million treated with APs demonstrated irreversibility, but, in the same symposium in the *American Journal of Psychiatry*, George Crane[10] argued that the defining characteristic of TD is the persistence of movements for months to years. The American Psychiatric Association weighed in with the publication of a task force report,[11] claiming that the symptoms of TD remain fairly static in a "vast majority of patients," but then stated that it is impossible to predict the outcome in patients who continue to take APs. *It was never clear to me how the prognosis could be so ill defined if the vast majority don't worsen!* Similarly, George Simpson insisted[12] that nearly all patients improve, even with continued low-dose treatment, but Gardos and Cole[13] concluded that the effects of withdrawal studies were so inconsistent that no clear conclusions were possible.

Clinicians—and, indeed, patients and families—were quickly faced with a major clinical and ethical problem: how to deal with a patient who had developed TD but still needed AP treatment. The answers spanned virtually all the possibilities. One author recommended low-dose APs,[14] but, in another volume, the same author wrote that no treatment with APs was advisable,[15] while a prominent psychopharmacologist, Ross Baldessarini, stated[16] that continued use of an AP once TD developed was "essentially irrational." In a 1985 letter to members of the American Psychiatric Association,[17] John Kane and other prominent academicians wrote that it was not possible to identify which patients were at risk, although studies we'll review in a moment had clearly established a higher risk in women, older patients, and those with significant cognitive impairment. In these groups, rates of TD developed at double or triple the oft-quoted rate of 15% to 20%. Even the lower rate obviously amounted to more than "a few patients," a claim found in Nancy Andreasen's best-selling book, *The Broken Brain.*[18]

Despite this hodgepodge of contradictory information and opinion, and despite growing evidence of high rates of TD in some groups, Baldessarini and Cohen in 1986 published an editorial[19] in the *American Journal of Psychiatry* claiming that TD is a "putative menace," the dangers of which have been exaggerated by those holding alarmist views of a condition they deemed disabling or irreversible in only a small number of patients. Yet only one year earlier, after concluding that TD was "a much worse problem than originally believed," the *FDA had issued an order*[20] *requiring that a black-box warning be placed on all APs*—although it had been 30 years since the condition was first described!

I took note of these contradictions in a letter to the *American Journal of Psychiatry*[21] and cited another paper by Dr. Baldessarini,[16] in which he had voiced concerns about the cosmetic and vocational impact of TD, as well as impairment in self-care, swallowing, and dexterity. I also voiced concern about the physiological consequences of TD, including breakdown of muscle tissue and the subsequent development of myoglobinuria, which in turn can lead to severe renal disease. In addition, patients can develop short, gasping respirations (respiratory TD) and gastrointestinal symptoms including stomach cramps and diarrhea (gastrointestinal TD), with both syndromes secondary to the effects of APs on smooth muscle.

Nevertheless, in a reply to my letter, Baldessarini and Cohen[22] continued to maintain that the majority of patients showed gradual improvement or remission, that the prevalence rate was stable at 15% to 20%, and that the life-threatening reactions to TD were not necessarily the direct result of TD. Once again, there was no acknowledgment of the very high prevalence rates in some groups or the fact that the baseline prevalence rate was likely much higher, since *most studies were done while patients were taking APs—which can mask the very movements they cause!* This phenomenon appears to rest, at least in part, on the blockade of supersensitive DA receptors.

Given the doubts about TD by "key opinion leaders" in psychiatry, it shouldn't be surprising that TD either wasn't recognized or was misdiagnosed.[23] Despite the publicity about TD and the FDA warnings, a national survey of community mental health centers published in 1994 found that only 20% had formal screening policies, and 20% relied on simple clinical observations.[24]

Unfortunately, prevalence rates continued to climb, rising from 14.6% in studies done from 1960 to 1969 to 24% in studies published from 1970 to 1979.[3] Later studies found prevalence rates up to 45%,[25] although one always has to take into account rates of spontaneous dyskinesias (4%). As we have already noted, the higher rates coincided with the development and widespread use of high-potency APs, although it was not clear if dosing was a critical risk factor. In our review of the older literature on TD,[8] we found prevalence rates in mood disorders ranging from 30% to 83%, a rate higher than in schizophrenia. In women, the situation was worse, with one group noting that the mean prevalence in women was 41% higher than in men,[26] although not all studies found a gender difference.[27, 28] In mental retardation, prevalence rates ranged from 16% to 49%,[29] while in the older population, the rate was about 49%. In other work, the rate was even higher at over 60%.[30]

In addition, the optimism voiced by some with regard to reversibility was not fully justified. For example, Yassa and associates[31] found that over a two-year span, only 18% of those with TD improved while 16% worsened. In a study of AP withdrawal in patients who had developed TD, 30% remitted in one year, but TD persisted in 38%.[32] In another withdrawal study,[33] only 1 patient of 49 had a complete remission, but at one year, over 90% had at least a 50% reduction in dyskinetic movements.

We should remember this: across the world, and indeed in the United States, large numbers of patients continued to use FGAs,[33] in no small part due to the initial costs of SGAs. Indeed, a meta-analysis published in 2017[34] found that the *global mean prevalence of TD was 25.3% across 41 studies.* With current SGA treatment, the rate fell to 20.7% vs 30% with FGAs. If subjects were FGA-naïve, the rate fell to 7.2%!

While the costs of SGAs are going down as generics come on the market, we have to stress that the overall costs of SGAs *necessarily* include money aimed at monitoring and treating their metabolic complications.

Complications of TD

While the cosmetic effects of severe oral-facial movements are bad enough, patients with TD suffer from other problems, including structural brain changes. As far back as the 1980s, numerous investigators[35–37] stressed that TD can be accompanied by numerous anatomical changes, including degeneration of the caudate nucleus, ventricular enlargement, narrowing of the third ventricle, and sulcal enlargement. Waddington et al.[36] noted that 8 of 11 systematic studies had found various qualitative or quantitative changes in a host of brain structures in association with abnormal, involuntary movements, but, as one might expect, some had found no abnormalities,[37] at least in patients under 60 years of age.

Given such changes, it isn't surprising that many studies reported evidence of cognitive impairment.[36–40] In one interesting study,[39] a decline in cognition was the factor *most often* associated with the development of TD. Other studies demonstrated that TD and increasingly high doses of APs were associated with an increase in reaction time, a decrease in attention span, and low basal skin conductance,[41] as well as an impaired gag reflex,[42] disruption of speech patterns,[43] and trouble swallowing.[44] Another group[45] found that about 90% of patients with TD had not only cognitive impairment but also negative symptoms of schizophrenia (blunted affect, poverty of speech, poor motivation), whereas these symptoms were present in only 30% of those without TD.

On the positive side, an analysis[46] of the CATIE study *did not* find an association of cognitive impairment with TD; yet, in a post-hoc analysis of the CATIE study, Caroff and colleagues found that neurocognitive improvement in patients with TD was less than in those without TD.[47] This group also found that TD did not influence time to discontinuation nor were changes in psychotic symptoms different between the two groups.

Genetic Factors in Cognition

In 2016, John et al.[48] investigated genetic associations with TD and cognitive functions in schizophrenia vs controls in genetically distinct north Indian cohorts. They focused on the possible influence of microRNAs. MicroRNAs are non-coding RNA molecules that negatively regulate gene expression. The regulatory functions of microRNAs range from neurodevelopment to cognitive functions. Participants included 91 patients with schizophrenia who had been diagnosed with TD; 161 had no TD. Cognitive assessment focused on eight domains associated with schizophrenia while the genes investigated included 100 top-ranked candidate genes in schizophrenia. The authors found 5 single-nucleotide polymorphisms (SNPs) that were *nominally* associated with TD and 12 SNPs that were associated with one or more cognitive domains. Unfortunately, the samples were small, so the results cannot be used diagnostically.

In a 2017 genetic study,[49] the authors noted that the gene for dopamine beta-hydroxylase (DBH) is increased in people with schizophrenia who have TD, so they decided to study whether a DBH5′-insertion/deletion polymorphism could influence cognitive functions in patients with (345) and without (397) TD. Interestingly, the deletion polymorphism appeared to influence cognition in schizophrenia patients without TD but did not seem to play a role in susceptibility to TD and cognitive deficits. Those with schizophrenia and TD demonstrated poorer attention and immediate memory, consistent with previous studies.

As in the previous study, these results badly need replication in much larger samples. Neither study argues for routine genetic testing in the clinic.

TD and Mortality

Does TD result in a higher mortality rate? This would seem an obvious issue, but the literature has been surprisingly skimpy, with only seven independent studies of all-cause mortality published by 2000. Nevertheless, a meta-analysis[50] found a 40% increase in risk. However, the authors noted a host of problems in the individual studies, including the lack of explicit criteria for a diagnosis of TD in some studies, and follow-up periods ranging from 1.5 to 15 years. Six of the seven studies lacked data on inter-rater reliability, a major omission. The authors concluded that TD is a "weak" risk factor for a shortened life span but left open the possibility that TD may simply be a surrogate for another unknown "organic liability."

We attempted to correct a number of these shortcomings in a study[51] of mortality and TD at the Minneapolis VA Medical Center, where we followed 1,600 patients for an average of 1,446 days. We used raters repeatedly trained in the use of the DISCUS, another rating scale designed to enable a systematic description of abnormal movements.[52] (We had earlier demonstrated[53] that this scale was equivalent to the more widely used AIMS.[54]) In another novel approach, we obtained mortality data from the National Death Index and received definitive data on mortality on 1,200 patients, of whom 17% had died during the observation period.

Echoing the earlier meta-analysis, we found that TD was associated with 57% in the risk of mortality, *but*, when we controlled for the interaction of FGAs, SGAs, and age, we found that *TD itself was no longer statistically significant*. Instead, we found that patients who had taken *only* FGAs were twice as likely to die as those taking SGAs. In the age group from 53 to 65 years, the use of FGAs was associated with a seven-fold increase in mortality, consistent with studies described earlier in this volume.

The bottom line: Older patients taking FGAs have a shortened survival time. Not surprisingly, given the fact that this was a male-dominated sample with a mean age of 53 at last observation, 24% had died of cardiac disease, 20% from cancer, and another 8% from stroke. Death by suicide had occurred in almost 7%, a rate considerably lower than in many epidemiologic studies, but this was a comparatively small sample. There was no association between specific causes of death and TD status.

Why the Ambivalence?

I think most would agree that this combination of motor signs, cosmetic changes, subjective distress, and various physiologic changes would have been enough to spark a uniform and consistent approach to TD, but, as we have seen, that was not the case. Indeed, in 1975 a paper[55] appeared that entirely discounted the concept of drug-induced dyskinesias! The ambivalence surrounding AP-induced neurologic side effects is further illustrated by a meta-analysis[56] of studies investigating the relationship between AP dose and response, wherein about one third of trials published from 1966 to 1999 failed to describe AP-induced side-effects! Of the studies that did, only 19% did so in an acceptable manner.

Why did it take so long for the APA and the FDA to admit that APs were inducing serious and sometimes permanent movement disorders? After all, these were obvious in the earliest studies, but EPSE were considered essential to the therapeutic effects of APs. Indeed, EPSE were seen as indicators of a positive outcome. This stance fit nicely with the growing collaboration between Pharma and psychiatry, an association that resulted in Big Pharma becoming the principal funding agent[57] for research, publication, and academic status—but, in the interest of being fair and balanced, I need to acknowledge other issues, particularly the presence of movement disorders in people with *no* prior AP exposure.

Movement Disorders in Antipsychotic-Naïve Patients

Emile Kraepelin's 1919[58] description of abnormal motor movements in dementia praecox (schizophrenia) could easily be cut and pasted into a study of TD in 2020. Other studies[59] of patients in the pre-neuroleptic era indicated that 15% to 28% of patients demonstrated abnormal movements, similar to rates found after the introduction of chlorpromazine. Despite the lower rates of TD found in the SGA era, two papers published in 2018 have focused on spontaneous dyskinesia, TD,[60] and other motor abnormalities found in psychoses,[61] noting some of the concerns discussed in this chapter. We should emphasize that many of the older studies focused on older, institutionalized patients with a wide variety of diagnoses and, not surprisingly, found an increasing prevalence with age and chronicity, with rates ranging from 53 to 67%.

Yet in a study of spontaneous dyskinesia (SDK) at the famous Chestnut Lodge,[62] age was not a factor, although this relatively young population had been ill for at least two years. The authors found that 15% had a definite oral-facial dyskinesia and 28% had evidence of motor abnormalities. Although the Chestnut Lodge study attracted a great deal of interest, in part because of the very rich clinical records and long-term follow-up, very little was said about the length of treatment with ECT and/or insulin coma, although the authors claimed that neither highly invasive treatment was associated with dyskinesias. How could they be so certain?

Another serious methodologic problem: the lack of a matched, healthy control group in at least 15 studies of abnormal movements in neuroleptic-naïve patients.[63] These unmatched studies reported various levels of abnormal movements, in contrast to six well-matched studies, in which few significant differences were found. Gervin et al[59] cited five key studies of SDK published from 1982 to 1996, with rates varying from 0% to 52%! In a review[64] comparing movement disorders in AP-naïve patients with schizophrenia to rates in first-degree relatives and healthy controls, the authors found that dyskinesia was 3.5 times more likely to occur in schizophrenia while EPSE was five times more likely. Interestingly, dyskinesia in first-degree relatives was 38% higher than in controls, and EPSE was twice as likely.

It seems reasonable to conclude that Kraepelin was correct in 1912: Both dyskinesia and parkinsonism can be found in antipsychotic-naïve patients with schizophrenia and their first-degree relatives, suggesting that abnormalities in the motor system, especially the basal ganglia, are part of the overall pathology associated with schizophrenia. Indeed, later studies found that blinded raters could *predict* which children in families would later develop schizophrenia by observing motor abnormalities in family videos.[65-67]

Despite the methodological problems, we must emphasize that these findings do not excuse APs from a causal role in the development of TD. For example, in a study of 386 older patients, *duration of AP exposure was the strongest predictor of TD*, with rates increasing from 16% of those with less than three months exposure to 41% with more than ten years exposure.[30] These findings were buttressed by extensive training, ratings of reliability, and the use of multiple rating scales.

Although we have focused on TD and spontaneous dyskinesias, we should not neglect EPSE since parkinsonism is even more common than TD. Rates among AP-treated patients have varied, with early estimates ranging from 39%[68] to as high as 75% for akathisia.[69, pp. 140-173] As we have seen in Chapter 3, the risk of EPSE continues to haunt the newer APs, including risperidone and aripiprazole. While patients with TD sometimes seem unaware of the movements, those with akathisia (motor restlessness) are acutely aware of their inability to sit still, the need to pace, and disturbances in concentration. I have seen instances where akathisia has been mistaken for mania or agitation and treated with higher dose of APs—exactly the wrong approach!

Bipolar Disorder, TD, and EPSE

We have been emphasizing the risks of neurologic side effects in schizophrenia, but given the increasingly frequent use of APs in bipolar disorder and, indeed, the explosion of this diagnosis in youth, what can we say about the risks in this group? We know from earlier studies that the point prevalence of TD in bipolar patients is as high as 41%,[70] but the older studies concentrated on FGAs. Recognizing this, Gao and associates[71] examined RCTS of *both FGAs and SGAs in bipolar disorder* and found that patients with bipolar depression were especially vulnerable to EPSE, with an NNH of only 5, meaning that only five patients would have to be treated with an AP to cause one additional case of parkinsonism compared with placebo. The authors compared rates among SGA-treated patients and found that only ziprasidone increased the rate of EPSE in both mania and schizophrenia. However, risperidone increased rates in mania while aripiprazole upped rates in mania and bipolar depression, and quetiapine upped rates in bipolar depression.

Taking a different approach, Gentile[72] examined 32 RCTS of SGAs, mood stabilizers, FGAs, and placebo in bipolar disorder and noted the frequency of EPSE. In olanzapine, risperidone, aripiprazole, and ziprasidone, rates were generally low, with the exception of aripiprazole, where akathisia and tremor were significantly increased vs placebo. In a 2011 meta-analysis[73] of efficacy and adverse events among four SGAs, haloperidol, and placebo, there were only small differences in efficacy, with clozapine taking first place and aripiprazole last place. As expected, EPSE were highest with haloperidol, but clozapine and olanazapine induced the most weight gain; however, risperidone and aripiprazole also led to considerable weight gain. In contrast to Gentile,[72] the authors[73] concluded that risperidone might rank first in terms of efficacy and acceptability, although acknowledging that several other studies had failed to find differences in efficacy in aripiprazole and olanzapine or between risperidone and aripiprazole! *Confusing, wouldn't you say?*

There is no doubt that EPSE impose a major burden on patients due to tremor, restlessness, muscle stiffness, cognitive impairment, and feelings of weakness/apathy. In addition, we sometimes forget that many studies have shown that parkinsonism is a predictor of TD.[74] Granted, there has been considerable variation in these figures due to any number of methodologic problems, including the lack of agreement on diagnostic criteria for TD, variations in the age group studied, rates of cognitive impairment, and changes in prescription patterns over the years. In addition, other drugs can cause parkinsonism, including serotonin reuptake inhibitors (SSRIs) such as fluoxetine, and in recent years, concerns have been raised about the association of mood stabilizers such as divalproex with parkinsonism.[75, pp. 103–139] We should also mention Reglan (metoclopramide), used for gastrointestinal disorders, since long-term use can result in dyskinesias in about 20% of patients. Reglan-induced dyskinesia can be as severe: witness a lawsuit heard by the U.S. Supreme Court in the case of a woman who developed disabling body-wide dyskinetic movements after exposure to generic metoclopramide.[76] The suit centered on the lack of a warning label, which was not required on the generic form until 2009 while she had begun the medication in 2001. The claimant was exactly correct in her assertion that the risks of dyskinesia with this agent had been documented well before 2001, indicating once again the lag between research and regulatory action by the FDA.

The primary lesson here, however, is that the prevalence of TD clearly rises with increasing exposure to APs. In addition, since EPSE predicts TD, and since both influence the course of schizophrenia, and since dyskinesia and parkinsonism can be found in the same patient and can exist prior to the use of any APs, there appear to be inextricable links between and among all of these conditions, making cause and effect a complex matter.

Clinical Ratings of Abnormal Movements

Complicating matters even further has been the reluctance of psychiatry to utilize advances in the detection of TD and parkinsonism. We have alluded at various points to the development of standardized rating scales used by clinicians, but they all are similar in that they depend entirely on clinical observation and self-reports from patients in order to diagnose and gauge the severity of the movements. (For a brief review of 14 scales and references, see Taksh, 2006.[77])

While the use of such scales lends an air of scientific respectability to the studies that employ them, numerous studies have established that these scales are marked by varying degrees of reliability due to variations in the patient, the rater, rater training, and sometimes weak inter-rater reliability.[78–80] In addition, while most scales call for the rater to judge movement severity, there is *no evidence* of a linear relationship between clinical ratings of severity.[80] In plain English, this means that a movement rated as a 4 (severe) is not necessarily twice as bad as a movement rated as a 2 (mild). This, of course, calls into question the validity of all studies that claim to establish correlations between levels of severity and their relationship to whatever variable is being studied, be it age, gender, dose, diagnosis, duration of illness, presence of diabetes mellitus, cognition, or any of a host of moderators.

Instrumental Ratings

These well-known problems have led to the development of instruments designed to detect the early and more subtle changes in motor functions and to allow *objective* measurements of tremor, rigidity, and dyskinesias. The ultimate goal has been to allow early intervention and corrective treatment before the changes become more severe and difficult to treat.[81] Objective measurements do away with the problems with clinical observations and also provide objective linear relationships with regard to severity, such that an instrumental rating of 4 is, in fact, twice the severity of the movement rated as 2. In addition, these methods are less susceptible to changes in the movements secondary to voluntary suppression by the patient. On the other hand, instrumental methods require investment in the instruments and software and additional training and can be more time consuming than simple clinical observation.[81]

Another issue: the lack of studies designed to compare the host of clinical rating scales with one another or comparisons of clinical rating scales with instrumental measurements. Given these issues, we did a three-way comparison of the Abnormal Involuntary Movement Scale (AIMS), the Dyskinesia Identification System Condensed User Scale (DISCUS), and instruments in 100 patients seen in our outpatient TD clinic.[53] Clinical raters were trained to a high degree of reliability, and patients were evaluated sequentially in a randomly assigned pathway. Our instruments were able to objectively measure tremor, dyskinetic hand movements, and rigidity.

The results were quite interesting. First, we found that the prevalence of TD when using the clinical scales was 28%, comparable to that found in other studies. *However, instrumental measurements revealed a prevalence of 61%, strikingly higher!* There was a clear mismatch between the AIMS and the instruments. For example, using an AIMS score of 3 or greater in one body area, the prevalence was 26%, but the rate doubled using instruments. On the other hand, ratings of tremor were similar whether using instruments or the clinical scales.

Remarkably, the most consistent predictor of parkinsonian/dyskinetic movements was cognition, as measured by the Mini-Mental Status Examination.[82] If limited to non-instrumental ratings, the combination of the total AIMS score and the MMSE score was the most informative. Unfortunately, the clinical use of instrument ratings has not been embraced by psychiatrists.

The primary lesson: Our dependence on clinical observation and clinical rating scales has no doubt resulted in *a serious underestimation* of the prevalence of abnormal motor movements, whether they be secondary to the illness, medications, or a combination.

TD and the Future

The advent of SGAs led many to predict that TD would become an interesting historical relic, even while investigators emphasized that dyskinesia and parkinsonism were reflections of the underlying pathology of major mental illnesses.[59, 65, 83] For example, in a study[84] of 100 neuroleptic-naïve psychotic patients, 34% had either parkinsonism or dyskinesia, with no relationship to age, gender, years of education, or family history of psychosis. These neurologic findings were associated with the length of untreated psychosis, obstetric complications, and poor premorbid adjustment. The authors emphasized that these motor changes are therefore "integral to the disease process." Pre-existing motor abnormalities also predicted a poor response to treatment.

Given such findings, why would TD/EPSE disappear? Indeed, one would expect that the underlying structural and metabolic brain changes in schizophrenia and bipolar disorder would continue to induce motor abnormalities, but at lower rates. It seems safe to say that if the patient is exposed *only* to SGAs, the risk of TD is lower than with FGAs.[34] I must add that we are largely ignorant of the consequences of long-term AP use in off-label conditions such as anxiety disorders, sleep disorders, and various forms of depression. We shall examine this shift in the chapter on psychiatric diagnosis, but I will mention here a seven-fold increase in the use of APs in youth for conduct disorders[85] and a doubling of APs for treatment of anxiety disorders in adults.[86]

We also have to stress that the use of SGAs to treat mood disorders—especially bipolar disorder—is rapidly increasing, yet people with depression are known to be more susceptible to the development of TD, especially where the patient has had multiple depressive episodes. Given that additional SGAs have received FDA approval for the treatment of mania and depression, and, since both disorders are more common than schizophrenia, will this ever-expanding list of disorders treated with APs significantly increase the population risk for TD?

Such data indicates that we should continue to closely monitor patients for TD as well as ESPE. For example, many patients now taking SGAS have been exposed to FGAs for years and may or may not have TD, but certainly are at risk, despite switching to SGAs. We also tend to forget that patients in underdeveloped countries may not be able to afford the very expensive SGAs, although this may be less of a problem in the future, since current SGAs are becoming generic and thus more available.

We mentioned in Chapter 2 doubts about the differences in prevalence of neurologic side effects when comparing FGAs with SGAs. Indeed, a secondary analysis of patients in the CutLass-1 study[87] found *no significant differences* in the rate of ESPE and TD when patients randomized to SGAs were compared with those taking FGAs at the end of one year. The investigators in CutLass-1 had expected significant improvement in those patients switched to SGAs, but it did not happen. The authors stressed that *limiting APs to SGAs may not serve patients well, especially given SGA-induced metabolic problems*. Indeed, they emphasize that splitting APs into FGAs and SGAs represents a "spurious dichotomy."[87, p. 387]

Although interest in TD has dropped among clinicians, it's of interest that in 2018 the *Journal of Neurological Sciences* published a special issue on "Tardive Syndromes and their Management," with several reviews of their pathophysiology and treatment,[88] with a focus on new FDA-approved drugs. In addition, we have the two historical reviews of TD and other motor disorders in psychoses,[60, 61] both worth reading.

Treatment of TD

Historically, the treatment of TD remained elusive, despite hundreds of studies on multiple drugs, including benzodiazepines, amantadine, levetiracetam, and botulinum toxin.[89] Fortunately, in 2017, the FDA approved two inhibitors of the vesicular monamine transporter (VMAT2) for treatment of

TD in adults. These drugs, valbenazine[90] (Ingrezza) and deutetrabenazine[91] (Austedo), decrease levels of dopamine at the synapse, as well as dopamine receptor stimulation, consistent with the long-held concept that TD is a hyperkinetic movement disorder—although imaging studies failed to show a difference in the number of D2 receptors and D2 binding in patients with and without TD.[92] Clearly, the pathophysiology of TD remains elusive.[93]

While I applaud the approval of these agents for TD, I note that the decrease in scores on the primary rating scale was only 3.2[90] and 3.0[91] points, enough to be statistically significant vs placebo, but if the patient has a very high baseline score, the drop may not be clinically obvious. We also have no immediate answer as to treatment of TD in youth. As Meyer has noted,[93] we still need additional advances in treatment and understanding the pathophysiology.

For those interested in additional information on the many clinical rating scales mentioned herein and elsewhere, please see the following: Guy W, 1976,[94] Sprague, RL et al.,1984,[95] Simpson GM et al.,1970,[96] Barnes TR, 1989,[97] Chouinard G et al., 1980,[98] and Simpson GM et al., 1979.[99]

Genetics of TD

Research in this area has focused on candidate genes: that is, genes underlying the receptors and neurotransmitters in the dopamine pathway, GABA, serotonin, and pharmacogenetic factors, but the results have been inconsistent.[100] On the other hand, a more optimistic review by Zai et al. in 2018[101] identified a list of promising genes associated with the aforementioned pathways, including the DRD_2, DRD_3, $VMAT_2$, HSPG2, three serotonergic genes, and SOD_2. The authors noted a number of shortcomings in the field, including a lack of research on epigenetics and whole-genome sequencing studies. They concluded that preclinical and genetic studies, despite their shortcomings, continue to support the dopamine hypotheses of TD, although studies cited earlier in this chapter point to other possibilities.[48, 49]

Clinical Notes

1. While the advent of SGAs has led to fewer cases of TD and EPSE, these neurological side effects can still occur and must be diagnosed and treated. Patients need to be educated regarding the nature of the movements and the need to report them quickly. The industry is correct in calling attention to the risks of TD in television and print advertisements.
2. Prescribers should be trained in how to assess TD and EPSE.
3. Note that the typical irregular movements of TD are *not in any way different* from the movements in other dyskinetic movement disorders such as Huntington's chorea, Sydenham's chorea, and a number of metabolic disorders. *Do not assume* that APs are responsible until a differential

diagnosis has been accomplished via the use of laboratory studies and, if necessary, imaging studies.

4. APs are not the only drugs that can induce dyskinesias. Stimulants are among them and need careful attention, given the epidemic of ADHD. Metaclopramide (Reglan) is another drug and, interestingly enough, SSRIs.

5. Avoid the use of APs in non-psychotic disorders. Unfortunately, they are being prescribed for insomnia, anxiety, misbehavior, irritability, and depression, conditions for which many options are available, including various forms of psychotherapy. Should the prescriber recommend APs, ask for an account of the goals and side effects and the scientific basis for the recommendation.

6. At this point, genetic studies are not likely to be helpful, given the problems with replication and the lack of clinical utility. Some evidence indicates that pharmacogenetic tests may be helpful, since the body has a set of hepatic enzymes (CYP450) that influence the metabolism of drugs, with slow metabolizers accumulating excessively high blood levels and ultra-rapid metabolizers washing the drug out too quickly.

7. The use of APs in children and adolescents is especially risky, given extensive evidence demonstrating that the metabolic and other side effects are more frequent and more severe. Why children ages two to eight are given APs is not at all clear, but this should be strongly discouraged.

8. While we have emphasized adverse effects, several well-done studies have shown a positive effect on life span, with lower rates of mortality than one finds in non-users. However, combing APs with benzodiazepines (Ativan, Valium) is not recommended due to increased mortality rates.

References

1. Delay J, Deniker P. Trente-huite cas de psychosis traits par la cure prolongee et continue de 4568. *Annals Medical Psychology* 1952;110:365.

2. Schonecker M. Trente-huit cas de psychoses traits par la cure prolongee et continue de 4658 R. *Nervenartz* 1957;28:35.

3. Lehmann HE, Hanrahan GE. Chlorpromazine: new inhibiting agent for psychomotor excitement and manic states. *Archives of General Psychiatry* 1954;17:153–162.

4. Whitaker RW. *Mad in America. Bad Science, Bad Medicine, and the Enduring Mistreatment of the Mentally Ill.* Perseus Publishing, Cambridge MA, 2002.

5. Winkelman, Jr NW. An appraisal of chlorpromazine. General principles for administration of chlorpromazine, based on experience with 1,090 patients. *American Journal of Psychiatry* 1957;113:961–977.

6. Healy D. *The Creation of Psychopharmacology.* Harvard University Press, Cambridge MA and London, 2002.

7. Rollin HR. The dark before the dawn. *Journal of Psychopharmacology* 1990;4:109–114.

8. Dean CE, Borchardt CM. Tardive dyskinesia: the risk-benefit ratio and the clinician's dilemma. *Integrative Psychiatry* 1992;3:225–240. (This journal is out of print. I have copies.)

9. Kline NS. On the rarity of "irreversible" oral dyskinesias following phenothiazines. *American Journal of Psychiatry* 1968;124(suppl):48–64.

10. Crane GE. Tardive dyskinesia in patients treated with major neuroleptics: a review of the literature. *American Journal of Psychiatry* 1968;124 (suppl):40–48.

11. Baldessarini RJ, Cole JO, Gardos G, et al. *Tardive Dyskinesia: Report of the APA Task Force on Late Neurologic Side Effects of Antipsychotic Drugs. Task Force Report 18.* American Psychiatric Association, Washington DC, 1980.

12. Simpson GM. Tardive dyskinesia: a commentary. In: *Tardive Dyskinesia: From Dogma to Reason.* Editors: Casey DM, Gardos G. American Psychiatric Press, Washington DC, 1986.

13. Gardos G, Cole JO. Neuroleptics and tardive dyskinesia in non-schizophrenic patients. In: *Tardive Dyskinesia: From Dogma to Reason.* Editors: Casey DE, Gardos G. American Psychiatric Press, Washington DC, 1986.

14. Casey DE, Toenniessen LM. Neuroleptic treatment in tardive dyskinesia: can it be developed into a clinical strategy for long-term treatment? In: *Modern Problems in Pharmacopsychiatry (New Directions in Tardive Dyskinesia Research), 1983.* Editors Bannet J, Belmaker RH, Basel S, Karger AG, Chapter 21:65–79.

15. Casey DE. Nondopaminergic treatment approaches. In: *Dyskinesia Research and Treatment.* Editors: Casey DE, Chase T, Chrisensen AV, Gerlach J. Psychopharmacology, Supplement 2. Springer-Verlag, Berlin, Heidelberg, 1985, pp. 137–144.

16. Baldessarini RJ. Clinical and epidemiological aspects of tardive dyskinesia. *Journal of Clinical Psychiatry* 1985;46:8–13.

17. Kane JM, Jeste DV, Casey DE, et al. Letter to APA members. *American Psychiatric Association,* July 1985.

18. Andreasen NC. *The Broken Brain. The Biological Revolution in Psychiatry.* Harper & Row, New York, 1984.

19. Baldessarini RJ, Cohen BM. Regulation of psychiatric practice. *American Journal of Psychiatry* 1986;143:750–751.

20. Neuroleptics to carry FDA class warning. *Psychiatric News,* May 17, 1985.

21. Dean CE. Tardive dyskinesia: a serious side-effect? *American Journal of Psychiatry* 1987;144:261–262.

22. Baldessarini RJ, Cohen BM. Drs Baldessarini and Cohen reply. *American Journal of Psychiatry* 1987;144:262.

23. Hansen TE, Brown WL, Weigel RM, et al. Under-recognition of tardive dyskinesia and drug-induced parkinsonism by psychiatric residents. *General Hospital Psychiatry* 1992;14:340–344.

24. Benjamin S, Munetz MR. CHMC practices related to tardive dyskinesia screening and informed consent for neuroleptic drugs. *Hospital and Community Psychiatry* 1994;45:343–346.

25. Kane JM, Smith JM. Tardive dyskinesia: prevalence and risk factors, 1959–1979. *Archives of General Psychiatry* 1982;39:473–481.

26. Kane JM, Woerner M, Borenstein M, et al. Integrating incidence and prevalence of tardive dyskinesia. *Psychopharmacology Bulletin* 1986;22:254–258.

27. Jeste DV, Iager AC, Wyatt RJ. The biology and experimental treatment of tardive dyskinesia and related movement disorders. In: *American Handbook of Psychiatry* (Biological Psychiatry), Volume 2. Editors: Berger PA, Brodie HKH. Basic Books, New York, 1986.

28. Morgenstern H, Glazer WM. Identifying risk factors for tardive dyskinesia among long-term outpatients maintained with neuroleptic medications. *Archives of General Psychiatry* 1993;50:723–733.

29. Kalachnik J. Tardive dyskinesia and the mentally retarded: a review. In: *Advances in Mental Retardation and Developmental Disabilities, vol 2.* Editor: Breuning S. JAI Press, Greenwich CT, 1983.

30. Glazer WM, Morgenstern H. Predicting the long-term risk of tardive dyskinesia in outpatients maintained on neuroleptic medications. *Journal of Clinical Psychiatry* 1993;54:133–139.

31. Yassa R. Tardive dyskinesia: a two-year follow-up study. *Psychosomatics* 1984;25:852–855.

32. Gaultieri CT, Schroeder SR, Hicks RE, et al. Tardive dyskinesia in young mentally retarded individuals. *Archives of General Psychiatry* 1986;43:335–340.

33. Glazer WM, Morgenstern H. Predictors of occurrence, severity and course of tardive dyskinesia in an outpatient clinic. *Journal of Clinical Psychopharmacology* 1988;8:10s–16s.

34. Carbon M, Hsieh C-H, Kane JM, et al. Tardive dyskinesia prevalence in the period of second-generation antipsychotic use: a meta-analysis. *Journal of Clinical Psychiatry* 2017;78:e264–e278.

35. Kaufmann CA, Jeste DV, Shelton RC, et al. Noradrenergic and neuroradiological abnormalities in tardive dyskinesia. *Biological Psychiatry* 1986;21:799–812.

36. Waddington JL, Youssef HA, Dolphin C, et al. Cognitive dysfunction, negative symptoms and tardive dyskinesia in schizophrenia: their association in relation to topography of involuntary movements and criterion of their abnormality. *Archives of General Psychiatry* 1987;44:907–912.

37. Kolokowska T, Williams AO, Ardern M, et al. Tardive dyskinesia in schizophrenics under 60 years of age. *Biological Psychiatry* 1986;21:161–169.

38. Wolf M, Ryan J, Mosnaim AD. Cognitive functions in tardive dyskinesia. *Psychological Medicine* 1983;13:671–674.

39. DeWolf AS, Ryan JJ, Wolf ME. Cognitive sequelae of tardive dyskinesia. *Journal of Nervous and Mental Disease* 1988;176:270–274.

40. Waddington JL, Youseff HA, Kinsella A. Cognitive dysfunction in schizophrenia followed-up over 5 years, and its longitudinal relationship to the emergence of tardive dyskinesia. *Psychological Medicine* 1990;20:835–842.

41. Spohn HE, Coyne L, Lacoursiere R, et al. Relationship of neuroleptic dose and tardive dyskinesia to attention, information-processing and psychophysiology in medicated schizophrenics. *Archives of General Psychiatry* 1985;42:849–859.

42. Craig TJ, Richardson MA. Swallowing, laryngeal dystonia and anticholinergics, *American Journal of Psychiatry* 1982;193:1083.

43. Geratt GR. Speech abnormalities in tardive dyskinesia. *Archives of Neurology* 1984;41:273–276.

44. Massengill R, Nashold B. A swallowing disorder denoted in patients with tardive dyskinesia. *Acta Otolaryngology* 1969;68:457–458.

45. Waddington JL, Youseff HA. Late onset involuntary movements in chronic schizophrenia: relationship of tardive dyskinesia to intellectual impairment and negative symptoms. *British Journal of Psychiatry* 1986;149:616–620.

46. Miller DD, McEvoy JP, Davis SM, et al. Clinical correlates of tardive dyskinesia in schizophrenia: baseline data from the CATIE schizophrenia trial. *Schizophrenia Research* 2005;80:33–43.

47. Caroff SN, Davis VG, Miller DD, et al. Treatment outcomes of patients with tardive dyskinesia and chronic schizophrenia. *Journal of Clinical Psychiatry* 2011;72:295–303.

48. John J, Bhatia R, Kuksal P, et al. Association study of MiRSNPs with schizophrenia, tardive d dyskinesia and cognition. *Schizophrenia Research* 2016;174:29–34.

49. Hui Han M, Yin GZ, et al. Association between DBH 19bp insertion/deletion polymorphism and cognition in schizophrenia with and without tardive dyskinesia. *Schizophrenia Research* 2017;182:104–109.

50. Ballesteros J, González-Pinto A, Bulbena A. Tardive dyskinesia associated with higher mortality in psychiatric patients: a meta-analysis seven independent studies. *Journal of Clinical Psychopharmacology* 2000;20:188–194.

51. Dean CE, Thuras PD. Mortality and tardive dyskinesia: a long-term study using the US national death index. *British Journal of Psychiatry* 2009;194:360–364.

52. Sprague RL, Kalachnik JE, Breuning SE, et al. The Dyskinesia Identification System-Coldwater (DIS-CO): a tardive dyskinesia rating system for the developmentally disabled. *Psychopharmacology Bulletin* 1984;20:328–338.

53. Dean CE, Russell JM, Kuskowski MA, et al. Clinical rating scales and instruments: how do they compare in assessing abnormal, involuntary movements? *Journal of Clinical Psychopharmacology* 2004;24:298–304.

54. Guy W. *ECDEU Assessment Manual for Psychopharmacology: Publication ADM 76–388.* US Department of Health, Education, and Welfare, 1976.

55. Turek IS. Drug-induced dyskinesia: reality or myth? *Diseases of the Nervous System* 1975;36:397–399.

56. Bollini P, Pampallona S, Orza MJ, et al. Antipsychotic drugs: is more worse? A meta-analysis of published randomized controlled trials. *Psychological Medicine* 1994;24:307–316.

57. Erhardt S, Appel J, Meinhardt CL. Trends in National Institutes of Health funding for clinical trials registered in ClinicalTrials.gov. *JAMA* 2015;314:2566–2577.

58. Kraepelin E. *Manic-Depressive Insanity and Paranoia.* Translated by Barclay RM. Edited by Robertson GM, E&S Livingstone, Edinburgh, 1919.

59. Gervin M, Browne S, Lane A, et al. Spontaneous abnormal involuntary movements in first-episode schizophrenia and schizophreniform disorder: baseline rate in a group of patients from an Irish catchment area. *American Journal of Psychiatry* 1998;155:1202–1206.

60. Caroff SN, Ungvari GS, Ownes DGC. Historical perspectives on tardive dyskinesia. *Journal of the Neurological Sciences* 2018;389:4–9.

61. Berrios GE, Markova IS. Historical and conceptual aspects of motor disorders in the psychoses. *Schizophrenia Research* 2018;200:5–11.

62. Fenton WS, Wyatt RJ, McGlashan TH. Risk factors for spontaneous dyskinesia in schizophrenia. *Archives of General Psychiatry* 1994;51:643–650.

63. Brockner S. Neurological symptoms with phenothiazines. *British Medical Journal* 1964;57:876.

64. Koning JPF, Tenback DE, van Os J, et al. Dyskinesia and parkinsonism in antipsychotic-naïve patients with schizophrenia, first-degree relatives and healthy controls: a meta-analysis. *Schizophrenia Bulletin* 2010;36:723–731.

65. Walker E. Developmentally moderated expressions of the neuropathology underlying schizophrenia. *Schizophrenia Bulletin* 1994;20:453–480.

66. Schiffman J, Walker EF, Ekstrom M, et al. Childhood videotaped social and neuromotor precursors of schizophrenia: a prospective evaluation. *American Journal of Psychiatry* 2004;161:2021–2027.

67. Mittal VA, Walker EF. Movement abnormalities predict conversion to Axis I psychosis among prodromal adolescents. *Journal of Abnormal Psychology* 2007;116:796–803.

68. Ayd F. A survey of drug-induced extrapyramidal reactions. *Journal of the American Medical Association* 1961;175:1054–1060.

69. Adler LA, Rotrosen J, Angrist B. Acute drug-induced akathisia. In: *Drug Induced Movement Disorders*, Second Edition. Editors: Factor SA, Lang AE, Weiner WJ. Blackwell Futura, Malden MA, 2005, pp. 140–173.

70. Hamra BJ, Nasrallah HA, Clancy J, et al. Psychiatric diagnosis and risk for tardive dyskinesia. *Archives of General Psychiatry* 1983;40:346–347.

71. Gao K, Kemp DE, Ganocy SJ, et al. Antipsychotic-induced extrapyramidal side effects in bipolar disorder and schizophrenia. *Journal of Clinical Psychopharmacology* 2008;28:203–209.

72. Gentile S. Extrapyramidal adverse events associated with atypical antipsychotic treatment of bipolar disorder. *Journal of Clinical Psychopharmacology* 2007;27:35–45.

73. Klemp M, Tvete IF, Skomedal T, et al. A review and Bayesian meta-analysis of clinical efficacy and adverse effects of 4 atypical neuroleptic drugs compared with haloperidol and placebo. *Journal of Clinical Psychopharmacology* 2011;31:698–704.

74. Jeste DV, Caligiuri MP, Paulsen JS, et al. Risk of tardive dyskinesia in older patients: a prospective longitudinal study of 266 outpatients. *Archives of General Psychiatry* 1995;52:756–765.

75. Friedman JH, Trieschmann ME, Fernandez HH. Drug-induced parkinsonism. In: *Drug Induced Movement Disorders*, Second Edition. Editors: Factor SA, Lang AE, Weiner WJ. Blackwell Futura, Malden MA, 2005.

76. Herb J. An Owatonna woman who developed a neurological disease has her claim against drugmakers argued at the US Supreme Court. *Minneapolis Star Tribune*, March 31, 2011, p. 1.

77. Taksh U. A critical review of rating scales in the assessment of movement disorders in schizophrenia. *Current Drug Targets* 2006;7:1225–1229.

78. Bergen JA, Griffiths DA, Rey JM, et al. Tardive dyskinesia: fluctuating patient or fluctuating rater. *British Journal of Psychiatry* 1984;144:498–502.

79. Caligiuiri MP, Lohr JB, Vaughn RM. Fluctuation of tardive dyskinesia. *Biological Psychiatry* 1995;38:336–339.

80. Caligiuri MP, Lohr JB. Fine force instability: a quantitative measure of neuroleptic-induced dyskinesia in the hand. *Journal of Neuropsychiatry* 1990;2:395–398.

81. Lohr JB, Caligiuri MP. Quantitative instrumental measurement of tardive dyskinesia: a review. *Neuropsychopharmacology* 1992;6:231–239.

82. Folstein MF, Folstein SE, McHugh PR. "Mini-Mental State," a practical method for grading the cognitive state of patients for the clinician. *Journal of Psychiatric Research* 1975;12:189–198.

83. Peralta V, Cuesta MJ. Neuromotor abnormalities in neuroleptic-naïve psychotic patients: antecedents, clinical correlates, and prediction of treatment response. *Comprehensive Psychiatry* 2011;52:139–145.

84. McCreadie RG, Srinivasan TN, Padmavathi R. Extrapyramidal symptoms in unmedicated schizophrenia. *Journal of Psychiatric Research* 2005;39:261–266.

85. Alessi-Severini S, Biscontri RG, Collins DM, et al. Ten years of antipsychotic prescribing to children: a Canadian-based population study. *Canadian Journal of Psychiatry* 2012;57:52–58.

86. Comer JS, Mojtabi R, Olfson M. National trends in the antipsychotic treatment of psychiatric outpatients with anxiety disorders. *American Journal of Psychiatry* 2011;168:1057–1065.

87. Peluso MJ, Lewis SW, Barnes TRE, et al. Extrapyramidal motor side-effects of first-and second-generation antipsychotic drugs. *British Journal of Psychiatry* 2012;200:387–392.

88. Hauser RA, Truong D. Special issue: tardive syndromes and their management. *Journal of Neurological Sciences* 2018. https://doi.org.1016/jns.2018.02.009.

89. Soares KV, McGrath JJ. The treatment of tardive dyskinesia: a systematic review and meta-analysis. *Schizophrenia Research* 1999;39:1–16.

90. Hauser RA, Factor SA, Marder SR, et al. KINECT 3: a phase 3 randomized, double-blind, placebo-controlled trial of valbenazine for tardive dyskinesia. *American Journal of Psychiatry* 2017;174:476–484.

91. Fernandez HH, Factor SA, Hauser RA, et al. Randomized controlled trial of deutetrabenazine for tardive dyskinesia: the ARM-TD study. *Neurology* 2017;88:203–210.

92. Mahmoudi S, Levesque D, Blanchet PJ. Upregulation of dopamine D3, not D2 receptors correlates with tardive dyskinesia in a primate model. *Movement Disorders* 2014;29:1125–1133.

93. Meyer JM. Future directions in tardive dyskinesia research. *Journal of the Neurological Sciences* 2018;389:76–80.

94. Guy W. ed: *ECDEU Assessment Manual for Psychopharmacology: Publication ADM 76–338.* US Department of Health, Education, and Welfare, Washington DC, 1976.

95. Sprague RL, Kalachnik JE, Breuning SE, et al. The dyskinesia indentification system-Coldwater ((DIS-CO): a tardive dyskinesia rating system for the developmentally disabled. *Pharmacological Bulletin 2004* 1984;20:328–338.

96. Simpson GM, Angus JWS. A rating scale for extra-pyramidal side-effects. *Acta Psychiatrica Scandinavica* 1970;212(suppl 44):11–19.

97. Barnes TR. A rating scale for drug-induced akathisia. *British Journal of Psychiatry* 1989;154:672–686.

98. Chouinard G, Ross-Chouinard A, Annable L, et al. The extra-pyramidal symptom rating scale. *Canadian Journal of Neurological Sciences* 1980;7:233.

99. Simpson GM, Lee JH, Zoubek B, et al. A rating scale for tardive dyskinesia. *Psychopharmacology* 1979;64:171–179.

100. Alkelai A, Greenbaum L, Heizen EL, et al. New insights into tardive dyskinesia genetics: implementation of whole-exome sequencing research. *Progress in Neuropsychopharmacology & Biological Psychiatry* 2019. https://doi.org.10.1016/j.pnpbp.109659.

101. Zai CC, Maes MS, Tiwari AK, et al. Genetics of tardive dyskinesia: promising leads and ways forward. *Journal of the Neurological Sciences* 2018;389:28–34.

8 Antidepressants and Depression
Background and Biology

Introduction

> We have not far to look for suffering. It's in the streets, fills the air, lies upon our friends . . . So-consider one who suffers . . . perhaps a man in his middle fifties with a depressive character, normal to his friends, but constantly brushing away cobweb thoughts of suicide, one who is bored, finds no meaning in life, is ashamed. Consider one who suffers—anyone you know well. Consider perhaps yourself.
>
> Allen Wheelis, *How People Change*, Harper Colophon
> Books, pp. 3, 7–8, 1973

There is no doubt that depression remains among the most ubiquitous and damaging of all the psychiatric disorders, both with regard to personal suffering and costs to the health care system. Unfortunately, the prevalence of depression in the U.S. has increased over the past 25 years[1] and, indeed, doubled from 1992 to 2002.[2] In a national survey of adults carried out in 2012 and 2013, the ten-month prevalence of DSM-5 major depressive disorder was 10.4%, while the lifetime prevalence was 20.6%,[3] one-fifth of the population! By 2013, personal health care spending on depressive disorders reached $71 billion, ranking 6th among 150 conditions.[4] In contrast, spending on anxiety disorders was ranked 26th, schizophrenia 37th, and bipolar disorder 44th.

Despite the outpouring of money, and the advent of SSRIs in the 1990s, the World Health Organization in 1996 predicted that depression would be the second leading cause of disability by the year 2020,[5] an accurate forecast. But depression was not the only issue. By 2010,[6] 7.4% of *all* disability adjusted life-years (DALYS) were secondary to mental health and substance abuse disorders, with depression accounting for 40% of that total, and use of illicit drugs accounting for another 11%, anxiety 15%, and schizophrenia 7.4%. The same grouping resulted in 23% of years of life lost to premature mortality (YLLs). *The authors noted that the global burden of mental health and substance abuse disorders exceeded* those of HIV/AIDS, diabetes, tuberculosis, and transport injuries.[6, p1582] However, there was little evidence to suggest a global increase in the prevalence of mental disorders, but the prevalence of alcohol, cocaine, and opioid dependence increased markedly, with white, middle-aged males showing significant increases. It does not seem realistic to separate out substance use disorders from mental disorders, but we shall examine problems in the diagnostic system in Chapters 13 and 14.

Given this data, it may not be surprising to learn that *life expectancy in the U.S. began to fall in 2014 and did so for the next three years,*[7] *a remarkable finding.* All-cause mortality in adults ages 24 to 64 began to increase in the 1990s, rising from 328 deaths per 100,00 in 2010 to 348 deaths per 100,000 by 2017! Increases were found in all racial groups and were secondary to suicide, alcohol abuse, and a variety of organ system diseases. The greatest increases in mortality rates were found in the Ohio Valley states.

During this same era, Olfson et al. found a significant decline in the quality of life in the U.S. population,[8] while the suicide rate rose by 35% in adults ages 35 to 64, and by 60% among women ages 60 to 64.[9] In a ground-breaking study published in 2015, Case and Deaton[10] reported a marked increase in mortality secondary to suicide, chronic liver disease, and poisoning from drugs and alcohol among non-Hispanic whites ages 45 to 54. This was a significant reversal from years past and a phenomenon *not found* in other wealthy countries. (We shall take up the effects of socioeconomic inequality in a later chapter.)

Not surprisingly, the use of prescription drugs in the U.S. rose by 8% between 1999 and 2012, accompanied by an 8% increase in the use of five or more agents.[11] *The use of antidepressants more than doubled from 13 million people in 1996 to 27 million in 2005.*[12] Another study[13] found that the long-term use—at least 24 months—of ADs doubled from the turn of the century to 2010. Among adults 65 and older, per a 2017 study,[14] visits to primary care where ADs or benzodiazepines were prescribed increased from 9.9% in 2003 through 2005 to 12.3% in 2010 through 2012. In addition, the use of ADs expanded to include non-FDA-approved conditions such as insomnia, anxiety, and malaise and use as adjuncts to psychotic disorders.[15, 16] It seems reasonable to assume that these increases reflected an increased demand secondary to socioeconomic factors such as income inequality, increasing rates of poverty, and the decline of the middle class.[10, 17, 18]

In the meantime, questions began to arise regarding the efficacy of ADs, despite the demand and the popularity of the newer antidepressants, specifically serotonin reuptake inhibitors (SSRIS) and serotonin-norepinephrine reuptake inhibitors (SNRIS). Beyond efficacy, concerns were raised about their costs and side effects, especially sexual dysfunction, suicidality, and aggression. We shall examine these issues in subsequent chapters, but in this chapter, let's focus on some basics of ADs, including their development and mechanisms of action—but first, a question.

Did the Nature of Depression Change?

I find it striking that in the 1970s, staff at the National Institute of Mental Health (NIMH) observed that depression had the best possibility of recovery, with or without treatment,[19] and that patients almost always returned to their premorbid status.[20] Yet, over the ensuing years, data from the 30-year NIMH-sponsored Collaborative Depression Study (CDS) began to paint a starkly different picture. In one of their early papers, Keller et al.[21] noted that in five major university medical centers, 67% of patients with major depression had not recovered at eight weeks, and 38% still had severe symptoms! Remarkably, 31% of inpatients had received inadequate treatment, as did almost half the outpatients. In 2013, the summary publication[22] noted that in the CDS depressed population, *20% had failed to recover, no matter the treatment!* Of those who recovered, 40% relapsed by 2 years, 60% by 5 years, and 85% to 91% by 30 years.

These data, plus the studies on the increasing rates of depression cited earlier, have transformed our view of depression into a chronic, recurring illness. We have also seen increasing attention given to treatment-resistant depression (TRD), as defined by failure to respond to a minimum of two well-done trials of ADs. While the CDS data indicated that 20% fail to respond, current estimates indicate that TRD occurs in about 33% of people with major depression,[23] with a 76% increase in health care costs compared to people with non-treatment-resistant depression.[24] This has become such an important topic that we will review it in Chapter 12.

Antidepressants and Neurochemistry: The Early Years

Interest in the calming effects of antihistamines helped lead the way to chlorpromazine in the late 1940s, a development that spurred a search for structurally similar compounds. Geigy came upon G22355, a three-ring compound very similar to the structure of chlorpromazine, soon to be known as imipramine. It was marketed in Switzerland as Tofranil in 1957, following a number of clinical studies carried out by Roland Kuhn. Imipramine was the first tricyclic antidepressant (TCA), but about four years passed before it became established in clinical care.[25, pp. 51–57] Kuhn came to the United States to lecture on the drug and, in 1958, published the seminal paper on the treatment of depression with imipramine,[26] spurring the eventual development of amitriptyline (Elavil) in 1961, quickly followed by other TCAs. One year earlier, iproniazid had been marketed as an AD (Marsilid).[25, pp. 59–67] This agent was the first monoamine oxidase inhibitor (MAOI), a drug that led to multiple problems and its eventual withdrawal from the market. Nevertheless, a number of other MAOIs soon appeared, but they continue to be plagued by dietary restrictions and hypertensive crises.

While the MOAIs seem to have some grounding in neurochemistry, imipramine remained a mystery. In 1959, Pollack[27] noted that its mode of action was not clear but observed that it had some anticonvulsant effects and no hypothermic effects, but it might have some "slight peripheral anesthetic effects." He then claimed that imipramine did not increase norepinephrine or serotonin in the brain—a comment he no doubt regretted by 1968—but correctly stated that it was not a MAOI. Unfortunately, he also credited imipramine with a large margin of safety!

By 1964, Cole noted[19] that imipramine had been superior to placebo in 9 of 15 controlled trials, but the evidence for efficacy with MAOIs was somewhat in doubt. Interestingly, nothing was said about mechanisms of action, although considerable research was underway. This culminated in the development of the catecholamine hypothesis of affective disorders in 1965.[28] In this model, ADs block the reuptake of norepinephrine (NE) and serotonin (5-HTA) by binding to the protein transporters that carry the drugs into the presynaptic nerve endings, thus increasing levels of these neurotransmitters at the synapse, as countless television commercials have reminded us.

In Chapter 2, I reviewed the subsequent models of AD actions, including the permissive amine hypothesis, the cholinergic hypothesis, and a model focusing on a primary deficiency of 5-HTA (serotonin), so I refer the reader to that section and the citations. In contrast to the remarks by Pollak,[27] it had become obvious that *TCAs did not have a wide margin of safety*, given their blockade of histamine receptors, muscarinic cholinergic receptors, and alpha-adrenergic receptors, resulting in a host of side effects, including sedation, dry mouth, constipation, dizziness, fainting, and cardiotoxic effects. Indeed, overdoses of TCAs could be fatal, an issue we will visit later.

By 1980, literally thousands of studies had been done seeking to confirm or disprove the early models of AD pathophysiology, but the results were often contradictory, inconsistent, or not specific to depression. Indeed, Eric Nestler wrote in 1998 that while "Monoamines reigned supreme" from 1950 to 1980,[29] several decades of research had uncovered little in the way of direct evidence showing that depression is *caused* by specific abnormalities in NE, DA, or 5-HTA. Nor was there any fundamental reason to expect that abnormalities in monoamine pathways were the primary cause of depression,[29, p. 526] yet these doubts did not stop us from continuing the search for specific deficits in DA, NE, 5-HTA, and their transporters.

Nevertheless, given the mixed and often paradoxical results of these studies, there was some movement away from focusing on the cell surface (receptors/transmitters) and moving deeper into the cell, its intracellular signaling systems, and the hypothalamic-pituitary-adrenal axis (HPA) and its response to stress. Hundreds of studies were done on the HPA axis, particularly after Bernard Carroll and his group[30] in Ann Arbor found that stimulation of the HPA axis by dexamethasone was blunted in melancholic depression (i.e., dexamethasone failed to suppress secretion of plasma cortisol). Note that failure to suppress cortisol secretion is counted as a positive dexamethasone suppression test, or DST.

This very fine study assured clinicians that the DST was sensitive enough to identify melancholia in 67% of those with clinically diagnosed melancholia. Remarkably, the specificity was 96%: that is, only 4% of those with a positive DST were not clinically melancholic. In addition, the early studies indicated that should the DST fail to normalize with treatment, the patient might be at an increased risk of relapse. Moreover, clinical improvement appeared to dovetail nicely with gradual normalization of cortisol levels. A positive DST also correlated with a family history of depression. Taken together, this data appeared to validate the DST as a diagnostic test for melancholia.[30]

Ah, yes, these were heady times for psychiatrists! Suddenly we were all doing DSTs on everyday patients and feeling much more like scientists. At last, a laboratory test that would be useful in predicting who would respond to an antidepressant! Sadly, it later became apparent that this test was not specific enough to be of value in clinical practice: that is, the test could be positive in 10% of non-depressed people. One group found that simply restricting caloric intake and sleep could result in a positive DST.[31] Not willing to give up, investigators began combining the DST with other putative biological markers, still hoping for the diagnostic silver bullet. One group,[32] for example, coupled the DST with rapid eye movement (REM) latency and two other biologic tests and found that almost 92% could be correctly classified as endogenous (melancholic) depressives by at least one marker.

A major problem, however, was a growing appreciation of the many confounding factors that could influence the outcome of the DST, including age, gender, subtype of depression, early life stress, duration of stressors, and hospitalization status.[33] Not surprisingly, investigators have moved on to other biologic hypotheses, of which there is no end in sight, since none have been consistently reliable, sensitive, or specific.

Later Biochemical Hypotheses: From Serotonin to Sigma Receptors

Although a number of prominent investigators continued to emphasize the futility of seeking answers to the mysteries of depression in a deficiency or excess of a single neurotransmitter or receptor, many continued to do so, particularly after the astounding success of fluoxetine (Prozac), the first of the SSRIs and the only drug ever to grace the covers of four national news magazines! Within three years of its approval by the FDA in December of 1987, fluoxetine was prescribed more often than any other drug by psychiatrists, and by 1994, it was the second most prescribed drug in the world.[34] Indeed, some claimed that it was a miracle drug, capable not only of treating multiple disorders, but also of enhancing the functioning of non-depressed people. Indeed, Edward Shorter noted that such a phenomenon would not have been possible had not psychiatry become so entangled in the Pharma corporate culture.[34, p. 324] Small wonder that this success set off an avalanche of articles and books, including "The Medicalization of Unhappiness," by Ronald Dworkin,[35] Peter Kramer's famous "Listening to Prozac,"[36] and many others, some positive, others intensely critical—but the flood of SSRIs proceeded, with even more focus on 5-HTA. We now have at least 23 SSRIs, SNRIs, and closely related variations.

The development of these drugs paralleled the focus on the *blockade* of serotonin receptors by SGAs, and, interestingly enough, some found that the 5-HT2c receptor was blocked by fluoxetine and other ADs.[37] Yet more controversy over the role of 5-HTA emerged in 2008 with the publication of a major review by Cowen,[37] who postulated that the enthusiasm over 5-HTA stemmed from a marketing myth rather than a pathophysiologic mechanism. The author pointed to the many inconsistencies found in neurochemical studies and noted, for example, that lowering levels of 5-HTA in normal people does not induce depression. In addition, genetic studies aimed at finding variations at the locus for the gene encoding 5-HTA had produced mixed results.

Despite the scientific concerns, interest in 5-HTA and fluoxetine sparked national campaigns aimed at fostering awareness of depression and its symptoms, with events such as a National Depression Screening Day, a Depression Awareness Recognition Treatment program, and others.[38] In August 1995, one research organization launched an advertising campaign emphasizing that depression is caused by a chemical imbalance in the brain,[39] spurring investigators to continue their search for what that imbalance might entail, including several proteins that nurture the growth and functions of neurons.

Brain-Derived Neurotropic Factor and Neurogenesis

Brain-derived neurotrophic factor (BDNF) and nerve growth factor (NGF) are proteins that foster the growth and health of neurons. There is clear evidence that stress lowers levels of BDNF, especially in the hippocampus, while some studies have found hippocampal atrophy in depression.[40, 41] Indeed, studies have found that BDNF stimulated growth of serotonergic neurons in the brains of adult rats.[42] In rodents, infusion of BDNF into the hippocampus resulted in antidepressant-like effects, but this can be prevented by knocking out the gene coding for BDNF.[43] In 2003, Santarelli et al.[44] stressed that hippocampal neurogenesis appears necessary for the behavioral effects associated with ADs.

As often happens, matters quickly became more complicated, with evidence indicating that the effects of BDNF depend on the brain area injected.[45] Indeed, infusion of BDNF into the ventral tegmentum/nucleus accumbens *increases depressive-like behaviors*, while a Val66-Met66 polymorphism in a gene encoding BDNF dampens BDNF signaling but does not make one more vulnerable to depression.[46] Other work uncovered the existence of at least four other neurotrophic agents.[47] In addition, other psychotropic agents, including APs,[48] mood stabilizers, and lithium[49] exert neuroprotective effects.

Complicating matters, a wide range of non-drug factors can affect neurogenesis, including exercise, sleep disruption, and inflammation.[50] Unfortunately, like the dexamethasone suppression test, levels of BDNF should not be used as a diagnostic tool or biomarker. Finally, Krishnan and Nestler concluded that the BDNF hypothesis is "too simplistic."[46, p. 897]

Acid-Sensing Ion Channels (ACICs) and Sigma Receptors

In another and somewhat more exotic approach to the origins of depression, Wemmie et al. began to focus on acid-sensing ion channels (ACICs). ACICs are found in the cell membrane, and are encoded by three genes.[51] ACICs are important to synaptic plasticity, memory, and modulation of pain and may be important in the pathophysiology of strokes—an interesting observation, given the relationship between depression and strokes, a topic I will discuss later. With regard to depression, ACICs are found in a number of brain structures important to depression, including the amygdala and the nucleus accumbens, among others. In rodents, inhibition of ACICs by medications, or by knocking out the genes, leads to robust antidepressant-like behaviors *not* dependent on the loss of 5-HTA. Naturally, some have posited that ACIC inhibitors might be another method of improving depression in humans.[52] However, ClinicalTrials.gov did not list any studies on ACICs and depression as of February 8, 2020.

Sigma Receptors

Sigma-1 receptors are present in neurons and oligodendrocytes in the hypothalamus, hippocampus, substantia nigra, and Purkinje cells in the brain.[53] They are involved in learning, memory, cell differentiation, release of dopamine and serotonin, and drug dependence.[54] Interestingly, sigma-1 knockout mice display deceased mobility in the forced-swim test, a classic rodent model of depression,[55] while sigma agonists have antidepressant effects.[56] A specific agonist, in combination with venlafaxine, acted synergistically in the forced-swim test while several antagonists reversed the effects of venlafaxine.[57] Of additional interest: SSRIs have a higher degree of affinity for sigma-1 receptors than do TCAs, but whether this is clinically meaningful is not clear. After all, SSRIs and TCAs are equally effective, albeit with different side effects.

While the studies just cited focused on the possible therapeutic effects of drugs and sigma receptors in treating depression, a 2019 review[57] emphasized alcohol and cocaine addiction as areas where ligands of the receptors might have value. The authors also cited one study[58] wherein an RCT of a cyclic amide (MN-101) that binds to sigma-2 and 5-HT2a receptors showed promise in treating the negative symptoms of schizophrenia. However, the focus of the review[57] was on the treatment of Parkinson's disease, Alzheimer's disease, neuropathic pain, amyotrophic lateral sclerosis, and ischemic stroke. ClinicalTrials.gov did record several trials of sigma agonists on February 8, 2020, but no results have been posted.

Beyond Biochemistry: The Limbic-Cortical Neural Network Model

The limbic-cortical network has been championed for some years by Dr. Helen Mayberg, who reported in 1997[59] that *responders to ADs* were characterized by hypermetabolism in the rostral anterior cingulate gyrus while non-responders were hypometabolic, with rates of metabolism measured by PET scans. No other brain area was involved, and *no clinical characteristics* appeared to be relevant. However, cingulate metabolism did not correlate with severity of depression, cognitive   performance, or motor speed. The authors posited that the anterior cingulate is a "bridge linking dorsal and ventral pathways" that seem necessary for the integration of cognitive, mood, autonomic, and motor behaviors. Unfortunately, the authors did not obtain any endocrine or biochemical data.

In 2003, Mayberg[60] reviewed the literature on limbic-cortical circuits, stating that modulation of these dysfunctional pathways is critical to remission, no matter the treatment. Eight years later, she and Paul Holtzheimer[61] described the development of deep brain stimulation (DBS), with the list of brain areas targeted for DBS expanding from the cingulate to the nucleus accumbens, the inferior thalamic peduncle and habenula, and the ventral anterior internal capsule/ventral striatum. Nevertheless, they concluded *that "treatments are no more effective today than they were 50–70 years ago,"* and the neurobiology of depression is largely unknown—startling statements after 60 years of biological research! But the search continued, with a publication in 2019 noting that our interest in limbic-cortical circuits has expanded *beyond depression* to include autism spectrum disorder, schizophrenia, and non-affective psychotic disorders.[62]

We should note as well that the present focus on the default mode network (DMN), a set of areas of the brain that include the medial prefrontal cortex, the posterior cingulate cortex, medial temporal lobes, lateral temporal-parietal areas, and the posterior inferior parietal lobule. The DMN is normally inhibited when people are engaged in a focused task performance and activated when engaged in more internally directed activities such as daydreaming or maladaptive depressive rumination.[63] Normalization of DMN activity has been shown with the successful treatment of depression *and* schizophrenia.[63, 64]

We shall have more to say about neural networks and the genetics of depression in subsequent chapters, but it is clear that models of depression and antidepressant mechanisms are limited only by the creativity and imagination of investigators. These have ranged from demon possession to a psychoanalytic model of anger turned inward to ego-dependent learned helplessness, altered cognition with negative expectations, separation, trauma, bereavement in childhood, and on to multiple biochemical models, intracellular signaling and the devastating effects of poverty.[18, 65, 66]

Clinical Notes

1. The significant increase in depression and suicidality in the U.S. deserves more attention, particularly with regard to deaths of despair, as noted by Case and Deaton.[10] I strongly recommend their new book, *Deaths of Despair and the Future of Capitalism,*[68] for additional details and discussion of this phenomenon.

2. While the biology of depression and the mechanisms underlying the effects of ADs have yielded a great deal of knowledge regarding brain structure and function, research must shift to a more holistic approach, encompassing the socioeconomic context in which depression arises and the methods by which it is treated.

3. Do not be misled by advertisements touting the effects of an AD on additional receptors or combinations of receptors. While of academic interest, these discoveries have not yielded any substantial improvements in efficacy.

4. The advent of a new AD should lead the reader to ask several questions: Has the new drug been compared with an older AD? This almost never occurs until much later, so none of us can accurately assess whether the cost of the new drug is justified. History suggests it is not. Is the cost of the new AD justified? It is not likely that the new drug is more effective than the less expensive, older agents. What about non-drug strategies? As we shall see, there are a number of well-validated forms of psychotherapy.

At this point, let's move to the next chapter and examine ADs in more detail, including the debates over efficacy, the magnitude of the placebo effect, predictors of outcome, comparisons between ADs and psychotherapeutic approaches, the use of ADs in pregnancy, and adverse events. We certainly don't need more of the same ADs. By the year 2000, we had tricyclics, tetracyclics, and MAOIs,[67] then SSRIs, SNRIs, and others, but with no increase in efficacy. We have now become enthusiastic over non-invasive and invasive brain stimulation and a host of "novel" approaches.

References

1. Mojtabai R, Olfson M, Han B. National trends in the prevalence and treatment of depression in adolescents and young adults. *Pediatrics* 2016;138:pii, e20161878.

2. Compton WM, Conway KP, Stinson FS, et al. Changes in the prevalence of major depression and comorbid substance abuse in the United States between 1991–1992 and 2001–2002. *American Journal of Psychiatry* 2006;163:141–147.

3. Hasin DS, Sarvet AL, Meyers JL, et al. Epidemiology of adult DSM-5 major depressive disorder and its specifiers in the United States. *JAMA Psychiatry* 2018;75:336–346.

4. Dieleman JL, Baral R, Birger M, et al. US spending on personal health care and public health 1996–2013. *JAMA* 2016;316:2627–2646.

5. Murray CJL, Lopez AD. *The Global Burden of Disease: A Comprehensive Assessment of Mortality and Disability from Diseases, Injuries, and Risk Factors in 1990 and Projected to 2020*. Harvard University Press, Cambridge MA, 1996.

6. Whiteford HA, Degenhardt L, Rehm J, et al. Global burden of disease attributable to mental and substance abuse disorders: finding from the global burden of disease study 2010. *The Lancet* 2013;382:1575–1586.

7. Woolf SH, Schoomaker H. Life expectancy in the United States, 1959–2017. *JAMA* 2019;322(20):1996–2016. Doi:10.1001/jama.2019.16932.

8. Olfson M, Wall M, Liu SM, et al. Declining health-related quality of life in the U.S. *American Journal of Preventive Medicine* 2018;54:325–333.

9. Centers for Disease Control. Suicide among adults aged 35–64 years—United States, 1992–2012. *Morbidity and Mortality Weekly Report* 2013;62:321.

10. Case A, Deaton A. Rising morbidity and mortality in midlife among white non-Hispanic Americans in the 21st century. *Proceedings of the National Academy of Sciences* 2015;112:15078–15083.

11. Kantor ED, Rehm CD, Hass JS, et al. Trends in prescription drug use among adults in the United States from 1992–2012. *JAMA* 2015;314:1818–1831.

12. Olfsen M, Marcus SC, Druss B, et al. National patterns in antidepressant medication patterns. *Archives of General Psychiatry* 2009;66:848–856.

13. Motjtabai R, Olfson M. National trends in long-term use of antidepressant medications: results from the US national health and nutrition examination survey. *Journal of Clinical Psychiatry* 2014;75:169–177.

14. Maust DT, Blow FC, Wiechers IR, et al. National trends in antidepressant, benzodiazepine, and other sedative-hypnotic treatment of older adults in psychiatric and primary care. *Journal of Clinical Psychiatry* 2017;78:e363–e371. Doi:10.4088/JCP.16m10713.

15. Dean CE. The death of specificity in psychiatry: cheers or tears? *Perspectives in Biology and Medicine* 2012;55:443–460.

16. Dean CE. Psychopharmacology: a house divided. *Progress in Neuro-Psychopharmacology & Biological Psychiatry* 2011;35:1–10.

17. Piketty T. *Capital in the Twenty-First Century.* Translated from the French by Arthur Goldhammer. Belknap Press, Harvard University Press, Boston, 2013.

18. Wilkinson R, Pickett K. *The Spirit Level: Why Greater Equality Makes Societies Stronger.* Bloomsbury Press, New York, 2009.

19. Cole J. Therapeutic efficacy of antidepressant drugs: a review. *American Journal of Psychiatry* 1964;131:448–455.

20. Cole J. Depression. *American Journal of Psychiatry* 1974:131:204–205.

21. Keller MB, Lavori PW, Klerman GL, et al. Low level and lack of predictors of somatotherapy and psychotherapy received by depressed patients. *Archives of General Psychiatry* 1986;43:458–511.

22. Keller MB, Bell WH, Endicott J, et al. *Clinical Guide to Depression and Bipolar Disorder. Findings From the Collaborative Depression Study.* American Psychiatric Publishing, Washington DC and London, 2013. An excellent summary!

23. Cai Q, Sheehan JJ, Wu B, et al. Descriptive analysis of the economic burden of treatment resistance in a major depressive episode. *Current Medical Research and Opinion* 2019. https//doi.org/10.1080/03007995.2019.1671087. Article FT0500/1671087.

24. Amos TB, Tandon N, Lefebvre P, et al. Direct and indirect cost burden and change of employment status in treatment-resistant depression: a matched cohort study using a US commercial claims data base. *Journal of Clinical Psychiatry* 2018;79. Doi:10.10.4088/JCP.17m11725.

25. Healy D. *The Antidepressant Era.* Harvard University Press, Cambridge MA and London. First paperback edition, Harvard University Press, 1999. Fourth printing, 2003.

26. Kuhn R. The treatment of depressive states with G2255 (imipramine hydrochloride). *American Journal of Psychiatry* 1958;115:459–464.

27. Pollack B. Clinical findings in the use of Tofranil in depressive and other psychiatric states. *American Journal of Psychiatry* 1959;116:312–316.

28. Schildkraut JJ. The catecholamine hypothesis of affective disorders: a review of supporting evidence. *American Journal of Psychiatry* 1965;122:509–522.
29. Nestler EJ. Antidepressant treatments in the 21st century. *Biological Psychiatry* 1998;44:526–533.
30. Carroll BJ, Feinberg M, Greden JF, et al. A specific laboratory test for the diagnosis of melancholia: standardization, validation, and clinical utility. *Archives of General Psychiatry* 1981;38:15–22.
31. Mullen PE, Linsell CR, Parker D. Influence of sleep disturbance and calorie restriction on biological markers of depression. *The Lancet* 1986;2(8515):1051–1055.
32. Ansseau M, Scheyvaerts M, Doumant A, et al. Concurrent use of REM latency, dexamethasone suppression, clonidine, and apomorphine tests as biological markers of endogenous depression: a pilot study. *Psychiatry Research* 1984;12:261–272.
33. Burke HM, Davis MC, Otte C, et al. Depression and cortisol responses to psychological stress: a meta-analysis. *Psychoneuroendocrinology* 2005;30:846–856.
34. Shorter E. *A History of Psychiatry*. John Wiley & Sons, New York, 1997.
35. Dworkin RW. The medicalization of unhappiness. *The Public Interest*, Summer 2001, pp. 85–89.
36. Kramer PD. *Listening to Prozac. A Psychiatrist Explores Antidepressant Drugs and the Remaking of the Self*. The Viking Press, New York, 1993.
37. Cowen PJ. Serotonin and depression: pathophysiologic mechanism or marketing myth? *Trends in Pharmacological Sciences*. Doi:10.1016/j/tips.2008.05.004.
38. Brugha TS. Depression undertreatment: lost cohorts, lost opportunities? *Psychological Medicine* 1995;25:3–6.
39. Duffy JF. A flaw in chemistry, not character. *Psychiatric Times*, August 1995, p. 14.
40. Duman RS, Monteggia LM. A neurotrophic model for stress-related mood disorders. *Biological Psychiatry* 2006;59:1116–1127.
41. Martinowich K, Manji H, Liu B. New insights into BDNF function in depression and anxiety. *Nature Neuroscience* 2007;10:1089–1093.
42. Mattson MP, Maudsley S, Martin B. BDNF and 5-HT: a dynamic duo in age-related neuroplasticity and neurodegenerative disorders. *Trends in Neurosciences* 2004;37:589–597.
43. Shirayama Y, Chen AC, Nakagawa S, et al. Brain-derived neurotrophic factor produces antidepressant effects in behavioral models of depression. *Journal of Neuroscience* 2002;22:3251–3261.
44. Santarelli L, Saxe M, Gross C, et al. Requirement of hippocampal neurogenesis for the behavioral effects of antidepressants. *Science* 2003;301:805–809.
45. Berton O, McClung CA, DiLeone RJ, et al. Essential role of BDNF in the mesolimbic dopamine pathway in social defeat stress. *Science* 2006;311:864–868.
46. Krishnan V, Nestler EJ. The molecular neurobiology of depression. *Nature* 2008;455(7215):894–902.
47. Baudry A, Mouillet S, Launay J-M, et al. New views on antidepressant action. *Current Opinion in Neurobiology* 2011;21:858–865.
48. Lieberman JA, Bymaster FP, Meltzer HY, et al. Antipsychotic drugs: comparison in animal models of efficacy, neurotransmitter regulation, and neuroprotection. *Pharmacological Reviews* 2008;60:358–403.
49. Young LT. Neuroprotective effects of antidepressant and mood-stabilizing drugs. *Journal of Psychiatry and Neuroscience* 2002;27:8–9.
50. Lucassen PJ, Meerlo P, Naylor AS, et al. Regulation of adult neurogenesis by stress, sleep disruption, exercise, and inflammation: implications for depression and antidepressant action. *European Neuropsychopharmacology* 2010;20:1–17.

51. Wemmie JA, Price MP, Welsh MJ. Acid-sensing ion channels: advances, questions, and therapeutic opportunities. *Trends in Neuroscience.* Doi:10.1016/j. tins.2006.06.06.014.
52. Coryell MW, Wunsch AM, Haenfler JM, et al. Acid-sensing ion channel-1-a in the amygdale, a novel therapeutic target in depression-related behavior. *Journal of Neuroscience* 2009;29:5381–5388.
53. Dhir A, Kulkarni SK. Involvement of sigma-1 receptors modulation in the antidepressant action of venlafaxine. *Neuroscience Letters* 2007;420:207–208.
54. Bermack JE, Debonnel G. The role of sigma receptors in depression. *Journal of Pharmacological Science* 2005;97:317–336.
55. Sabino SV, Cottone P, Parylak SL, et al. Sigma-1 receptor knockout mice display a depressive-like phenotype. *Behavioral Brain Research* 2009;198:472–478.
56. Wang J, Mack AL, Coop A, et al. Novel sigma (sigma) receptor agonists produce antidepressant-like effects in mice. *European Neuropsychopharmacology* 2007;17:708–716.
57. Schmidt HR, Kruse AD. The molecular function of O' receptors: past, present, and future. *Trends in Pharmacological Sciences* 2019;40. https://doi.org.10.1016/j. tips.2019.07.006.
58. Davidson M, Saoud J, Staner C, et al. Efficacy and safety of MIN-101, a 12-week randomized, double-blind, placebo-controlled trial of a new drug in development for the treatment of negative symptoms in schizophrenia. *American Journal of Psychiatry* 2017;174:1195–1202.
59. Mayberg HS, Brannan SK, Mahuurin RK, et al. Cingulate function in depression: a potential predictor of treatment response. *NeuroReport* 1997;8:1057–1061.
60. Mayberg HS. Modulating dysfunctional limbic-cortical circuits in depression: towards development of brain-based algorithms for diagnosis and optimized treatment. *British Medical Bulletin* 2003;65:193–207.
61. Holtzheimer PE, Mayberg HS. Stuck in a rut: rethinking depression and its treatment. *Trends in Neuroscience* 2011;34:1–9.
62. Kalin NH. Prefrontal cortical and limbic circuit alterations in psychopathology. *American Journal of Psychiatry* December 2019;176:12, Ajp.psychiatryonline.org.
63. Willner P, Scheel-Krüger J, Belzung C. The neurobiology of depression and antidepressant action. *Neuroscience and Biobehavioral Reviews* 2013. http://dx.doi. org/10.1016/j.neubiorev.2012.12.007.
64. Dodell-Feder D, DeLisi LE, Hooker CI. The relationship between default mode network connectivity and social functioning in individuals at familial high-risk for schizophrenia. *Schizophrenia Research* 2014;156:87–95.
65. Akiskal HS, McKinney, Jr WT. Overview of recent research in depression. Integration of ten conceptual models into a comprehensive clinical frame. *Archives of General Psychiatry* 1975;32:285–305.
66. Dean CE. Social inequality, scientific inequality, and the future of mental illness. *Philosophy, Ethics, and Humanities in Medicine* 2017;12:10. Doi:10.1186/s13010-107-0052-x.
67. López-Muñoz F, Álamo C, Juckel G, et al. Half a century of antidepressant drugs. On the clinical introduction of monoamine oxidase inhibitors, tricyclics, and tetracyclics. Part I: monoamine oxidase inhibitors. *Journal of Clinical Psychopharmacology* 2007;27:555–559.
68. Case A, Deaton A. *Deaths of Despair and the Future of Capitalism.* Princeton University Press, Princeton and Oxford, 2020.

9 Antidepressants

Do They Work? If So, When, How Often, and at What Costs?

Introduction

The introduction of imipramine (Tofranil) in 1958[1] marked a new phase in the treatment of depression, although only twelve people attended Roland Kuhn's introduction of the drug at the Second International Congress of Psychiatry in 1957.[2, p. 261] Indeed, the use of psychotropic drugs and the early enthusiasm over a new biological psychiatry met with considerable resistance, despite conditions in the asylums. In fact, just as the antidepressants (ADs) and antipsychotics (APs) were coming into vogue, books began to appear[2, pp. 274–275] that were harshly critical of psychiatry, including *The Myth of Mental Illness* by Thomas Szasz in 1960,[3] Erving Goffman's *Asylums* in 1961,[4] and Ken Kesey's great novel *One Flew Over the Cuckoo's Nest* in 1962.[5] Nevertheless, the marketing of imipramine (Tofranil) was quickly followed by additional tricyclic antidepressants (TCAs), including amitryptyline (Elavil) in 1961, and later by second-generation antidepressants, serotonin reuptake inhibitors (SSRIs), and serotonin-norepinephrine reuptake inhibitors (SNRIs) in the late 1990s and subsequently. The development of the latter two groups led to a rapid increase in the use of antidepressants but also to questions regarding their superiority to the older drugs and whether they were significantly superior to placebo. The very high initial costs of SSRIs and SNRIs raised additional concerns about their risk–benefit ratio. I shall explore these issues in detail.

Early Studies: Looking Good!

In 1958 Roland Kuhn published a study[1] on imipramine (Tofranil) which was notable for its size (500 subjects) and observations on which patients responded best. On the other hand, his paper mimicked the same problems found in the early studies on chlorpromazine,[6] including the absence of informed consent, no placebo controls, no rating scales or diagnostic studies, and vague data on response rates. Nevertheless, Kuhn made several interesting observations, noting first that imipramine's mode of action was "completely unknown."[1, p. 459] He also claimed that the effects of imipramine were "striking" in those patients whose movements were slowed (today's psychomotor retardation) and who felt much worse in the morning but better by evening (today's diurnal rhythm).

Clearly, some of these patients were severely depressed with somatic delusions and pervasive feelings of guilt, but even these symptoms improved, as did suicidality. These observations led to a question still debated today: Do ADs work preferentially well in patients with severe depression? This question rests in part on Kuhn's enthusiasm for the concept of an endogenous-reactive split in depression, a concept holding that endogenous depression arises from a combination of biochemical and genetic factors, whereas reactive depression is secondary to social and environmental stressors. He concluded that endogenous depression responds best to imipramine, setting a precedent that would be followed for decades, despite mounting evidence to the contrary.

In marked contrast to the commonly held but probably incorrect rule of today that ADs require two to three weeks to work, Kuhn wrote that patients respond within two to three days, "as a rule,"[1, p. 464] although in some instances one to four weeks may be needed, and, in some patients, there is no response. Regrettably, no percentages were given. However, he wrote that in many cases, recovery was complete,[1, p. 460] but patients relapsed rapidly after the medication is stopped—although it can be "cured" again with resumption of the drug. Therefore, the treatment is essentially symptomatic. We have a semantic problem here, since a purely symptomatic response is quite at odds with the term "cure." Not even the most ardent defender of ADs today would use the word "cure"; instead, the goal is remission.

With regard to side effects, Kuhn noted the absence of serious complications, a finding at variance with later observations but similar to statements made by Lehmann and Hanrahan[6] in their studies on chlorpromazine—although they viewed parkinsonian symptoms and apathy not as side effects, but as goals of therapy. It's also interesting that some patients received imipramine by injection (did they object?) yet he observed little in the way of significant dizziness or fainting. However, he did note dry mouth and tachycardia, as well as sweating and constipation, consistent with the anticholinergic effects of imipramine—a concern with all the TCAs. Kuhn also wrote that imipramine did not work well in schizophrenia and organic diseases and that it might precipitate a manic episode in those with manic-depressive illness, thus anticipating decades of research on the risks of ADs in bipolar disorder.

In 1959, a more detailed review of imipramine was published by Pollack,[7] based on the treatment of 273 patients with a variety of diagnoses. Pollack came to several of the same conclusions as had Kuhn, finding a greater response in those with endogenous depressions, especially in those with depression marked by psychomotor slowing.[7, p. 314] The overall treatment response was 72% in various forms of depression. (We shall see later that a 72% response rate, if found today, would be cause for celebration!)

Not only did Pollack provide response rates, but he also included a detailed table of side effects, noting that tremor, sweating, and dizziness occurred in about 10% of patients, but only five patients had side effects severe enough to warrant stopping the drug. Interestingly, he emphasized the phenomenon of sudden falls in those aged 60 and older, a side effect not previously described. There was *no* mention of cardiovascular problems. Pollack further noted that imipramine does "not increase norepinephrine or serotonin in the brain,"[7, p. 312] a claim not supported by any cited evidence, but perhaps the first to cast doubt on what would later become the catecholamine theory. He also emphasized a wide margin of safety for the drug, a statement few would support today.

The Advent of Controlled Studies

By the mid-1960s, a number of placebo-controlled trials of antidepressants had been carried out, prompting a narrative review by Jonathan Cole from the NIMH.[8] The available ADs included imipramine, amitryptyline, and several monamine oxidase inhibitors (MAOIs), including tranylcypromine (Parnate) and phenelzine (Nardil). Iproniazide (Marsilid) and others had already been withdrawn from the market, largely due to liver toxicity and concerns over hypertensive crises. The studies on MAOIs were less extensive and marked by decidedly mixed results. The data was most extensive for imipramine, as one might expect. In a forerunner to the contemporary debate, Cole found that imipramine was superior to placebo in 9 of the 15 controlled trials carried out in hospitalized patients but *failed to show an advantage in the other 6*. The data were mixed with regard to head-to-head comparisons of imipramine, amitryptyline, and MAOIs. Interestingly, ECT was given to a subgroup of these women, but imipramine achieved comparable results. (Why was ECT given in this particular group, since the women were reacting to stress?)

Other reviews in the 1960s and 1970s noted that about *one third of studies found no difference between ADs and placebo*.[9, 10] In an attempt to reconcile the inconsistencies found in these early studies, Cole wrote in 1964[8] that depression has "*the best prognosis for eventual recovery with or without treatment*." Ten years later, he remained optimistic, stating that depression is quite treatable, and the patient almost returns to a reasonably satisfactory pre-illness adjustment, although it is potentially lethal and a significant public health problem.[11, p. 204] I am not convinced that a disease reputed to be easily treatable and marked by spontaneous remissions and a return to premorbid functioning should simultaneously be described as lethal and a major public health problem!

As we noted in Chapter 8, data from the Collaborative Depression Study[12] clearly undercut the optimism of Cole and others, given the mounting evidence of chronicity and recurrence. We also noted in Chapter 8 the disturbing increase in the prevalence of depression and rates of suicide in the

United States, despite decades of research in depression with increasingly elegant biochemical/genetic/imaging/studies and a flood of new ADS and behavioral therapies. Yet the results with the newer ADs have been no better than those with the older ADs.[13] The effect sizes have hovered around 0.30, and, according to a review in 2019,[14] remission rates have been in the range of 37% to 43%. Why? One immediate question: Are ADs, in fact, effective? The question seems odd, given their popularity and extraordinary costs when first marketed. Nevertheless, let's take a look at some relevant studies, starting with comparisons of ADs with active placebos or older antidepressants.

Study Methodology: The Focus on Active Placebos

In 1989 Greenberg and Fisher reviewed 16 studies of ADs compared with placebo[15] and found a median difference of 21% in response rates. They also posed a specific methodological question: Would this modest difference hold up if a new AD was compared with an older AD or active placebo? With an active placebo, patients would experience more side effects vs an inactive placebo and thus help preserve the blind. Greenberg et al. then decided to examine effect sizes (ES) in studies where a new AD had been compared with an older AD *and* placebo. They found 22 studies and subjected them to a meta-analysis.[16] The results were striking.

The average ES for the older, standard AD was 0.19, and for the new drug 0.25. These effect sizes are quite low. The active drugs were better than placebo by only 0.2 SDs (standard deviations). The active drug produced an eight-point average improvement in the rating scales, such that *the average patient taking placebo was better off than 42% of those taking an AD!* The results were no different for outpatients vs inpatients and no different for age groups or gender. Note that self-ratings by patients showed no advantage of drug over placebo, raising the question of clinician bias.

A major problem with this study: The new ADs were limited to trazodone (Desyrel), amoxapine (Asendin), and maprotiline (Ludiomil). On the other hand, this was the era of *second-generation ADs* that had been hyped as much-improved successors to the TCAs, due to their alleged lack of side effects. Unfortunately, amoxapine was found to cause parkinsonian side effects while maprotiline induced seizures. Neither is used today, while trazodone is generally used for insomnia. In any case, this paper was one of the first to call attention to the importance of clinician bias, study design, and the crucial role of appropriate blinding.

Taking note of the Greenberg study, Russell Joffe and his associates[17] followed up with another meta-analysis of studies involving *an active comparator drug and placebo*. This study had an advantage in that several still-current SSRIs were studied, including fluoxetine (Prozac), paroxetine (Paxil), and fluvoxamine (Luvox). The database was expanded to 49 studies, 10% of which took place on inpatient units. The mean ES for active drugs was 0.49

compared with placebo, meaning that almost 70% of those taking medication were better off than those taking placebo. The reader will notice that the ES in this study is twice that found by Greenberg and associates, a very substantial difference! Did the inclusion of SSRIs make a difference? Probably not. The more significant factor appeared to be the inclusion of studies that used objective diagnostic criteria, in comparison to older studies using criteria developed prior to the introduction of the DSM-III in 1980. The use of objective criteria was associated with a better response. Unfortunately, the authors did not analyze patient self-reports. We should also take into account the fact that all the early studies included *only published reports, an omission that can significantly bias the data in favor of positive outcomes.*[18, 19] We shall have more to say about this later, and whether check-list diagnostic criteria are objective.

The Increase in Placebo Response Rates and Drug-Placebo Differences

Another problem with the drug vs placebo studies has been the growing response rates to placebo over the past three to four decades. In 2002, Walsh et al. published a widely cited study in *JAMA*,[20] in which they reviewed 75 studies of ADs published between 1981 and 2000 and found that placebo response rates averaged almost 30% but varied between 12% and 52%. The average response rate with ADS was 50% but *varied between 32% and 70%. If we take the extremes in this data, we could show that ADs are either very effective or less effective than placebo!* In addition, response rates to both ADs and placebo were positively correlated with year of publication, but the increase in the placebo response rate was even more statistically impressive. In fact, year of publication was the only significant predictor of placebo response. The authors could not say with certainty why the placebo response rate grew over time but speculated that patients with milder depressions were enrolling in studies and were more likely to be placebo responders. (Indeed, there have been concerns raised about the phenomenon of the "professional patient," who repeatedly volunteers for studies, no matter the issue.)

Another creative approach[21] to this problem confirmed that the response rate to ADS was about 50% vs 30% with placebo, but the authors noted a neglected problem. It seems that studies have assumed that all placebo responders would respond to ADs, but this is an assumption never confirmed. The point: If a significant number of placebo responders are antidepressant non-responders, the drug-placebo differences would be much greater!

It's probably no exaggeration to say that Irving Kirsch and his colleagues have been major players in the placebo wars that began in 1998 with their article "Listening to Prozac but hearing placebo."[22] The authors claimed that 75% of what ADs accomplish is duplicated by placebo. Similar results were found by other investigators.[23, 24] Kirsch and his collaborators[25] then analyzed data from RCTs submitted to the FDA on six ADs (fluoxetine, sertraline, paroxetine, venlafaxine, nefazodone [no longer on the market], and citalopram) developed between 1987 and 1999. They made the startling claim that these highly touted and very expensive ADs had led to only a two-point drop on the Hamilton Rating Scale for Depression compared with placebo. Put another way, *placebo was responsible for 80% of the antidepressant effect!* (Please note that the usual score on the HAM-D is about 25, indicting a moderately severe depression.)

The problem here is that no clinician—and, for that matter, no patient—would be able to clinically discern such a small change in depressive symptoms. In addition, a drop from 23 to 21 in a given patient, while conceivably besting placebo and thus counted as a responder, would mean the patient still had serious depressive symptoms! From another perspective, 22 of the 47 trials did not demonstrate a drug-placebo difference. On the bright side—from an industry perspective—no trial found that placebo was superior to drug. A further, albeit neglected finding: *Higher doses were no more effective than lower doses, echoing what we found with APs.* Kirsch et al. also noted[25] that the FDA reviewers hoped to have trials with at least a 70% completion rate, since that would enable them to better generalize the results to the larger population, but only *4 of the 47 RCTs met that goal.* The actual dropout rates were similar to what we've described with SGAs, in that a little more than 60% of patients in both the placebo and medication groups failed to complete the trial.

As one might expect, the key opinion leaders in psychiatry were not happy with his results, not to mention Pharma.

One major response was written by Michael Thase,[26] a psychopharmacologist at the University of Pittsburgh, who admitted that multiple studies had shown similar results. He nonetheless insisted that antidepressants have modest effects, even while calling attention to an earlier paper of his in which he noted *that some 50% of RCTs done by the industry were negative and that most of these had not been published!*[27] Had the negative trials been published, the data would yield a 10% difference between drug and placebo, consistent with the Kirsch et al. data. Another Kirsch et al. critic[28] noted that some people may be helped substantially by ADs and that the Kirsch et al. paper contained claims that were exaggerated and misleading, given the fact of individual variability.

Blockbuster Meta-Analytic Studies

While the debate continued over methodology and placebo response rates, ever-larger meta-analytic studies cast even more doubt over whether the development of new ADs had produced better efficacy. Among the first to raise our collective eyebrows was a 1993 meta-analysis of 63 RCTs that compared the efficacy and acceptability of TCAs with SSRIs.[29] (Only 20 of the 63 RCTs had data sufficient for a meta-analysis.) The older TCAs and related drugs showed a "small but non-significant benefit" over SSRIs. In the trials for which data had to be imputed, no significant differences were found. Remarkably, the pooled dropout rate for SSRIs was 32.3% vs 33.2% with TCAs, *much in contrast to the marketing hype stressing the greater tolerability of SSRIs*. The authors concluded[29, p. 683] that SSRIs had no significant advantages over the older drugs, whether with regard to efficacy or acceptability. Much to the horror of Pharma, they concluded that the routine use of selective serotonin reuptake inhibitors as the first-line treatment of depressive illness is not warranted. Sound familiar? Didn't we just find essentially the same message with regard to SGAs vs FGAs?

Yet meta-analytic studies continued to multiply, driven in part by growing concerns over the costs of ADs. Enough studies had accumulated by 2001 that another British investigator, Ian Anderson,[30] did an overview of 108 meta-analytic studies but focused on those that had compared ADs against one another, rather than ADs against placebo. He concluded that *SSRIs are as effective as TCAs*; that venlafaxine (Effexor) is superior to SSRIs; and that SSRIs are better tolerated than TCAs but have more gastrointestinal side-effects and cause more stimulation, an observation that proved problematic in the case of fluoxetine and assaultive behaviors (more on this later).

On the other hand, I have to admit that the early meta-analytic studies had some problems, including the lack of access to unpublished studies and the failure to use intent-to-treat analyses. (Note: An intent-to-treat analysis means that efficacy is determined in all the subjects who began the study, as opposed to determining efficacy in those who completed the study.) Bech and his group[31] therefore analyzed the Eli Lilly database on fluoxetine (a compilation of 69 RCTs) but did some winnowing due to problems with diagnostic criteria and other issues. That left 30 trials, published and unpublished, involving 4,000 patients. They looked at both completers and the intent-to-treat population. In the latter group, only *13.6%* showed improvement superior to placebo, giving a very low effect size. The most striking finding: *Fluoxetine was not superior to TCAs!*

Yet for all the concerns about cost and the lack of improvement in efficacy, SSRIs and SNRIs have dominated the market for years, no doubt due in part to the side effects of TCAs. That being the case, a meta-analysis[32] in 2009 didn't include the older agents and instead concentrated on 117 RCTs of 12 new-generation ADs: fluoxetine, sertraline, paroxetine, fluvoxamine, citalopram (Cylexa), mirtazapine (Remeron), bupropion (Wellbutrin), duloxetine (Cymbalta), escitalopram (Lexapro), venlafaxine, and two ADs not marketed in the U.S.: milnacipran and reboxetine. The study was unusual since it obtained not just data on direct comparisons of the drugs, but indirect comparisons as well. (The formal term for this is a multiple-treatments meta-analysis.) In addition to published studies, the authors obtained 15 unpublished studies from drug companies.

The *most efficacious* were mirtazapine, venlafaxine, sertraline, and escitalopram while the best tolerated were escitalopram, citalopram, sertraline, and bupropion. Taking into account the balance between efficacy and acceptability, the authors concluded that *escitalopram and sertraline might be the best choices for the acute treatment of major depression.* They did not undertake a formal economic analysis, but only escitalopram and duloxetine were still on patent and presumably more expensive. However, Ioannidis[33] noted that in the registration trials of sertraline, *only one was positive, while three negative studies had not been published,* again raising the issue of publication bias. In addition, most differences between drugs were clinically trivial. He added that research on ADs is totally under industry control, lending more uncertainty to the conclusions. Another critic[34] noted that a communications agency working for the manufacturer of sertraline had developed a list of studies to be assigned, presumably to key opinion leaders, perhaps introducing bias in the results.

In 2018, Cipriani et al. published an even larger network meta-analysis of 522 trials,[35] now including RCTs and head-to-head comparisons of 21 antidepressants, including TCAs. *While all ADs were superior to placebo,* the two most efficacious drugs were agomelatine (not available in the U.S.) and *amitriptyline, the second-oldest TCA and a drug marked by severe side effects.* (What does this say about the funds invested in psychopharmacology? Where is the payoff?) Escitalopram followed, then mirtazapine, paroxetine (Paxil), venlafaxine, and vortioxetine. *Among the least efficacious: fluoxetine,* fluvoxamine, reboxetine, and trazodone. The most tolerable included agomelatine, citalopram, escitalopram, and others. Not surprisingly, amitriptyline, clomipramine, duloxetine, and fluvoxamine had the highest dropout rates. With regard to the efficacy of amitriptyline, Anderson,[30] in his meta-analysis in 2001, also found it superior to SSRIs, but the side effects were severe.

We shall return to the Kirsch et al. studies later, but let's turn to a problem that plagues us even today: publication bias.

Publication Bias

The concerns raised by Kirsch and his group regarding publication bias were supported by a much larger analysis[18] of the FDA data on 74 RCTs of 12 antidepressants; over 12,000 patients were included. The drugs included all the major players. The FDA had found that 38 of the 74 studies had positive results. To no one's surprise, 37 of the 38 were published. In marked contrast, of the 36 studies with either questionable or negative results, only 3 were published as not positive. *Worse, 11 of the 36 negative studies were published with a positive spin,* in marked contrast to the FDA evaluation! This resulted in 94% of the 51 published studies being viewed as positive, in contrast to the FDA's view that only 51% were positive. Two other findings are worth noting:

- Studies found positive by the FDA were 12 times more likely to be published than studies found negative.

- In the published articles, the ES for each drug was greater than the ES found by the FDA, with a median inflation of 32%.

Given the results just reviewed, one strongly suspects that the 10% difference in drug-placebo efficacy is too high, and the NNT cited by Dr. Thase is too low.[26] In any case, psychiatrists and patients are not getting unbiased data on which to base decisions about ADs. Unfortunately, the problems with publication bias continue, as shown by Duyx et al.[36] in a 2017 meta-analysis demonstrating that positive studies are much more likely to be published. A variety of tactics have been employed in gaining publication, including spinning the results in abstracts and titles, omitting or altering the protocol-specified primary outcome, and adding well-known investigators as authors, despite their lack of involvement in the research.[37]

Mental health professionals, patients, families, and the government should demand honest and complete reporting of study results, methodology, and sources of bias. Current practices are simply unacceptable.

Barriers to Better Antidepressants

In addition to publication bias, what are the other barriers? Indeed, if such practices continue, of what value are the studies? And what of the trials themselves? Are they being conducted correctly? One would think so, given that numerous articles and guidelines have provided investigators with methodologically sound approaches.[38–40] Are they being followed? One attempt at answering this question can be found in a study by Steiner and Joffe,[38] who did a painstaking review of 69 RCTS of ADs. They were principally concerned with whether the trials provided data of sufficient quality such that the results could be included in a meta-analysis. Unfortunately, *none* of the RCTs met all the criteria set forth by their guidelines. Now, some might say that the proposed criteria are too demanding, but even where the criteria called only for the inclusion of the final sample size and values for the means and standard deviations (SDs), only 13% of the studies qualified!

Sadly, in another detailed review of methodology 10 years later, Ioannidis[41, p. 8] listed many of the same problems and bluntly added that lies are not the way to make scientific progress! Many of the problems are commonplace, including small sample sizes, lack of an active comparator, no systematic assessment of study blindedness, short-term studies, selective reporting, the lack of solid evidence for using a 50% drop in a rating scale as the measure of responsiveness, and excluding "real-world" patients,[42] in part due to safety rules established by the FDA. Yet, in a rather unique study in the Netherlands, van der Lem et al.[43] divided 1,653 patients into those who would be eligible for an AD trial and those not eligible and found *no difference in outcome!* (Like other groups, they found that 17% to 25% would be eligible for enrollment in a trial.) Unfortunately, the response rates were very low: *only 28% responded, and 21% remitted.*

Do Antidepressants Work Only in Severe Depression?

A fundamental assumption is that a given AD should be effective for most patients who have a major depressive disorder. This is clearly the dream of Pharma, which, after all, hopes to profit from the $10 million or so necessary to bring an AD to market and make that profit in the shortest possible time. Company-sponsored studies and marketing strategies are designed with that goal in mind, so in most instances, the company has little motivation to break down the enrolled patients into smaller groups, some of which might have a better response to the drug than others. There seems little question but that the one-drug-fits-all approach, vital to the promotion of fluoxetine, may well lose valuable information along the way. On the other hand, the statistical power of an already small sample size becomes further compromised when the population is subdivided.

Nevertheless, several recent studies have focused on a particular subgroup with severe depression. We turn once again to the ubiquitous Irving Kirsch and his group,[44] who looked again at the clinical trial data submitted to the FDA for approval of the new ADS (see the list cited earlier). In this study, however, they restricted their analysis to the ADs that had complete data: fluoxetine, paroxetine, nefazodone, and venlafaxine. The drug-placebo difference was 1.80 points on the HAM-D—similar to their earlier findings—which was statistically significant but *did not* meet the three-point criteria set by the British National Institute for Clinical Excellence (NICE) for clinical significance.[40] The ES was 0.32, well below the NICE criterion of 0.50. Yet, as Kirsch and his group wrote, the mean change did not fairly describe the results, given that the degree of change varied widely. They therefore examined "moderator variables" that might influence the results, including type of drug, duration of treatment, and severity of depression at baseline.

Jackpot! The difference between drug and placebo increased as a function of initial severity, wherein the HAM-D score was about 28 (scores of 23 to 28 reflect very severe depression; from 19 to 22, severe depression). There was no difference in drug-placebo scores at moderate levels of depression, but, *when the HAM-D scores were at the upper end of severe depression, the drug-placebo difference was clinically significant.* However, those patients with a HAM-D score greater than 28 had less improvement than did those with scores of 23 to 28.

Making matters even more complicated, we have to recognize that the improvement in drug-placebo differences was *not* due to an increase in AD efficacy, but instead a fall-off in placebo response as severity increased. Kirsch et al.[44, p. e45] concluded that "there seems little evidence to support the prescription of antidepressant medication to any but the most severely depressed patients unless alternative treatments have failed to provide benefit." This recommendation has failed to have any clinical impact. In fact, recent evidence indicates that ADs are being used for an increasingly wide range of symptoms and illnesses, with little regard for FDA approval or severity of depression.[45]

Kirsch and his associates have not been alone in finding a relationship between severity and a greater differentiation between drug and placebo, but, as we have seen so often, the evidence is mixed. For example, Khan et al.[46] found more symptom change with ADs as baseline HAM-D scores increased, but this did not occur with placebo. However, Khan's group later examined trials sorted according to entry criteria and found that trials requiring a higher level of depressive symptoms did *not* have a better outcome.[47] Another investigation[44] pointed out several problems with these two studies, one being the preponderance of severely depressed patients, a population that stands in marked contrast to the 71% of patients in a community survey who had HAM-D scores of less than 22.

Given these issues, Fournier and colleagues[48] decided to investigate studies in which patients had a broad range of severity. They excluded studies using a placebo washout period. These criteria resulted in only six studies being accepted for the meta-analysis, three of which used imipramine (rarely used in today's world) and three of which used paroxetine, clearly limiting the generalizability of the findings. Yet their results were similar to those just reviewed, in that *superiority of drug over placebo increased with increasing severity of depression at baseline* and reached clinical significance at a baseline HAM-D score of 25.

They concluded that even in the face of these results, it is not possible to state with certainty whether ADS are more effective in the more severely depressed patients or whether the fall-off in placebo efficacy is more important. Nevertheless, the cumulative data suggests[48] that *we have moderate evidence that ADs produce greater benefits in those patients with severe depression.* As usual, contrary evidence is out there. For example, an analysis[49] of six SSRIs and two SNRIs approved for use in Sweden found that all drugs were superior to placebo, *independent of severity of depression.* In the UK, Wiles et al.[50] compared citalopram to reboxetine (a noradrenalin reuptake inhibitor) in an RCT and found no interaction between treatment and severity of depression, while Gibbons et al.,[51] in a synthesis of 20 RCTs of fluoxetine and venlafaxine, found no significant evidence that baseline severity was related to outcome.

Yet we do have to take into account those suffering from depression of lesser severity. As we shall see, the evidence also indicates that various forms of psychotherapy are available and effective. In addition, those critical of the Kirsch et al. studies[52, 53] point to problems common to such investigations, including the lack of "real-world" patients, the problems engendered by placebo responders, separating out the state of depression from baseline functioning, spontaneous improvement, and the lack of any independent means of validating the diagnosis—a recurrent and serious problem in psychiatry.

At this point, let's visit the problems associated with treatment of chronic or persistent depression, formerly called dysthymia. Is this a less severe form of depression? If so, does it respond to ADs?

Antidepressants in Dysthymia (Persistent Depressive Disorder)

Dysthymic disorder has now been labeled persistent depressive disorder (PDD) in DSM-5. The diagnostic criteria represent a consolidation of dysthymia and the DSM-IV chronic major depression,[54, p. 168] but I will use the term *dysthymia* to be consistent with the citations.

Whatever the term, it has been studied less frequently, as shown in a meta-analysis of RCTS,[55] wherein 177 trials focused on MDD but only 17 on dysthymia. While this form of depression has fewer and usually less severe depressive symptoms, patients can remain symptomatic for over a decade and often use higher rates of medical services and psychotropic drugs than the general population. In addition, some have found that the general psychological and social burden in dysthymia may exceed that found with MDD.[56]

Given these issues and given the mixed evidence of AD efficacy in dysthymia, a meta-analysis[55] found that the rate of placebo response in dysthymia was actually significantly *lower* than that found in MDD (30% vs 38%). Although depressive symptoms were graded as more severe in MDD, the response rates were no different: 52.4% for dysthymia and 54.3% for MDD. The NNT was quite low in both (4.4 for dysthymia; 6.1 for MDD), so it appears that ADS in are useful in dysthymia.

Drilling deeper into the many depressive subtypes, we find "minor depression," sometimes labeled subsyndromal or subthreshold depression.[56] In this pharmacological world of ours, not even the slightest deviation from normality escapes a diagnosis! On the other hand, although those with minor depression are required to have *only two depressive symptoms* "most of the time" for at least two weeks, there is evidence of impaired social function and a poorer quality of life—which led many to question the term "minor," now dropped from DSM-5.

In a meta-analytic study[57] of the efficacy of ADs and benzodiazepines in minor depression, the authors found only six studies that met their inclusion criteria. Moreover, the quality of the studies was poor. However, they found that the benefits of ADs did *not* exceed those of placebo, with a mean difference of only 2.2 points on the HAM-D, a difference that did not meet the NICE standard (3 points) for clinical relevance.[40] They concluded that depression exists on a continuum and returned to the theme played by Kirsch et al., insisting that severity plays a major role in AD response while psychological therapies may be helpful in minor depression.

Speaking of a return to older themes, Arnow et al.[58] found that classifying depression into melancholia, atypical, or anxious depression was of no help in predicting response rates to ADs. The reader may recall that the early success of imipramine was based on treating melancholia, but subsequent studies often failed to show a positive response.[59, 60]

The Levkowitz et al. study[55] is notable for providing evidence indicating that ADs can provide relief even in the case of lesser severity and fewer symptoms—at least, as assessed by rating scales. But the discerning reader will note that we have a major problem in that all such studies rely heavily on self-report, whether the psychiatrist or investigator is gathering a clinical history or using one of the many clinical rating scales routinely used in research. These scales offer a modicum of respectability in that they are well studied, offer a systematic method of assessing symptoms and symptom change, and offer room for observations of behavior. Nevertheless, the rating scales depend on the patient accurately reporting his or her current symptoms and past history. I shall have more to say about this in the chapter on psychiatric diagnoses, but I must insist that our current approach to assessment and diagnoses bears a remarkable resemblance to the approach used 60 years ago. Shameful!

Do Men and Women Differ in Their Response to Antidepressants?

Severity of depression is one factor that affects response rates, but a number of investigators have also focused on gender differences. This seems logical, since epidemiologic studies have shown a higher incidence of depression in women[61] as well as differences in symptoms, with women having more anxiety and somatic symptoms.[62] In addition, several fundamental gender differences have been shown in plasma levels of ADs, markers of the serotonin transporter, as well as a differential sensitivity to side effects (see Baca et al.[63] for a review). In 2019, another group[64] found that female mice seemed more sensitive than male mice to sertraline-induced changes in the serotonergic systems located in the hippocampus and prefrontal cortex. The authors cite other animal studies showing more depressive-like behaviors in rodents whose ovaries has been removed while estrogens prolonged time in the forced-swim test. (The Web of Science lists multiple bench studies aimed at clarifying the basic science of gender differences, for those interested.).

The results of clinical studies have been mixed. Some have suggested that women respond better to SSRIs than men,[62] but others have not.[65] Quitkin et al.[66] found that the response rates to TCAs and SSRIs were similar in men and women, but women had a better response to MAOIs! In another effort to settle this issue, Baca and his group[63] studied 239 patients with non-psychotic major depression who were randomized to sertraline or imipramine for eight weeks. The response rates to sertraline were 20% higher in women than men (72% vs 52%), with similar results in anxiety. In addition, the dropout rates with sertraline were much lower in women (11% vs 28%). Response rates in men did not differ between the two drugs. Unfortunately, this study was *open label*, so the results must be viewed with caution. The famous STAR★D trial found that remission was more likely in women but *also* in those with higher levels of education and income, those who were employed, and Caucasians.[67] (We should also note that STAR★D was also open-label for the patients and investigators, but not the outcome raters.)

In a 2014 review[68] of the gender issues, Weissman noted a number of problems, particularly the greater prevalence of women in studies of depression, in part secondary to their greater proclivity for seeking help from the health care system. This imbalance does affect the statistical power to detect moderators of outcome, especially in smaller studies. She went on to note the mixed results in a number of studies, noting the lack of definitive evidence regarding moderators. Given the mixed evidence, one notes that a 2018 review of 12 guidelines[69] aimed at the treatment of unipolar depression *did not include gender* as one of their focal points.

While the data on the gender differences remains controversial, there is little doubt that women are more frequent uses of ADs, as shown by the National Center for Health Statistics,[70] which noted that women are 2.5 times more likely to be taking ADs than men, except at ages 12 through 17. In women ages 40 through 59, 23% of women are taking ADs, the *highest* in any group by age or gender. In addition, women are more likely to take ADs than men at every level of depression severity, although rates increased in both genders as severity increased. Even at the level of mild depression, 24% of women and 11% of men are using ADs. *About 8% of men and women are taking ADs, even if no depressive symptoms are present!*

These data should raise concerns about not only the root causes of such massive use of ADs in the population, but also the risks of ADs generally, and specifically in women. Another issue: Do women experience depression differently from men? Using a new scale that includes possible "male-type" depressive symptoms,[71] men were found to experience more anger, irritability, substance abuse, and risks-taking behaviors—in additional to traditional symptoms—than did women. When this was taken into account, there was no difference in the prevalence of depression among men and women. However, these differences in symptoms would seem to call for different treatment approaches.

Antidepressants and Suicide: Helpful, Harmful, or Neutral?

In Chapter 8, we reviewed evidence showing that the prevalence of depression and the rates of suicide in the U.S. have risen substantially since the 1990s, so we will not repeat that here. Have antidepressants made a difference? One would think so, since the use of ADs doubled from 13 million people in 1996 to 27 million in 2005.[72] However, a major problem in untangling these relationships is the very low base rate of suicide: about 14 per 100,000, depending of the study, making prediction very difficult if not impossible.[73]

In 1990, a report from Massachusetts General Hospital raised the possibility that fluoxetine might induce suicidality.[74] Additional reports surfaced in the media describing instances of suicide and homicide among patients taking fluoxetine,[75] resulting in a number of lawsuits against Eli Lilly, the manufacturer, and a warning label added to the package insert in 1990. Yet similar concerns had arisen with other ADS, as noted by Avery and Winokur in 1978.[76] Multiple studies followed,[77] but case reports always found emergence of suicidality while RCTs did not. 1n 1991, a meta-analysis[78] of 17 RCTS comparing fluoxetine, TCAs, and placebo found that patients taking fluoxetine reported *less* suicidality than with TCAs or placebo, while another study found no association between SSRIs or other ADs and suicidality! Not surprisingly, the evidence continued to be mixed in a large number of subsequent reports.[79–81]

Nevertheless, the FDA in 2003[82] issued a public health advisory emphasizing the emergence of suicidality in pediatric patients. This was followed by a black-box warning in 2004 aimed at the use of ADs in children.[83] In a meta-analysis[84] by the FDA of 23 RCTs of ADs used in the treatment of in MDD, generalized anxiety disorder, ADHD social anxiety disorder, and obsessive-compulsive disorder, no trials reported a completed suicide. However, with SSRIs, a 66% increase in risk was found, but this rose to 95% for all ADs across all disorders. *Yet the risk difference for the primary outcome (suicidality) was 0.01, indicating that between one and three patients out of 100 being treated would have an increase in suicidality.* Now, this seems like a small risk, but on a population level—or to a family—this was worrisome and helped spur the black-box warning. Caution: Risk could not be determined past 16 weeks, given the trial lengths.

In 2006, the FDA conducted another meta-analysis[85] of 372 RCTs of the *newer* ADs used in adults, but the data was based on spontaneous adverse event reports from the trials, always a tricky approach since this depends on the accuracy of the reports, instead of a prospective follow-up. *For those ages 18 to 24, the risk of suicidality approached significance, with a 62% increase, but for adults aged 25 to 64, the risk was decreased, and in the geriatric group, the risk was even less.* As one might expect, the black-box warning was expanded to include the 18-to-24-year-old group. In a study[86] specifically aimed at the data within the FDA Adverse Reporting System, the authors found that TCAs have a significantly higher risk of events involving suicidality than do SNRIs and SSRIs. This was expected, given the cardiovascular toxicity of TCAs. Please note that the FDA has included in its warnings that *patients of all ages* should be closely observed for clinical worsening and the emergence of suicidality.

With regard to the risk associated with individual drugs in pediatric trials, venlafaxine was the only agent for which the risk was statistically significant,[84] while in two adult trials, paroxetine was associated with an increased risk (cited in Simon[87]). In another study, Simon et al.[88] calculated that the risk of a serious suicide attempt during the first six months of AD treatment is less than 1 in 300 in children and less than 1 in 1,000 in adults. *The risk of suicide was highest in the month before beginning an AD* and declined progressively afterward. Again, an increase in risk starting after initiation of treatment was found only with TCAs and trazodone.

Yet the studies continued, with good news coming from a 27-year observational study of 757 patients at five academic medical centers who had been exposed or not exposed to ADs.[89] Those exposed had a *20% drop in the risk of suicide attempts or completions.* Nevertheless, there were concerns about the practical impact of the FDA warnings. Indeed, after the warnings, prescription rates of ADs fell in all age groups, but more so in patients up to age 14, where a 30% decline in new scripts occurred.[90] Unfortunately, *the suicide rate in the U.S. among youth rose by 14% between 2003 and 2004,* the *largest increase ever recorded in a one-year period!*[90] Yet psychiatrists and other caregivers failed to follow up on compensatory measures, such as using more psychotherapy or increasing the frequency of office visits.[91]

Given the concerns about venlafaxine and paroxetine noted earlier, I should balance those concerns with data from a 2018 study,[92] in which the authors approached efficacy from a different perspective. Instead of simply examining the literature for the effect size, they analyzed the FDA registered trials of second-generation ADs for the *magnitude of the evidence load*, using a Bayesian meta-analysis. In other words, using a combination of the effect size and the evidence load might help differentiate between and among the ADs. In fact, the evidence load pointed to clear differences. While all ADs, except bupropion and vilazodone, had strong evidence for efficacy, the highest pooled effect size was found for venlafaxine, an AD that also had the highest evidence load, with paroxetine just below it. Note the contrast between these findings and those of Cipriani et al., also in 2018,[35] in which the efficacy of venlafaxine was ranked below amitriptyline, escitalopram, mirtazapine, and paroxetine. On the other hand, the present study[92] did not rank any of the older drugs.

Can Antidepressants Prevent Relapse?

Given the high relapse rate found by the Collaborative Depression Study, this is a critical question. Guidelines have recommended continuation of ADs for four to nine months after recovery, but, as a practical matter, considerable variation occurs. As one might expect, numerous studies that have examined this issue, such that by 2003 Geddes et al.,[93] were able to pool results from 37 RCTs involving 4,410 participants treated with TCAs, SSRIs, and/or psychotherapy for an average of 12 months, although six trials lasted two to three years. *The odds of relapse were reduced by 70%* in those who continued medication, with a relapse rate of 18%, vs 41% of those taking placebo. The reduction appeared to be independent of duration of treatment prior to randomization. However, 18% of those who continued medication dropped out of the study, vs 15% of those taking placebo. In a 2011 commentary, Davis et al.[94] cited multiple studies finding that ADs not only reduce relapse, but, over time, also reduce the number of depressive episodes, perhaps by as many as half. While that figure is somewhat speculative, any approach that can decrease the morbidity of MDD is welcome.

A 2019 Cochrane random-effects meta-analysis[95] of continuation and maintenance treatments for persistent depressive disorder found that relapse occurred in 13.9%, vs 33.8% with placebo, but *this did not hold if the analysis focused only on studies with a low risk of bias!* The body of evidence did not permit any conclusions regarding the effects of individual drugs, combinations of drug and therapy, or therapy alone. This is unfortunate, but the inclusion of non-randomized studies no doubt sank the study from the start. Why include such low-quality studies?

More Adverse Events

While mounting evidence suggests that ADs are helpful in many patients, we must remember that ADs and other psychotropic agents may be used in overdose and can be lethal. In the early years of AD development, TCAs were the leading cause of death by overdose.[96] Fortunately, SSRIs were considerably safer, but in an analysis of cases reported to the U.S. Poison Control Centers in 2000 through 2014,[80] the rate of serious outcomes associated with psychotropics rose in a linear fashion, with *serious outcomes doubling during those 15 years, while fatal outcomes increased by 32%.* Higher morbidity and mortality rates were reported with TCAs and MAOIs. Lithium was also associated with higher morbidity and mortality, as were quetiapine, olanzapine, bupropion, and carbamazepine. Population growth did not account for the outcome. This data is worrisome, but it is likely an underestimate, since reports to poison control centers are voluntary.

We also have an analysis of emergency room visits[97] from 2009 through 2011 for adverse events secondary to psychotropic medications, noting that visits associated with the use of ADs were far less common than those associated with APs, lithium, and stimulants. In 2019, a meta-analysis[98] of 45 meta-analytic studies that reported on adverse health outcomes associated with antidepressants initially found an association with the risk of suicide or suicide attempt in youth, preterm birth, low Apgar scores, and autism spectrum disorders. However, after sensitivity analyses that adjusted for confounding by indication, *none of these associations remained significant, indicating that the underlying illness was the principal player, not ADs.* The authors also emphasized highly suggestive evidence that ADs protect against suicidality in adults, prompting them to conclude that the benefits appear to outweigh the risks.

Nevertheless, some people will not feel comfortable taking ADs or cannot tolerate them. In this context, we should not forget that psychotherapeutic efforts should be considered. Among the best studied are cognitive behavioral therapy, interpersonal psychotherapy, problem-solving therapy, and psychodynamic therapy.[99] Psychotherapy is usually begun during the acute phase or continuation phase of treatment and then continued for preventative purposes, often in combination with medication. In recent years, we have seen intense interest in mindfulness-based interventions, including mindfulness-based cognitive therapy.[100] In a 2013 meta-analysis of seven psy-chotherapeutic interventions,[101] all were superior to wait-list controls, with impressive ESs of d = 0.62–0.92.

Nevertheless, I must emphasize that all these efforts will be limited by the socioeconomic problems faced by our patients and families. For example, after an investigation into the relationship between unemployment and MDD, the authors[102] found a high risk of major depression. Sustained MDD was also associated with an elevated risk of becoming unemployed while others have found that population density, income inequality, and deprivation increased the risk of non-affective psychotic disorders by 18% to 28%.[103] Others have noted a relationship between the decline of hospital beds for mental illnesses and the increase in suicide,[104] as well higher rates of suicide in less urban areas,[105] secondary to shortages of health care providers, greater social isolation, the economic recession, and more access to lethal means. We shall explore these issues in more detail in Chapters 14 and 15, as well as problems with the diagnostic criteria for major depression,[106] the markedly different clinical presentations,[107] and the different trajectories post treatment.[108]

Clinical Notes

1. Sadly, the development of newer ADs has not resulted in any substantial gains in therapeutic efficacy, despite their very high initial costs. The rate of improvement with active drug over placebo is probably in the 10%-25% range. ADs may be more helpful in preventing relapse than in treating an acute episode of depression, but evidence does support the effectiveness of ADs in adults and a protective effect against suicidality.

2. Patients, families, and mental health providers need to be aware of the markedly different pathways taken by people with depression. About 77% have only brief contact with professionals, while 3% have prolonged contact and treatment. To no one's surprise, the best predictors of prolonged contact include inpatient treatment of the first episode, being female, experiencing psychotic symptoms, and severity of the first episode.

3. We also see a remarkable number of differing symptom presentations, with one group finding some 1,000 different possibilities,[107] clearly complicating the choice of treatment and research approaches.

4. The SSRIs, SNRIs, and other, newer ADs have fewer cardiovascular events and fewer anticholinergic side effects but are associated with high rates of sexual dysfunction and, on occasion, signs of parkinsonism with tremors and restlessness. A small percentage may develop dyskinesia. Unfortunately, many psychiatrists are not aware of these adverse neurological events.

5. Psychiatrists underestimate the frequency of side effects. Patients should insist that their psychiatrists and other providers pay close attention to

their complaints, including sexual dysfunction. It appears that some prescribers are reluctant to ask about sexual dysfunction, which is common with SSRIs.

6. While ADs may lead to an increase in suicidality in youth, absolute rates of completed suicides remain very low. More definitive evidence would require studies of at least 150,000 patients, and that seems unlikely.

7. SSRI-induced motor restlessness (akathisia) may be mistaken for anxiety and, in rare cases, may lead to hostility and aggressive behaviors.

8. Genetic studies and biomarkers provide little in the way of helpful information, at least at this point. The exception may be in assessing the impact of drug-metabolizing enzymes on blood levels, side effects, and response rates, although debate continues over the clinical applicability of this information.

9. Patients, families, and providers should always consider alternatives to ADs, including cognitive behavioral therapy (CBT) and other forms of psychotherapy, as well as exercise. These approaches should be offered to those who cannot tolerate ADs or have other objections to medications. A number of studies have found that a combination of ADs and psychotherapy may be superior to either alone.

10. At this point, it is not possible to predict which people will respond to the various interventions now available, despite at least 1,000 treatment trials.[109] However, developing predictive data is a high priority.

In the next chapter, we will discuss the use of ADs in pregnancy, vascular events, and abnormal movements. Chapter 11 provides a more detailed discussion of alternatives to ADs, including ketamine, transcranial stimulation, hallucinogens, and "novel" approaches in treatment-resistant depression.

References

1. Kuhn R. The treatment of depressive states with G22355 (Imipramine hydrochloride). *American Journal of Psychiatry* 1958;115:459–464.
2. Shorter E. *A History of Psychiatry. From the Era of the Asylum to the Age of Prozac.* John Wiley & Sons, New York, Chichester, Brisbane, Toronto, Singapore and Weinheim, 1997.
3. Szasz T. *The Myth of Mental Illness.* Harper and Row, New York, 1960.
4. Goffman E. *Asylums: Essays on the Social Situations of Mental Patients and Other Inmates.* Doubleday, Anchor, New York, 1961.
5. Kesey K. *One Flew Over the Cuckoo's Nest.* The Viking Press, New York, 1962.
6. Lehmann HE, Hanrahan GE. Chlorpromazine: a new inhibiting agent, for psychomotor excitement and manic states. *AMA Archives of Neurology and Psychiatry* 1954;71:227–231.
7. Pollack B. Clinical findings in the use of imipramine in depressive and other psychiatric states. *American Journal of Psychiatry* 1959;116:312–317.
8. Cole JO. Therapeutic efficacy of antidepressant drugs: a review. *Journal of the American Medical Association* 1964;124:448–455.

9. Smith A. Studies on the effectiveness of antidepressant drugs. *Psychopharmacology Bulletin* 1969;5:1–53.

10. Morris J, Beck A. The efficacy of antidepressant drugs: a review of research (1958–1972) *Archives of General Psychiatry* 1974;30:667–674.

11. Cole JO. Depression. *American Journal of Psychiatry* 1974;131:204–205.

12. Keller MB, Bell WH, Endicott J, et al. *Clinical Guide to Depression and Bipolar Disorder. Findings From the Collaborative Depression Study.* American Psychiatric Publishing. Washington DC and London, 2013.

13. Holtzheimer PE, Mayberg HS. Stuck in a rut. Rethinking depression. *Trends in Neuroscience* 2011;34:1–5.

14. Liechsenring F, Steinert C, Ioannidis JPA. Toward a paradigm shift in treatment and research of mental disorders. *Psychological Medicine* 2019;49:2111–2117.

15. Greenberg RP, Fisher S. Examining antidepressant effectiveness: findings, ambiguities, and some vexing puzzles. In: *The Limits of Biological Treatments for Psychological Distress: Comparisons with Psychotherapy and Placebo.* Editors Fisher S, Greenberg RP. Erlbaum, Hillsdale NJ, 1989.

16. Greenberg RP, Bornstein RF, Greenberg MD, et al. A meta-analysis of antidepressant outcome under "blinder" conditions. *Journal of Consulting and Clinical Psychology* 1992;60:664–669.

17. Joffe R, Sorkolov S, Streiner D. Antidepressant treatment of depression: a meta-analysis. *Canadian Journal of Psychiatry* 1996;41:613–616.

18. Turner EH, Matthews AM, Linardatos E, et al. Selective publication of antidepressant trials and its influence on apparent efficacy. *New England Journal of Medicine* 2008;358:252–260.

19. Mathew SJ, Charney DS. Publication bias and efficacy of antidepressants. *American Journal of Psychiatry* 2009;166:140–145.

20. Walsh BT, Seidman SN, Sysko R, et al. Placebo response in studies of major depression: variable, substantial, and growing. *Journal of the American Medical Association* 2002;287:1840–1847.

21. Rihmer Z, Gonda X. Is drug-placebo difference in short-term antidepressant drug trials on unipolar major depression much greater than previously believed? *Journal of Affective Disorders* 2008;108:195–198.

22. Kirsch I, Saperstein G. Listening to Prozac but hearing placebo: a meta-analysis of antidepressant medication. *American Psychological Association. Prevention and Treatment* 1. Article 0029. http://journals.apa.org/prevention/volume1/pre0010002a.html.

23. Greenberg RP, Bornstein RF, Zborowski MJ, et al. A meta-analysis of fluoxetine outcome in the treatment of depression. *Journal of Nervous and Mental Disease* 1994;182:547–551.

24. Khan A, Warner HA, Brown WA. Symptom reduction and suicide risk in patients treated with placebo in antidepressant clinical trials: an analysis of the food and drug administration data base. *Archives of General Psychiatry* 2000;57:311–317.

25. Kirsch I, Moore TJ, Scoboria A, et al. The emperor's new drugs: an analyses of antidepressant medication data submitted to the U.S. food and drug administration. *Prevention & Treatment* 5. Article 23. www.journals.apa.org/prevention/volume5/pre0050023a.html.

26. Thase ME. Antidepressant effects: the suit may be small, but the fabric is real. *Prevention & Treatment* 5. Article 32, posted July 15, 2002. American Psychological Association.

27. Thase ME. How should efficacy be evaluated in randomized clinical trials for treatments of depression? *Journal of Clinical Psychiatry* 1999;60(suppl 14):23–31.

28. Salomone JD. Antidepressants and placebos: conceptual problems and research strategies. *Prevention and Treatment* 2002;5. Article 24, posted July 15, 2002.

29. Song F, Freemantle N, Sheldon TA, et al. Selective serotonin reuptake inhibitors: meta-analysis of efficacy and acceptability. *British Medical Journal* 1993;306:683–687.

30. Anderson IM. Meta-analytical studies on new antidepressants. *British Medical Bulletin* 2001;57:161–178.

31. Bech P, Cialdella P, Haugh MC, et al. Meta-analysis of randomized controlled trials of fluoxetine v. placebo and tricyclic antidepressants in the short-term treatment of major depression. *British Journal of Psychiatry* 2000;176:421–423.

32. Cipriani A, Furakawa TA, Salanti G, et al. Comparative efficacy and acceptability of 12 new-generation antidepressants: a multiple-treatments meta-analysis. *The Lancet* 2009. Doi.1016/S0140-6736(09)60046-5.

33. Ioannidis JPA. Ranking antidepressants. *The Lancet* 2009;373:1769–1760.

34. Jefferson T. Ranking antidepressants. *The Lancet* 2009;373:1759.

35. Ciprani A, Furukawa TA, Salanti G, et al. Comparative efficacy and acceptability of 21 antidepressant drugs for the acute treatment of adults with major depressive disorder: a systematic review and network meta-analysis. *The Lancet* 2018;391:1357–1366. http://dx.doi.org/10.1016/50140-6736(17)32802-7.

36. Duyx B, Urlings MJE, Swaen GH et al. Scientific publications favor positive results; a systematic review and meta-analysis. *Journal of Clinical Epidemiology* 2017;88:92–101.

37. Fong EA, Wilhite AW. Authorship and citation manipulation in academic research. *Public Library of Science* 2017. https://doi.org/10.1371/journal.pone.0187394.

38. Steiner DL, Joffe R. The adequacy of reporting randomized, controlled trials in the evaluation of antidepressants. *Canadian Journal of Psychiatry* 1998;43:1026–1030.

39. Moncrieff J. Are antidepressants overrated? A review of methodological problems in antidepressant trials. *The Journal of Nervous and Mental Disease* 2001;189:288–295.

40. National Institute for Clinical Excellence. *Depression. Management of Depression in Primary and Secondary Care.* Clinical Guideline 23. www.nice.org.uk/CGO23NICEguideline.

41. Ioannidis JPA. Effectiveness of antidepressants: an evidence myth constructed from a thousand randomized trials. *Philosophy, Ethics, and Humanities in Medicine* 2008;3:14. Doi:10.1186/1747-5341-3-14.

42. Zimmerman M, Mattia JI, Posternak MA. Are subjects in pharmacological treatment trials of depression representative of patients in routine clinical practice? *American Journal of Psychiatry* 2002;159:469–473.

43. van der Lem R, van der Wee NJA, van Veen T, et al. The generalizability of antidepressant efficacy trials to routine psychiatric out-patient practice. *Psychological Medicine.* Doi:10.1017/S0033291710002175.

44. Kirsch I, Deacon BJ, Huedo-Medina TB, et al. Initial severity and antidepressant benefits: a meta-analysis of data submitted to the Food and Drug Administration. *Public Library of Science Medicine* 2008;5(2):e45.

45. Dean CE. The death of specificity: cheers or tears? *Perspectives in Biology and Medicine* 2012;55:443–460.

46. Khan A, Leventhal RM, Khan SR, et al. Severity of depression and response to antidepressants and placebo: an analysis of the Food and Drug Administration Database. *Journal of Clinical Psychopharmacology* 2001;22:40–45.

47. Khan A, Schwartz K, Kolts RL, et al. Relationship between depression severity entry criteria and antidepressant clinical trial outcomes. *Biological Psychiatry* 2007;62:65–71.

48. Fournier JC, DeRubeis RJ, Hollon S, et al. Antidepressant drug effects and depression severity: a patient-level meta-analysis. *Journal of the American Medical Association* 2010;303:47–53.

49. Melander H, Salmonson T, Abadie E, et al. A regulatory *Apologia*—A review of placebo-controlled studies in regulatory submissions of new-generation antidepressants. *European Neuropsychopharmacology* 2008;18:623–627.

50. Wiles NJ, Mulligan J, Peters TJ, et al Severity of depression and response to antidepressants: GENPOD randomized controlled trial. *British Journal of Psychiatry* 2012;200:13–136.

51. Gibbons RD, Hur K, Hendricks-Brown C, et al. Benefits of antidepressants. Synthesis of 6-week patient-level outcomes from double-blind placebo-controlled randomized trials of fluoxetine and venlafaxine. *Archives of General Psychiatry* 2012;69:572–579.

52. Nutt DJ, Malizia AL. Why does the world have such a 'down' on antidepressants? *Journal of Psychopharmacology* 2008;22:223–226.

53. Parker G. The benefits of antidepressants: news or fake news? *British Journal of Psychiatry* 2018;454–455.

54. American Psychiatric Association. *Diagnostic and Statistical Manual of Mental Disorders*, Fifth Edition. American Psychiatric Association, Arlington VA, 2013.

55. Levokovitz Y, Tedeschini E, Papakostas GI. Efficacy of antidepressants for dysthymia: a meta-analysis of placebo-controlled randomized studies. *Journal of Clinical Psychiatry* 2011;72:509–514.

56. Pincus HA, Davis WW, McQueen LE. "Subthreshold" mental disorders. A review and synthesis of studies on minor depression and other "brand names." *British Journal of Psychiatry* 1999;174:288–296.

57. Barbui C, Cipriani A, Patel V et al. Efficacy of antidepressants and benzodiazepines in minor depression: systematic review and meta-analysis. *British Journal of Psychiatry* 2011;198:11–16.

58. Arnow BA, Blasey C, Williams LM, et al. Depression subtypes in predicting antidepressant response: a report from the iSPOT-D Trial. *American Journal of Psychiatry* 2015:iA–8. Doi:10.1176/appi.ajp.2015.14020181.

59. Zimmerman M, Coryell WH, Pfohl B, et al. The validity of 4 definitions of endogenous depression. Part 2. Clinical, demographic, and psychosocial correlates. *Archives of General Psychiatry* 1986;43:234–244.

60. Peselow ED, Sanfilipo MP, Difiglia C, et al. Melancholic/endogenous depression and response to somatic treatment. *American Journal of Psychiatry* 1992;149:1324–1334.

61. Kessler RC, Bergland P, Demler O, et al. The epidemiology of major depressive disorder: results from the National Comorbidity Survey Replication (NCS-R). *JAMA* 2003;289:3095–3105.

62. Silverstein B. Gender differences in the prevalence of clinical depression: the role played by depression with somatic symptoms. *American Journal of Psychiatry* 1999;156:480–482.

63. Baca E, Garcia-Garcia M, Porras-Chavarino A. Gender differences in treatment response to sertraline vs imipramine in patients with non-melancholic depressive disorders. *Progress in Neuropsychopharmacology & Biological Psychiatry* 2004;28:57–65.

64. Ma L, Xu Y, Jiang W, et al. Sex differences in antidepressant effect of sertraline in transgenic mouse models. *Frontiers in Cellular Neuroscience* 2019. Doi:10.3389/fncel.2019.00024.

65. Thase MA, Reynolds CF, Frank E, et al. Gender differences in response to treatments of depression. In: *Gender and Its Effects on Psychopathology*. Editor: Frank E. American Psychiatric Press, Washington DC, 2000.

66. Quitkin FM, Stewart JW, McGrath PJ, et al. Are there differences in between women's and men's antidepressant responses? *American Journal of Psychiatry* 2002;157:1848–1854.

67. Sinyor M, Schaffer A, Levitt A. The sequenced treatment alternatives to relieve depression (STAR*D) trial: a review. *Canadian Journal of Psychiatry* 2010;55:126–135.

68. Weissman MM. Treatment of depression: men and women are different? *American Journal of Psychiatry*, April 1, 2014. https://doi.org/10.1176/appi.ajp.2013.13121688.

69. Bayes AJ, Parker GB. Comparison of guidelines for the treatment of unipolar depression: a focus on pharmacotherapy and neurostimulation. *Acta Psychiatrica Scandinavica* 2018;137:459–471. Doi:10.1111/acps.12878.

70. Pratt LA, Brody DJ, Gu Q. Antidepressant use in persons aged 21 and over: United States 2005–2008. *NCHS Data Brief*, Number 76, October 2011.

71. Martin LA, Neighbors HW, Griffith DM. The experience of symptoms of depression in men vs women: analysis of the national comorbidity survey replication. *JAMA Psychiatry* 2013;70:1100–1106.

72. Olfsen M, Marcus SC, Druss B, et al. Trends in antidepressant use among adults in the United States from 1992–2012. *Archives of General Psychiatry* 2009;66:848–856.

73. Gilbert AM, Garno JL, Braga RJ, et al. Clinical and cognitive correlates on suicide attempts in bipolar disorder: is suicide predictable? *Journal of Clinical Psychiatry* 2011;72:1027–1023.

74. Teicher MH, Glod C, Cole JO. Emergence of intense suicidal preoccupation during fluoxetine (Prozac) treatment. *American Journal of Psychiatry* 1990;147:207–210.

75. Breggin PR, Breggin GR. *Talking Back to Prozac*. St. Martin's Press, New York, 1994.

76. Avery D, Winokur G. Suicide, attempted suicide, and relapse rates in depression. *Archives of General Psychiatry* 1978;35:749–753.

77. Mann JJ, Kapur S. The emergence of suicidal ideation and behavior during antidepressant pharmacotherapy. *Archives of General Psychiatry* 1991;48:1027–1033.

78. Beasley CM, Dornseief BE, Bosomworth JD, et al. Fluoxetine and suicide: a meta-analysis of controlled trials for the treatment of depression. *British Medical Journal* 1991;303:685–692.

79. Fergusson D, Doucette S, Glass KC, et al. Association between suicide attempts and selective serotonin reuptake inhibitors: systematic review of randomized controlled trials. *British Medical Journal* 2005;330:396–399.

80. Gunnell D, Saperia J, Ashby D. Selective serotonin reuptake inhibitors (SSRIs) and suicide in adults: meta-analysis of drug company data from placebo controlled randomized controlled trials submitted to the MHRA's safety review. *British Medical Journal* 2005;385. Doi:10.1136://bmj.330.7488.385.

81. Donovan S, Clayton A, Beeharry M, et al. Deliberate self-harm and antidepressant drugs. Investigation of a possible link. *British Journal of Psychiatry* 2000;177:551–557.

82. U.S. Food and Drug Administration: FDA public health advisory: reports of suicidality in pediatric patients treated with antidepressant medication for major depressive disorder (MDD) October 23, 2003. (Not available online.)

83. U.S. Food and Drug Administration. *Center for Drug Evaluation and Research: FDA Public Health Advisory and Suicidality in Patients Being Treated with Antidepressant Medications*, March 22, 2004. http://.www.fda.gov/cder/drug/antidepressants/Antide pressantsPHA.htm.

84. Hammand TA, Laughren T, Racoosin J. Suicidality in pediatric patients treated with antidepressant drugs. *Archives of General Psychiatry* 2006;63:332–339.

85. *United States Food and Drug Administration*. Clinical review: relationship between antidepressant drugs and suicidality in adults. www.fda.gov/ohrms/dockets/ad/06/briefing/2006-4272b1-01-FDA.pdf. Accessed November 20, 2019.

86. Gibbons RD, Segawa E, Karabatsos G, et al. Mixed-effects Poisson regression analysis of adverse reports events: the relationship between antidepressants and suicide. *Statistics in Medicine* 2008;27:1814–1833.

87. Simon GE. How can we know whether antidepressants increase suicide risk? *American Journal of Psychiatry* 2006;163:1861–1863.

88. Simon GE, Savarino J, Operskalski B, et al. Suicide risk during antidepressant treatment. *American Journal of Psychiatry* 2006;163:41–47.

89. Leon AC, Solomon DA, Chunshan L, et al. Antidepressants and risks of suicide and suicide attempts: a 27-year observational study. *Journal of Clinical Psychiatry* 2011;72:580–586.

90. Gibbons RD, Brown CH, Hur K, et al. Early evidence on the effects of regulators's suicidality warnings on SSRI prescriptions and suicide in children and adolescents. *American Journal of Psychiatry* 2007;164:1356–1363.

91. Morrato EH, Libby AM, Orton HD, et al. Frequency of provider contact after FDA advisory on risk of pediatric suicidality with SSRIs. *American Journal of Psychiatry* 2008;165:42–50.

92. Monden R, Roest AM, van Ravenzwaaij D, et al. The comparative evidence base for the efficacy of second generation antidepressants in the treatment of depression in the US: a Bayesian meta-analysis of food and drug administration reviews. *Journal of Affective Disorders* 2018;235:393–398.

93. Geddes JR, Carney SM, Davies C, et al. Relapse prevention with antidepressant drug treatment in depressive disorders: a systematic review. *The Lancet* 2003;361:653–661.

94. Davis JM, Giakas WJ, Qu J, et al. Should we treat depression with drugs or psychological interventions? A reply to Ioannidis. *Philosophy, Ethics, and Humanities in Medicine* 2011;6:8. www.peh-med-com/content/6/1/8.

95. Machmutow K, Jansen A, Kriston L, et al. Comparative effectiveness of continuation and maintenance treatments for persistent depressive disorders in adults (Review). *Cochrane Database of Systematic Reviews* 2019;(5). Art.No: CD012855.

96. Nelson JC, Spyker DA. Morbidity and mortality associated with medications used in the treatment of depression: an analysis of cases reported to U.S. poison control centers, 2000–2014. *American Journal of Psychiatry* 2017;174:438–450.

97. Hampton LM, Daubresse M, Chang H-Y, et al. Emergency department visits by adults for psychiatric medication adverse events. *JAMA Psychiatry* 2014. Doi:10.1001/jamapsychiatry.2014.436.

98. Dragioti E, Solmi M, Favaro A, et al. Association of antidepressant use with adverse health outcomes. A systematic umbrella review. *JAMA Psychiatry* 2019;76:1241–1255. Doi:10.1001/jamapsychiatry.2019.2859.

99. *Practice Guideline for the Treatment of Patients with Major Depressive Disorder*, Third Edition. American Psychiatric Association, Washington, DC, October 2010.

100. Metcalf CA, Gold AK, Davis BJ, et al. Mindfulness as an intervention for depression. *Psychiatric Annals* 2019;49:16–20.
101. Barth J, Munder T, Gerger H, et al. Comparative efficacy of seven psychotherapeutic interventions for patients with depression: a network meta-analysis. *Public Library of Science* 10(5);e1001454.
102. Jefferis BJ, Nazareth I, Marston L, et al. Associations between unemployment and major depressive disorder: evidence from an international, prospective study (the predict cohort). *Social Science and Medicine* 2011;73:1627–1634.
103. Kirkbride JB, Jones PB, Ulrich S, et al. Social deprivation, inequality, and the neighborhood-level incidence of psychiatric outcomes in East London. *Schizophrenia Bulletin* 2012;40:169–180.
104. Bastiampillai T, Sharfstein SS, Allison S. Increase in U.S. suicide rates and the critical decline in psychiatric beds. *JAMA* 2016;316:2591–2592.
105. Kegler SR, Stone DM, Holland KM. Trends in suicide by levels of urbanization—United States, 1995–2015. *MMWR Morbidity Mortality Wkly Report* 2017. Published online March 17, 2017. Doi:10.15585/mmwr.mm6610a2.
106. Kendler KS, Gardner, Jr CO. Boundaries of major depression: an evaluation of DSM-IV criteria. *American Journal of Psychiatry* 1998;155:172–177.
107. Fried EI, Nesse RM. Depression is not a consistent syndrome. An investigation of unique symptom patterns in the STAR*D study. *Journal of Affective Disorders* 2015;172:96–102.
108. Musliner KL, Munk-Olsen T, Laursen TM, et al. Heterogeneity in 10-year course trajectories of moderate to severe major depressive disorder. A Danish National Register-based study. *JAMA Psychiatry* 2016;73:346–353.
109. Cuijpers P, Stringaris A, Wolpert M. Treatment outcomes for depression: challenges and opportunities. *The Lancet*, Published online February 17, 2020. https://doi.org/10.1016/S2215-0366(20)30036-5.

10 Antidepressants and Adverse Events

Falls and Fractures, Vascular Events, Risks in Pregnancy, and Abnormal Movements

Introduction

Leaving aside the issue of AD-induced suicidality, what are the other problems, common and uncommon, with ADs? We noted earlier the remarkable historical similarity between the adverse effects found with ADs and APs and further emphasized that the industry simply traded one set of side effects for another. To recap: The older TCAs (tertiary amines), such as imipramine and amitryptyline, are strongly associated with sedation, dry mouth, constipation, weight gain, tachycardia, cardiac conduction defects, and arrthymias, secondary to their blockade of muscarinic cholinergic, alpha-adrenergic, and histamine receptors. Some improvement was seen with the secondary amines (desipramine and nortriptyline), ADs that are metabolites of imipramine and amitriptyline, respectively. The secondary amines are less potent at the relevant receptors and therefore cause less sedation and dizziness and fewer problems with blood pressure, dry mouth, and constipation. Next came the SSRIs and SNRIs, which are associated with even fewer anticholinergic and antihistaminic side effects and are generally safer in overdose. Nevertheless, SSRIs continue to be associated with arrhythmias, other cardiovascular problems, fractures, and SSRI-induced sexual dysfunction, nausea, and diarrhea. As we shall see, multiple studies have demonstrated evidence of AD-associated risks to infants whose mothers have been treated with ADs, although questions have been raised about the validity of the associations.

As one can see, there are a number of rather non-specific and common side effects with all classes of ADs and APs, some of which can be found with placebo, including headache, dizziness, dry mouth, weight gain, and gastrointestinal problems such as nausea and diarrhea. So, we have an ever-changing picture of side effects—some better, some worse—but, as we have stressed, very little evidence of an increase in efficacy with the newer APs and ADs. In addition, studies have clearly shown that clinicians fail to evaluate side effects in a systematic fashion, despite evidence that the presence of side effects is a critical factor in the refusal of patients to continue medications.[1] Indeed, when patients and doctors are systematically compared with regard to reporting side effects, *patients report at a rate 20 times higher than do their physicians.*[2] Even when patients rate side effects as "very bothersome," they still report at a rate twice that of the physicians.

Antidepressants and Serious Adverse Events: Falls and Fractures

Some of the risks with ADs are significant. For example, in a five-year observational study of depression in 60,000 patients ages 65 and older,[3] all classes of ADs were associated with an increased risk of adverse events. SSRIs were associated with a *66% increased risk of falls* while certain SSRIs (citalopram, fluoxetine, escitalopram) resulted in a 52% increase in the risk of hyponatremia. Some of the newer ADs (nefazodone, mirtazapine, bupropion) had the highest risk of overall mortality, as well as attempted suicide, stroke, and transient ischemic attacks (TIAs).

All classes of ADs were associated with a 26% to 64% increase in the risk for fractures. The authors admit that these risks have to be put into perspective since they could not adjust for all the variables that might have affected outcome. The investigators did not determine whether or to what extent ADs were being used to treat symptoms such as pain or sleep disturbances, but this is relevant to a study[4] in the U.S. that found a large increase in the rate of AD prescriptions written by non-psychiatrists for office visits that were *unaccompanied* by a psychiatric diagnosis. The increase was quite striking, rising from 59% in 1996 to almost 73% in 2007. Interestingly, and perhaps alarmingly, this group of patients was older and had increased rates of DM and heart disease when compared with non-users of ADs, all of which could set the stage for an increased rate of adverse events.

We should stress, too, that other medications significantly increase the risks of falls in the older population. For example, in a meta-analysis[5] of studies involving 79,000 patients and nine classes of drugs, the use of benzodiazepines resulted in a 41% increase in the risk of falls, with ADs in second place at 39%. The good news was that APs did *not* show an increased risk after adjustment for confounders. However, whether polypharmacy played a role in these results was not clear. In a case-control study[6] of people 50 years and older, *SSRIs had the strongest association with osteoporotic fractures* (45%), with wrist fracture being the most common. Benzodiazepines resulted in a much weaker association at 10%. APs were not associated with an increased risk, but higher doses of SSRIs and benzodiazepines were associated with a higher risk, as we have emphasized repeatedly. Surprisingly, polypharmacy was not associated with an increased risk. Lithium, for all of its problems with side effects, was associated with a lower risk of fractures. With regard to psychiatric diagnoses, the highest rate of fractures was found in those with substance abuse, with a 72% increase in risk; schizophrenia came in at 61%.

The evidence for increased fractures with increasing age was reinforced in 2019 by a nationwide study[7] in Denmark of 204,000 people taking ADs vs another 200,000 not taking ADS. The mean age was 80 years; 63% were women. Interestingly, AD users had twice as many hip fractures in the year *prior* to taking ADs *and* in the year after (2.8% vs 1.1% and 3.5 % vs 1.3%, respectively). The highest odds ratios were found across all ADs, in men and women, and in all age groups during the 16-to-30-month period *before* beginning use! (Note that SSRIs made up 62% of the ADs.) The odds ratio also increased with higher doses, but this varied with the time frame. The authors suggested that the increased risk of hip fractures depended, at least in part, on co-morbid conditions, and confounding by indication (e.g., ADs) would be more likely to be prescribed, given the need for treatment.

SSRIs and Bleeding

Although SSRIs are by far and away the most prescribed group of ADs, a number of case reports have called attention to SSRI-induced bleeding.[8] Several processes have been implicated, but the key issue is an SSRI-induced reduction in serotonin uptake by platelets. This decreases the ability of platelets to aggregate and thus prevent bleeding.[9] Other mechanisms involve a decrease in platelet binding, a decrease in some of the 14 platelet surface markers that are important in clotting, and the influence of a polymorphism in the promoter region of the gene coding for the serotonin transporter.[10]

These reports stimulated additional studies designed to compare the incidence of upper gastrointestinal (UGI) bleeding with SSRIs vs controls. For example, in 2008, de Abajo et al. compared the use of SSRIs in patients who had suffered UGI bleeding with 10,000 controls who had no such history.[11] The risk of bleeding in patients using SSRIS was triple that found in non-users, but, if aspirin had been taken with the SSRI, the risk was 7 times greater. The use of non-steroidal anti-inflammatory agents (NSAIDs), such as ibuprofen, led to a *15 times greater risk*. From another perspective, 5% of those taking an SSRI developed UGI bleeding. These figures were comparable to those reported by Dalton et al.[12] in Denmark, who also found a significant increase in risk when SSRIs were combined with aspirin or NSAIDs. Yet others have found no association between SSRI use and bleeding[13] and no increase when SSRIs were combined with NSAIDs,[14] although some have found that SSRIs that are more potent in blocking the reuptake of serotonin carry a higher risk of bleeding.[15]

As we have noted in multiple conditions, studies have not been consistent, but caution is warranted.

The post-partum period is another time of risk, with Heerdink et al.[16] finding a 47% increase in the risk of hemorrhage in women who were taking SSRIs on the delivery date. Once again, the absolute risk was somewhat less alarming, with bleeding occurring in 4% of SSRI users vs 2.8% of non-users. Note that non-SSRIs also carried an increased risk. The perioperative period[17] also carries an 9% increased risk of bleeding in patients taking SSRIs and an increased risk of in-hospital mortality. In addition, there was a 22% increase in the risk of readmission at 30 days. After sensitivity and propensity analyses, the results remained the same. Obviously, the use of SSRIs might be a marker for poor functional status, chronic pain, and severe mood disorders, all of which can affect survival. The risks were similar for SSRIs and SNRIs.

De Abajo and associates[11] noted that 11 epidemiologic studies have been done on this subject, with *most showing an increased risk, but of different magnitudes.* Before we get too alarmed, we should note that 2,000 patients would need to be treated with an SSRI to induce one case of UGI bleeding.[11, p. 800] Yet if an SSRI is combined with an NSAID, the number needed to harm (NNH) drops to 250. If antacids (proton pump inhibitors) are used in combination with an SSRI and an NSAID, the number NNH rises to 5,000, indicating a protective effect of antacids.

SSRIs and Stroke

Here we enter exceedingly complex territory, since depression itself is an independent risk factor for stroke,[18, 19] and the presence of depression in post-stroke patients has been associated with an increase in mortality, with depressed patients being three to eight times more likely to die during follow-up periods of varying lengths.[20–22]

On the other hand, ADs have been associated not only with bleeding and hemorrhagic stroke[21] but also with vasoconstriction of cerebral arteries and ischemic stroke.[23] Wu and colleagues[24] found a 48% increase in the risk of stroke in patients who had taken an AD in the two weeks prior to the stroke, with a higher risk in ADs having more affinity for the serotonin transporter, echoing the study of Meijer et al.[15] The risk of CNS hemorrhage in controlled observational studies of exposure to SSRIs revealed an increased risk across case-controlled studies, cohort studies, and case-crossover studies, with relative risks ranging from 1.34 to 4.24, but the authors noted that the absolute risk is "likely to be very low."[24, p. 1862]

Yet the data is not consistent, in that other studies have found no association between SSRIs and the risk of stroke.[25–27] Nevertheless, a review of the cardiovascular side effects of the new ADs and APS concluded that SSRIs and SGAs, as well as TCAs, have clinically important effects on cardiac functioning, largely by inhibiting vascular sodium, calcium, and potassium channels, thus invalidating the more optimistic assumptions about their safety.[28]

A Critical Question

What to do in the case of a patient who has suffered a stroke but is simultaneously depressed? Do the risks of AD treatment outweigh the benefits? Several studies have provided data on which to make an informed decision. For example, Jorge and associates[29] studied 104 post-stroke patients who were pseudo-randomly assigned to treatment with nortryptyline, fluoxetine, or placebo for 12 weeks starting in the early recovery period.[29] I say pseudo-randomly since those who had suffered a hemorrhagic stroke were not permitted to have fluoxetine, and those with heart block were not randomized to nortryptyline —both clinically reasonable decisions. Oddly enough, the patients were not required to be clinically depressed in order to be randomized, although the title of the study was "Mortality and Poststroke Depression." Thus, non-depressed patients might or might not receive drug or placebo.

The results demonstrated that 59% of those receiving full dose ADs were alive at nine years, compared with 36% of those who had taken placebo, a significant difference. But here is the most striking finding: *Taking an AD increased survival time at nine years regardless of whether the patient had been depressed or not!* This was true after controlling for age, type of stroke, and diabetes mellitus. Yet the authors admit they had not obtained psychiatric follow-up beyond two years post stroke, so there was no information on later-developing problems, if any.

A considerably larger study by Ried et al.[30] took a somewhat different approach, comparing veterans who (a) had been prescribed an SSRI at some point in the six-month period prior to the stroke, (b) had been prescribed an SSRI within one year post stroke, (c) had been prescribed an SSRI during both time periods, and (d) had not been given an SSRI. The authors also noted the presence or absence of a depression diagnosis prior to or after the stroke. The groups were compared on socioeconomic status, degree of co-morbid conditions, marital status, admission to an ICU, and whether ventilation or intubation was needed. The results were complicated, but a diagnosis of depression, both before and after a stroke led to a 35% greater likelihood of death. A shortened survival time was also associated with older age, lower socioeconomic status, more co-morbid conditions, and use of intubation and/or mechanical ventilation, all of which would naturally be associated with a shortened survival time.

But here are the odd results: *It appeared that death was more likely if an SSRI had been given for depression only before the stroke. If given both before and after the stroke, there was a protective effect* in the year following the stroke. The authors[30] proceeded to call for initiation of SSRI treatment in the depressed post-stroke patient but cautioned that *if the patient had been given an SSRI before the stroke, the risk of mortality was greater!* These results seem bizarre and leave one with no clear understanding of how to proceed. As the reader can see, SSRIs are held to simultaneously increase the risk of bleeding and cerebral vascular disease and, in some instances, decreasing post-stroke mortality!

Making matters even more complicated, the use of antiplatelet therapy (ASA, clopidogrel, and others) has become the standard of care following myocardial infarction (MI) yet some 20% of these patients are depressed and frequently given SSRIs.[31] As these authors indicate, some early studies did not find an increased risk with a combination of SSRIs and single-agent antiplatelet therapy, but since the evidence was uncertain, they did an observational study from 1997 to 2008 of 27,000 patients who had suffered an MI and were discharged taking antiplatelet therapy. The study endpoints included death, a bleeding episode, recurrent MI, or end of study. Compared with use of ASA alone (15%), here are the increases in risk:

*   ASA + SSRI: 42%
*   Clopidigrel + SSRI   230%
*   Dual antiplatelet + SSRI   57%, compared with dual antiplatelet therapy
                               alone

While some have found an association between bleeding risks and the potency of SSRI-induced reuptake blockade of serotonin,[16, 32] no such association was found in this study[31]—although the concept seems intuitively reasonable, since SSRIs can reduce the platelet content of serotonin by some 99%.[32] One would think that agents such as paroxetine and fluoxetine—with their very potent reuptake blockade—would be more likely to induce bleeding.[33] However, a nested case-control study in the United Kingdom looked at the risk of hemorrhagic stroke with both SSRIs and TCAs and found *no association* with either group.[34]

Some additional perspective can be found in an editorial by David Juurlink,[35] who cites studies showing a 200% increase in the risk of bleeding when ASA is combined with warfarin and a 400% increase with a combination of warfarin, ASA, and clopidogrel. Yet such combinations may be necessary, and of course, the addition of an SSRI may be necessary to treat depression, despite the risks. Jurrlink reminds us that *the absolute risk is probably low*, as we have seen earlier in this section.

Remarkably, none of these papers bother to note that non-SSRIs remain available (although they have their own adverse events) or that non-drug treatments are available, including CBT and other forms of psychotherapy. Clearly, we are in need of long-term controlled studies with much larger numbers of patients, but, for obvious reasons, recruitment would be very difficult. In the meantime, the risks of bleeding with SSRIs should be discussed in detail with prospective patients, particularly if they are being treated with antiplatelet therapy.

Antidepressants in Pregnancy

Here we have another serious problem, since depression is found in 12% to 25% of pregnancies, [36, 37] with about 8% taking an AD.[38, 39] Unfortunately, stopping the AD results in high rates of relapse.[40] Yet, as we shall see, various authors have reported multiple problems in the children of mothers exposed to ADs in pregnancy, including prematurity, low birth weight, pulmonary hypertension, and others.[41] Perhaps the greatest concern is the rate of congenital birth defects, especially cardiac defects.

Before proceeding, we should stress that congenital malformations occur in 1% to 3% of infants born in the general population,[42] so the primary question becomes whether ADs or other moderators elevate the risk to a significant degree. As will become evident, the data is not entirely consistent.

In a meta-analysis of prospective cohort studies of malformations involving 12 newer antidepressants (TCAs and MAOIs were excluded),[43] the number of exposed and non-exposed women was 1,774. About half the studies originated in the Motherisk program in Toronto, with a much more comprehensive level of care than found in many communities in the U.S. The relative risk of congenital malformations was 1.01 (CI = 0.57–1.80), indicating *no risk above the baseline of 1% to 3%*. No single AD stood out as a significant risk. However, there were limitations to the study, including the lack of data on birth weight, head circumference, premature births, or other difficulties suffered by the mother or the child. A similar result was found in a 2014 study[44] of almost one million Medicaid enrollees, in which there was no "substantial risk" of cardiac malformations, despite exposure to SSRIs.

In contrast, a retrospective but much larger nationwide study in Denmark of all pregnancies from 1997 through 2009 (n = 848,786) utilized national registers and exposure to five SSRIs in the first trimester, with the focus on cardiac malformations.[45] Continuous exposure was defined as use of an SSRI for least one month prior to conception and lasting through day 84. Paused exposure was defined as the use of an SSRI 3 to 12 months prior to conception, but no exposure during the first trimester.

The odds of a major malformation was 1.33, clearly exceeding the baseline rate. There was no association with dose, while paused or continuous treatment had little effect on the results. There was no association with TCAs or other ADs, but, as we have stressed, TCAs carry other very substantial risks, in addition to their common side effects.

The authors correctly noted that a number of prior studies had enrolled considerably smaller samples, and while one update of data in Sweden[45] found an increased rate of cardiovascular malformations with paroxetine, recall bias may have affected the results. Yet we should stress that the FDA and Health Canada have warned that *first-trimester use of paroxetine has led to a higher rate of major congenital malformations than have other ADs* (see Williams[46] for a review). Paroxetine doubled the risk, compared with a 39% increase for citalopram, 48% for sertraline, and 42% for more than one type of AD. There was no increase in risk with amitryptyline, bupropion, and fluoxetine, but note contrary results in the data listed earlier.

While the odds ratios (ORs) in some studies seem alarming, I must stress that the *absolute risk of AD-associated major malformations is quite low*.[42, 43] For example, the population risk of atrial septal defects is 0.26%, meaning that even if the risk of this defect is doubled with an SSRI, the absolute risk would be 1 in 1,000 births.[42] In an editorial,[47] Steiner noted that the population risk of major birth defects in the U.S. is about 2% to 3% and that *no* study has shown a higher level of risk with ADs—but see the results just discussed.

Antidepressants in the Late Stages of Pregnancy

We have just focused on the risks of AD exposure early in pregnancy, but what about complications associated with second- or third-trimester exposure? Unfortunately, a number of medications (anticonvulsants, benzodiazepines, APs, opiates) have resulted in neonatal respiratory problems, withdrawal symptoms, and the so-called "floppy infant syndrome."[46] In a 2012 study out of Sweden in which medical and medication registers were used,[48] the authors gathered data on virtually all deliveries (n = 14,284; live births = 15,045) and the use of SSRIs and other psychotropic drugs, with the goal of comparing neonatal complications in never-exposed infants, those exposed to SSRIs only, and those exposed to SSRIs plus other psychotropics in the second or third trimester.

Almost 5% of all live-birth infants were exposed to psychotropic drugs, of which 6.9% were born preterm, for an adjusted risk increase of 39%. *If exposed during both the second and third trimester, the risk of neonatal complications grew to 68%. If exposed to SSRIs, the increase in risk was 39%*, whether used singly or in combination with other psychotropics. With regard to other neonatal complications, exposure to *any* CNS-active drug was associated with a 51% increase in the risk for respiratory difficulties, a 49% increase in the risk for neonatal hypoglycemia, and a 33% increase in risk for a low Apgar score. *Exposure to SSRIs alone led to an 82% increase in risk for neonatal complications* while the combination of SSRIs and other CNS drugs was associated with a 2.5 times greater risk vs no exposure. The authors noted that 11% of infants exposed to CNS-active drugs had complications, considerably lower than the 30% figure found by another group,[49] perhaps due to the lack of information on "minor" difficulties such as jitteriness or problems with feeding.

In an Australian study of neonatal complications after maternal SSRI use,[50] women with a psychiatric disorder and SSRI use had over twice the risk of preterm delivery or low birth weight and a 92% increase in the risks of hospital admission. Yet in mothers with a psychiatric illness but no SSRI use in pregnancy, there was *no* increase in the risk of neonatal complications, but the mothers still had a 21% increase in the risk of a hospital admission. However, the authors had no information regarding the severity of the psychiatric disorders. They further noted that utilization of drug-dispensing records can underestimate exposure by as much as 25%—a criticism that could be leveled at many epidemiologic studies.

An earlier register-based study was done in British Columbia[51] of all live births in a 39-month period from 1998 to 2001; 14% of the mothers had diagnoses of depression during pregnancy, with SSRI use doubling to 5%. *Maternal use was associated with low birth weight and higher rates of respiratory distress*. In this instance, the authors did account for the severity of the depression. Indeed, their findings were contrary to the common notion that AD treatment should lower the rate of neonatal complications! As with many other studies, the authors could not control for extent of licit or illicit drug use, smoking, socioeconomic conditions, or co-morbid psychiatric disorders.

A somewhat different approach was used in the Netherlands by Marroun et al.,[52] who used fetal ultrasonography in each trimester to help assess the effects of use of SSRIs among 7,696 women. Only 1.3% used SSRIs, although 7% had depressive symptoms and did not use SSRIs. Mothers with prenatal depression had infants with decreased body and head growth, but prenatal use of SSRIs was also associated with reduced head growth; these infants were also at increased risk of preterm birth. However, the authors cautioned that factors other than SSRI use might be causal, including smoking, use of alcohol or illicit drugs, and malnutrition.

Cautionary Notes

None of these studies had information on blood levels of the ADs or other agents, an unfortunate omission, but one that is common in such large-scale register studies. The trade-off lies in sacrificing detail for statistical power. The health care systems in Sweden, Norway, Finland, Canada, and Australia differ considerably from those in the U.S. with regard to the availability of prenatal care, so it isn't clear if these results can apply to the United States. In addition, the support systems in the Nordic countries are quite extensive, access to higher education is more affordable, and the population is more homogeneous. Indeed, one has to wonder if the results wouldn't be considerably worse in the United States. Finally, we have to acknowledge the presence of contrary studies. For example, at least ten studies have *not* found an association between AD exposure and low birth weight, and seven have found no association with preterm delivery.[53]

Persistent Pulmonary Hypertension

Concerns have also been raised about the association of SSRIs and persistent pulmonary hypertension (PPH) in the newborn. Fortunately, the condition is rare, occurring in 1.9 infants per 1,000 live births, with mortality rates varying from 10% to 20%, but affected infants are at risk for developmental delay, hearing deficits, and motor disabilities.[54] Symptoms include cyanosis, grunting, and labored breathing, no doubt alarming to all concerned. There are multiple risk factors for PPH, including prematurity, hypoxia, sepsis, maternal smoking, male gender, C-section, and others, making conflicting studies almost inevitable. Nevertheless, the FDA in July of 2006 issued a public health advisory on PPH.[55] Guidelines developed by the APA and the American College of Obstetrics and Gynecology have recommended continued but judicious use of SSRIs if other treatments are not available.[56]

Nevertheless, research continued to indicate problems. For example, a study[57] in 2011 of 1.6 million infants in Norway, Denmark, Finland, Iceland, and Sweden found that the rate of PPH doubled when SSRIs were used after week 20 of gestation, but rates were similar among the individual SSRIs (sertraline, paroxetine, fluoxetine, and citalopram). *However, the absolute risk was small: 3 in 1,000 infants vs 1.2 in those not exposed.*

In a thorough review[54] of the risk factors and pathophysiology of PPH, including the impact of elevated serotonin blood levels on blood vessels, the authors observed that in the six major studies of PPH, only 50 infants were found to have PPH in the population of 25,000 exposed to SSRIs. They also cited three studies that found no association, perhaps not too surprising in view of its rarity. They concluded that the risk-benefit ratio for SSRIs should include consideration of (a) the rather weak evidence base for the association of SSRIs and PPH, (b) the fact that women stopping ADs during pregnancy have about a 68% chance of relapse, and (c) that maternal suicide is the leading cause of death in the 12 months after delivery.

Interestingly, the FDA reversed its stance on PPH in 2011,[58] advising health care professionals *not* to alter their current clinical approach to treating depression during pregnancy. The FDA stated that it is premature to claim a link between use of SSRIs and PPH.

Are There Long-Term Effects of Intrauterine Exposure to Antidepressants?

Several studies have attempted to answer this question, one being a four-to-five-year follow-up[59] in Denmark of children whose mothers were (a) exposed to ADs during pregnancy, (b) had untreated prenatal depression, or (c) had no prenatal depression and no AD exposure. Parents filled out a questionnaire aimed at eliciting problems at ages four to five. By this rather limited measure, AD exposure was *not* associated with either behavioral or emotional difficulties compared with the other groups.

Nulman et al.[60] compared depressed women who had been treated with venlafaxine or SSRIs during pregnancy against depressed women left untreated and against non-depressed healthy women. This rather complex study in Toronto found that children exposed to maternal depression and venlafaxine or SSRIs had similar full-scale IQs, but their IQs were significantly lower than the children born to the healthy controls. In addition, children exposed to maternal depression had higher rates of problematic behaviors, but these were *not statistically significant.*

It seemed clear that use of ADs during pregnancy did not predict IQ or behaviors in children tested at ages three through seven. Yet we still do not know the full extent of prior treatment or lack thereof in these depressed women, despite the exclusionary criteria. Duration of pharmacotherapy ranged from six to nine years in the depressed groups, but what did treatment include? Did no one have psychotherapy, benzodiazepines, or antipsychotics? Still, the authors did take note of the socioeconomic status of the mothers—most were medium or higher—which did not differ among the groups.

Another group[61] focused on internalizing behaviors (depression, anxiety, isolation) among four-year-old children of depressed/anxious mothers taking SSRIs during pregnancy and compared them with children of non-depressed, healthy mothers. Unfortunately, there were only 22 children in the exposed group and 14 in the non-exposed group. Of the 22 exposed children, only 13 were exposed only to SSRIs while the rest had also taken a benzodiazepine. As in the study just cited, exposure in utero to psychotropics was *not* associated with internalizing behaviors. *Instead, such behaviors were associated with increasing levels of maternal depression and anxiety.* Caution: the very small patient population makes any definitive conclusion impossible. Indeed, the authors stated they did not find a direct correlation.[61, p. 1032]

In contrast, we find a study[62] in California of 298 children with autism spectrum disorders (autism, Asperger's syndrome, pervasive developmental disorder), their mothers, and 1,500 control children. Interestingly, there was *a two-fold increase in the risk of ASD with maternal exposure to SSRIs during the year prior to delivery*, but no association with maternal diagnoses of depression, anxiety, bipolar disorder, schizophrenia, or others. After adjustment for all demographic factors and mental health history, the two-fold risk with SSRIs remained. The strongest association was found when SSRIs were used during the first trimester, but the increase in risk was "modest," a statement not likely to be accepted by the mothers.

Given the massive publicity and fears/concerns about ASD, we should note that only 20 of the case mothers had used an AD in the year prior to delivery, compared with 50 control mothers (6.7% vs 3.3%). Only 13 case mothers had used an SSRI, *so the data is actually based on very few cases, despite the statistical risk.* Perhaps more importantly, the authors failed to collect data on the use of antipsychotics and mood stabilizers.

What might be the link, if any, between the pathophysiology of ASD and SSRIs? Croen et al.[62, p. 1110] have provided a good review, citing studies that have found increased levels of serotonin (5-HTA) in the blood of patients with ASD but decreased levels in the brain, in addition to decreased levels of certain 5-HTA receptors. Others have reported that early exposure to SSRIs can lead to behavioral problems found in mice that are deficient in the serotonin transporter, but, if the transporter is deficient, one would think that blood levels of 5-HTA would be increased since less is being metabolized. Maternal stress can also lower 5-HTA levels and change brain development, with deficits in spatial learning and memory. Whether breast feeding by mothers taking ADs plays a role is unclear. In an interesting analysis[63] of AD levels in mothers, breast milk, and nursing infants, paroxetine, sertraline, and desipramine yielded undetectable levels in infants, but citalopram and fluoxetine produced elevated levels of 17% and 22%, respectively, compared with maternal levels averaging 10%. The authors caution that an undetectable level does not necessarily mean that an ADs has no effect on brain development. They further recommended nortryptyline, sertraline, and paroxetine as "preferred choices" in women who are breast feeding, but the recommendation for paroxetine seems outdated in view of the data we reviewed earlier.

Mothers, Medications, and Depression: Problems?

First, it's important to note the lack of long-term studies, meaning studies of at least five years. Nor are they likely since they would require a very large number of subjects, would require years to accomplish, and would be faced with the enormous task of adjusting for a huge number of complicating factors, including exposure to other drugs (illicit or not), life experiences, socioeconomic status, education, cognitive abilities, and the development of medical and psychiatric illnesses, many of which have their own neurological and cognitive complications.

However, the debate continues. In 2005, a commentator in *The Lancet*[64] recommended careful consideration of non-pharmacologic interventions in pregnancy (CBT and other forms of psychotherapy) and more research into the effects of SSRIs on fetal development, but a review[65] published in the *American Journal of Obstetrics and Gynecology*, concluded that the benefits of ADs in pregnancy and during breast feeding *far outweigh the risks*, whether with regard to birth defects, PPH, the neonatal adaption syndrome, or any post-natal complications. This was underscored by a 2019 systematic review[66] of exposure to ADs *in utero*, in which the authors stressed that questions remain as to the validity of the associations between exposure, higher rates of preterm birth, and neurodevelopmental problems. A complicating factor: A study in Sweden[67] found that almost 39% of women with depression or another illness for which treatment was recommended refused pharmacological intervention, leading an editorialist to caution against making fear the decisive factor in making a decision.[68] Nonetheless, the stakes are high in pregnancy, and one must understand the concerns, especially for mothers and families.

Do Antidepressants Induce Neurologic Side Effects?

As we shall see, a great deal of attention has been given to SSRI-induced neurologic side effects, but the issue of TCA-induced parkinsonism and dyskinesia has been given less attention. Yet reviews in 1997[69] and 2005[70] cited multiple reports of TCA-associated akathisia (motor restlessness), dystonias (severe muscle spasms), and dyskinesias, as well as one case of a neuroleptic malignant-like syndrome in a woman taking desipramine. The authors also cited a case report of akathisia in a woman taking tranylcypromine, as well as several other reports of tranylcypromine-associated oral dyskinesias.

However, little in the way of systematic investigation has been reported, and there had been no long-term controlled studies of these phenomena, but the general conclusion was that the risk of neurologic complications with TCAs and MAOIs was far lower than with APs.

The story is somewhat different with SSRIs. In 1979, Melzter and associates described[71] a patient taking fluoxetine who developed dystonia and muscle rigidity, along with an increase in prolactin levels, both of which are usually associated with APs. During the next 20 years, additional cases were published (see Arya[72] for an early review and citations), leaving little doubt that SSRIs could induce a variety of abnormal motor movements. Another lengthy review in 1997[73] summarized the literature to that point, noting SSRI-induced tremor, rigidity, akathisia, oral dyskinesias, choreoathetoid movements, an akinetic-rigid syndrome, masked facies, and myoclonus (muscle jerking).

The cumulative data led to an editorial by Ronald Pies in the *Journal of Clinical Psychopharmacology*[74] with the provocative title "Must We Now Consider SRIs Neuroleptics?" However, Dr. Pies pointed out that based on the number of patients exposed, for example, to fluoxetine, only 1 in 100 to 1 in 1,000 treated patients would develop akathisia, and fewer than 1 in 1,000 would develop a dystonia.

The primary clinical point: Neurologic side effects have been found with a broad range of psychotropic agents ranging from the oldest FGAs to the SGAs and from the TCAs to the newest SSRIs. Similarly, lithium has been famous for decades as a cause of tremor, but it can also induce dyskinetic movements that can be quite severe with high blood levels, as in the case of an overdose. More attention has been paid recently to other mood stabilizers—especially divalproex—that can induce parkinsonism, impair cognition, induce EEG changes, and, in several studies, cause new-onset but reversible cerebral atrophy.[75, 76] A study[77] of 201 patients in an epilepsy clinic found 45% with postural tremor and other signs of parkinsonism in almost 5%. *The odds of parkinsonism were five times higher with divalproex* than other anticonvulsants. However, the authors caution that the risk of parkinsonism drops dramatically when alternative causes are present, which might account for the 92% rate found in an earlier study.[73]

Given the many side effects of ADs and the continuing debate over efficacy and whether ADs have any significant positive effect in those with other than severe depression, the reader needs to know that alternatives do exist and, in some cases, are clearly helpful. Several widely touted therapeutic advances for treatment-resistant depression are based on questionable data and considerable risk, but the need for progress in this area is obvious.

Clinical Notes

1. ADs and benzodiazepines carry an increased risk of fractures, including hip fractures, which, of course, are quite serious. This is especially relevant with older patients, many of whom may be taking multiple

central nervous system drugs. Patients and families need to be educated regarding the risk, and consider alterative treatments.

2. Substantial evidence points to an increased risk of bleeding with SSRIs, especially when combined with ibuprofen or other NSAIDs, as well as aspirin. However, the absolute risk is low.

3. It appears that SSRIs increase the risk of stroke, but depression itself can lead to a shorter survival time, whether before or after a stroke. Remarkably, SSRIs have been found to increase bleeding risk but may also decrease post-stroke mortality! A meta-analysis in 2019[79] found an increased risk of intracranial hemorrhage with SSRIs, but emphasized that the risk was greater in studies marked by bias, pointing once again to problems with study methodology.

4. Similarly, a recent study[80] of stroke in the elderly found a higher risk of SSRIs in patients with a high baseline risk of bleeding and in patients with depression. Patients and families need to remember that non-drug therapy is often helpful for depression and should be strongly considered if the patient is reasonably cognitively intact and capable of cooperating. I strongly advise extensive consultation in such patients.

5. The absolute risk of congenital malformations associated with use of SSRIs is quite low. Most studies have found no increase beyond what is found in the general population. However, I would not recommend the use of paroxetine in pregnancy. Remember psychotherapy!

6. Any CNS drug can lead to neonatal complications, such as respiratory distress and neonatal hypoglycemia. This includes APs as well as ADs. Evidence suggests that SSRIs may reduce head growth and result in preterm birth, but multiple other risk factors may be present. The risk of persistent pulmonary hypertension is low, and the FDA has now recommended *not* changing one's approach to the treatment of depression in pregnancy based on this concern.

7. The field is badly in need of long-term, non-biased investigations on whether the use of prescription drugs in pregnancy and in children/ adolescents can result in long-term behavioral changes. The evidence at this point is slim, and the studies have been relatively short term.

8. A 2019 systematic review[78] of health outcomes with AD use noted convincing evidence for the association of AD use and the risk of suicide attempt or completion among children and adolescents, preterm birth, and autism spectrum disorders, *but the associations were not supported after sensitivity analysis, which adjusted for confounding by indication.* The need for sensitivity analyses in all such studies is obvious.

9. Careful attention needs to be given to the neurologic side effects of SSRIs and other ADs.

References

1. Hu XH, Bull SA, Hunkeler EM, et al. Incidence and duration of side-effects and those rated as bothersome with selective serotonin reuptake inhibitor treatment

for depression: patient report vs physician estimate. *Journal of Clinical Psychiatry* 2004;65:959–965.

2. Zimmerman MA, Ruggero CJ, Attiullah N, et al. Underrecognition of clinically significant side effects in depressed patients. *Journal of Clinical Psychiatry* 2010;71:481–490.

3. Coupland C, Dhiman P, Morriss R, et.al. Antidepressant use and risk of adverse outcomes in older people: population-based cohort study. *British Medical Journal* 2011. Doi:10.1136/bmj.d4551.

4. Mojtabai R, Olfson M. Proportion of antidepressants prescribed without a psychiatric diagnosis is growing. *Health Affairs (Millwood)* 2008;30:1434–1442.

5. Woolcott JC, Richardson KJ, Wiens MO, et al. Meta-analysis of the impact of 9 medication classes on falls in elderly persons. *Archives of Internal Medicine* 2009;169:1952–1960.

6. Bolton JM, Metge C, Lix L, et al. Fracture risk from psychotropic medications: a population-based analysis. *Journal of Clinical Psychopharmacology* 2008;28:384–391.

7. Brännström J, Lövheim H, Gustafson Y, et al. Association between antidepressant drug use and hip fracture in older people before and after treatment initiation. *JAMA Psychiatry* 2019;76:172–179.

8. Turner MS, May DB, Arthur RR, et al. Clinical impact of selective serotonin reuptake inhibitors therapy with bleeding risks. *Journal of Internal Medicine* 2006. Doi:10.111/j.1365-2796.2006.01720.x.

9. Butler J, Leonard BE. The platelet serotonergic system in depression and following sertraline treatment. *International Journal of Psychopharmacology* 1988;3:343–347.

10. de Abajo FJ. Effects of serotonin reuptake inhibitors on platelet function: mechanisms, clinical outcomes and implications for use in elderly patients. *Drugs and Aging* 2011;28:345–367.

11. de Abajo FJ, Garcia-Rodriguez LA. Risk of upper gastrointestinal bleeding associated with selective serotonin reuptake inhibitors and venlafaxine therapy. Interaction with nonsteroidal anti-inflammatory agents and effect of acid-suppressing agents. *Archives of General Psychiatry* 2008;65:795–803.

12. Dalton SO, Johansen C, Mellemkjaer L, et al. Use of selective serotonin reuptake inhibitors and risk of upper gastrointestinal tract bleeding: a population-based cohort study. *Archives of Internal Medicine* 2003;163:59–64.

13. Dunn NR, Pearce GL, Shakir SA. Association between SSRIs and upper gastrointestinal bleeding. SSRIs are no more likely than other drugs to cause such bleeding. *British Medical Journal* 2000;320:1405–1406.

14. Tata LJ, Fortun PJ, Hubbard RB, et al. Does concurrent prescription of selective serotonin reuptake inhibitors and non-steroidal anti-inflammatory drugs substantially increase the risk of upper gastrointestinal bleeding? *Alimentary Pharmacological Therapeutics* 2005;22:175–181.

15. Meijer WE, Heerdink ER, Nolen WA, et al. Association of risk of abnormal bleeding with degree of serotonin reuptake inhibition by antidepressants. *Archives of Internal Medicine* 2004;164:2367–2370.

16. Heerdkink ER. Antidepressants and post-partum haemorrhage. *British Medical Journal* 2013;347:15194. Doi:10.1136/bmj.15194.

17. Auerbach AD, Vittinghoff E, Mascelli J, et al. Perioperative use of selective serotonin reuptake inhibitors and risks for adverse outcomes of surgery. *JAMA Internal Medicine* 2013;173:1075–1081.

18. Ramasubbu R, Patten SB. Effect of depression on stroke morbidity and mortality. *Canadian Journal of Psychiatry* 2003;48:250–257.

19. Surtees PB, Wainwright NW, Luben RN, et al. Psychological distress, major depressive disorder, and risk of stroke. *Neurology* 2008;70:788–794.

20. Everson SA, Roberts SE, Goldberg DE, et al. Depressive symptoms and increased risk of stroke mortality over a 29-year period. *Archives of Internal Medicine* 1998;158:1133–1138.

21. Nilsson FM, Kessing LV. Increased risk of developing stroke for patients with major depressive disorder: a registry study. *European Archives of Clinical Psychiatry and Clinical Neuroscience* 2004;254:387–391.

22. Smoller JW, Allison M, Cochrane BB, et al. Antidepressant use and incident cardiovascular morbidity and mortality among post-menopausal women in the women's health initiative study. *Archives of Internal Medicine* 2009;169:2128–2139.

23. Singhal AB, Caviness VS, Begleiter AF, et al. Cerebral vasoconstriction and stroke after the use of serotonergic drugs. *Neurology* 2002;58:130–133.

24. Wu C-S, Wang S-C, Cheng Y-C, et al. Association of cerebrovascular events with antidepressant use: a case-crossover study. *American Journal of Psychiatry* 2011. Doi:10.1176/appi.ajp.2010.10071064.

25. Hackam DG, Mrkobrada M. Selective serotonin reuptake inhibitors and brain hemorrhage. *Neurology* 2012;79:1862–1865.

26. Bak S, Tsiropoulos I, Kjaersgaard O, et al. Selective serotonin reuptake inhibitors and the risk of stroke: a population-based case-control study. *Stroke* 2002;33:1465–1473.

27. Barbui C, Percudani M, Fortino I, et al. *International Clinical Psychopharmacology* 2005;20:169–171.

28. Pacher P, Kecskemeti V. Cardiovascular side effects of new antidepressants and antipsychotics: new drugs, old concerns? *Current Pharmaceutical Design* 2004;10:2463–2475.

29. Jorge R, Robinson RG, Arndt S, et al. Mortality and post-stroke depression: a placebo-controlled trial of antidepressants. *American Journal of Psychiatry* 2003;160:1823–1829.

30. Ried LD, Jia H, Cameon R, et al. Selective serotonin reuptake inhibitor treatment and depression are associated with post-stroke mortality. *Annals of Pharmacotherapy* 2011;45:888–897.

31. Labos C, Dasgupta K, Nedjar H, et al. Risk of bleeding associated with combined use of selective serotonin reuptake inhibitors and antiplatelet therapy following acute myocardial infarction. *Canadian Medical Association Journal* 2011;183:1835–1843.

32. Javors MA, Houston JP, Tekill JL, et al. Reduction of platelet serotonin content in depressed patients treated with either paroxetine or desipramine. *International Journal of Neuropsychopharmacoloogy* 2000;10:35–38.

33. Castro VM, Gallagher PJ, Clements CC, et al. Incident user cohort study of risk for gastrointestinal bleed and stroke in individuals with major depressive disorder treated with antidepressants. *British Medical Journal Open* 2012;2(2):e000544. Doi:10.1136/bmjopen.

34. Douglas I, Smeeth L, Irvine D. The use of antidepressants and the risk of hemorrhagic stroke: a nested case control study. *British Journal of Clinical Pharmacology* 2011;71:116–120.

35. Juurlink DN. Antidepressants, antiplatelets and bleeding: one more thing to worry about? *Canadian Medical Association Journal* 2011;183:1819–1820.

36. O'Hara MW. Social support, life events, and depression during pregnancy and puerperium. *Archives of General Psychiatry* 1986;43:569–573.

37. Kitamura T, Shima S, Sugawara M, et al. Psychological and social correlates of the onset of affective disorders among pregnant women. *Psychosomatic Medicine* 1993;23:967–975.

38. Cooper WO, Will ME, Pont SJ, et al. Increasing use of antidepressants in pregnancy. *American Journal of Obstetrics and Gynecology* 2007;196:544.e1–545.e1.

39. Andrade SE, Raebel MA, Brown J, et al. Use of antidepressant medications during pregnancy: a multi-site study. *American Journal of Obstetrics and Gynecology* 2008;194. e1–195.e1.

40. Cohen LS, Altschuler LL, Harlow BL, et al. Relapse of major depression during pregnancy in women who maintain or discontinue antidepressant treatment. *Journal of the American Medical Association* 2006;295:499–507.

41. Toh S, Mitchell AA, Louik C, et al. Selective serotonin reuptake inhibitor use and risk of gestational hypertension. *American Journal of Psychiatry* 2009;166:320–328.

42. Einarson TR, Einarson A. New antidepressants in pregnancy and rates of major malformations: a meta-analysis of prospective comparative studies. *Pharmacoepidemiology and Drug Safety* 2005;14:823–827.

43. Jimenez-Solem E, Andersen JT, Petersen M, et al. Exposure to selective serotonin reuptake inhibitors and the risk of congenital malformations: a nationwide cohort study. *British Medical Journal Open* 2012;2:e001148. Doi:10.1136/ bmjopen-2012-00148.

44. Huybrechts KF, Palmsten K, Avorn J, et al. Antidepressant use in pregnancy and the risk of cardiac defects. *New England Journal of Medicine* 2014;370:2397–2407.

45. Reis M, Kallen B. Delivery outcome after maternal use of antidepressants: an update using Swedish data. *Psychological Medicine* 2010;40:1723–1733.

46. Williams M. Paroxetine (Paxil) and congenital malformations. *Health and Drug Alerts, Canadian Medical Association Journal* 2005;173:1320–1321.

47. Steiner M. Prenatal exposure to antidepressants: how safe are they? *American Journal of Psychiatry* 2012;169:1130–1132.

48. Källén B, Reis M. Neonatal complications after maternal concomitant use of SSRI and other central nervous system active drugs during the second or third trimester of pregnancy. *Journal of Clinical Psychopharmacology* 2012;32:608–614.

49. Levinson-Castiel R, Merlob P, Lindner N, et al. Neonatal abstinence syndrome after in utero exposure to selective serotonin reuptake inhibitors in term infants. *Archives of Pediatric and Adolescent Medicine* 2006;160:173–176.

50. Grzeskowiak LI, Gilbert AL, Morrison JL. Neonatal outcomes after late-gestation exposure to selective serotonin reuptake inhibitors. *Journal of Clinical Psychopharmacology* 2012;32:615–621.

51. Oberlander TF, Warburton W, Misri P, et al. Neonatal outcomes after prenatal exposure to selective serotonin reuptake inhibitor antidepressants and maternal depression using population-based linked health data. *Archives of General Psychiatry* 2006;63:898–906.

52. El Marroun H, Jaddoe VWV, Hudziak JJ, et al. Maternal use of selective serotonin reuptake inhibitors, fetal growth, and risk of adverse birth outcomes. *Archives of General Psychiatry* 2012;69:706–714.

53. Ross LE, Grigoriadis S, Mamisashvili L, et al. Selected pregnancy and delivery outcomes after exposure to antidepressant medication. A systematic review and meta-analysis. *JAMA Psychiatry* 2013;70:436–443.

54. Occhiogrosso M, Omran SS, Altemus M. Persistent pulmonary hypertension of the newborn and selective serotonin reuptake inhibitors: lessons from clinical and translational studies. *American Journal of Psychiatry* 2012;169:134–140.

55. US Food and Drug Administration: Increased risk of Neonatal Persistent Pulmonary Hypertension. 2006. www.fda.gov/Drugs/DrugSafety/default.htm.

56. Yonkers K, Wisner K, Oberlander D, et al. The management of depression during pregnancy: a report from the American Psychiatric Association. *General Hospital Psychiatry* 2009;31:403–413.

57. Keiler H, Artama M, Engeland A, et al. Selective serotonin reuptake inhibitors during pregnancy and the risk of persistent pulmonary hypertension in the newborn: population based cohort study from the five Nordic countries. *British Medical Journal* January 12, 2011;344:d8012. Doi:10.1136/bmj.d.8012.

58. *FDA MedWatch*, December 14, 2011. Selective serotonin reuptake inhibitor antidepressants (SSRIS): drug safety communication-Use during pregnancy and potential risk of persistent pulmonary hypertension of the newborn.

59. Pedersen LH, Henriksen TB, Bech BH, et al. Prenatal antidepressant exposure and behavioral problems in early childhood—a cohort study. *Acta Psychiatrica Scandanavica* 2012. Doi:10.1111/acps.12032.

60. Nulman I, Koren G, Rovet J, et al. Neurodevelopment of children following prenatal exposure to venlafaxine, selective serotonin reuptake inhibitors, or untreated maternal depression. *American Journal of Psychiatry* 2012;169:1165–1174.

61. Misri S, Reebye P, Kendrick K, et al. Internalizing behaviors in 4-year-old children exposed in utero to psychotropic medications. *American Journal of Psychiatry* 2006;163:1026–1032.

62. Croen LA, Grether JK, Yoshida CK, et al. Antidepressant use during pregnancy and childhood autism spectrum disorders. *Archives of General Psychiatry* 2011;68:1104–1112.

63. Weissman AM, Levy BT, Hartz AJ, et al. Pooled analysis of antidepressant levels in lactating mothers, breast milk, and nursing infants. *American Journal of Psychiatry* 2006;161:1066–1078.

64. Ruchkin V, Martin A. SSRIs and the developing brain. *The Lancet* 2005;365:451–453.

65. Koren G, Nordeng H. Antidepressant use during pregnancy: the benefit-risk ratio. *American Journal of Obstetrics and Gynecology* September 2012;207:157–163.

66. Fitton CA, Steiner MFC, Aucott L, et al. In utero exposure to antidepressant medication and neonatal and child outcomes. *Acta Psychiatrica Scandinavaca* 2019. Doi:10.1111/acps.13120.

67. Wolgast E, Lind-Astrand L, Lilliecreutz C. Women's perspectives of medication use during pregnancy and breast-feeding—a Swedish cross-sectional questionnaire study. *Acta Obstetrical and Gynecologoical Scandinavaca* 2019;98:857–865.

68. Pedersen LH. Editorial. To treat or not to treat: do not let fear decide whether to use medication during pregnancy. *Acta Obstetrical and Gynecological Scandinavaca* 2019;98:821–822.

69. Gill HS, Lindsay CL, Risch SC. Extrapyramidal symptoms associated with cyclic antidepressants treatment: a review of the literature and consolidating hypotheses. *Journal of Clinical Psychopharmacology* 1997;17:377–389.

70. Moro-de-Casillas ML, Riley DE. Antidepressants. In: *Drug-Induced Movement Disorders*, Second Edition. Editors: Factor SA, Lang AE, Weiner WJ. Blackwell Futura, Malden MA, 2005, pp. 373–407.

71. Meltzer HY, Young M, Metz J, et al. Extrapyramidal side effects and increased serum prolactin following fluoxetine, a new antidepressant. *Journal of Neural Transmission* 1979;45:165–175.

72. Arya DK. Extrapyramidal symptoms with selective serotonin reuptake inhibitors. *British Journal of Psychiatry* 1994;165:728–733.

73. Caley CF. Extrapyramidal reactions and the selective serotonin reuptake inhibitors. *The Annals of Pharmacotherapy* 1997;31:1481–1489.

74. Pies R. Must we now consider SRIs neuroleptics? *Journal of Clinical Psychopharmacology* 1997;17:443–445.
75. Armon C, Shin C, Miller P, et al. Reversible parkinsonism and cognitive impairment with chronic valproate use. *Neurology* 1996;47:626–635.
76. Masmoudi K, Gras-Champel V, Bonnet I, et al. Parkinsonism and cognitive impairment associated with chronic valproate therapy. *Therapie* 2000;55:629–634.
77. Zadikoff C, Munhoz RP, Asante AN, et al. Movement disorders in patients taking anticonvulsants. *Journal of Neurology, Neurosurgery, and Psychiatry* 2007;73:147–151.
78. Dragioti E, Solmi M, Favaro A, et al. Association of antidepressant use with adverse health outcomes. *JAMA Psychiatry* 2019;76:1241–1255.
79. Jensen MP, Ziff O, Banerjee G, et al. The impact of selective serotonin reuptake inhibitors on the risk of intracranial haemorrhage: a systematic review and meta-analysis. *European Stroke Journal* 2019;4:144–152. Doi:10.1177/23969873|9827211.
80. Schäfer W, Prink C, Kollhorst B, et al. Antidepressants and the risk of hemorrhagic stroke in the elderly: a nested case-control study. *Drug Safety* 2019;42:1081–1089. https://doi.org/10.1007/s40264-019-00837-y.

11 Treatment-Resistant Depression

Combining and Switching Antidepressants, Adding Antipsychotics, and on to Neurotherapeutics

Introduction

We noted earlier a consensus in the 1970s that depression was not only relatively uncommon but also had the best possibility of recovery in comparison to other major mental disorders.[1] However, the 30-year NIMH-sponsored collaborative depression study[2] revealed that 33% of people with depression failed to improve after four treatments, and at least 20% failed to recover, despite multiple treatments. Unfortunately, recurrence was substantial. Keep in mind that these poor results took place in the context of a flood of new antidepressants, depression awareness campaigns, and additional emphasis on psychotherapeutic approaches. Given these data, many began to question the efficacy of ADs generally and whether SSRIs were any more effective than their predecessors, a topic we discussed in detail in Chapter 9. So, what to do about treatment-resistant depression? Let's examine the rapidly increasing options, including psychotropic drug combinations, anti-inflammatories, antidiabetic agents, non-invasive brain stimulation, the various forms of transcranial magnetic stimulation, deep brain stimulation, and irreversible neurosurgical procedures. Despite these developments, in 2019 many have continued to criticize the lack of progress in treating depression[3] and have urged a paradigm shift in our approach to mental disorders,[4] including a shift away from underperforming big ideas,[5] about which I will say more later.

Combining Antidepressants

Psychiatrists never tire of combining drugs from the same or different classes, hoping to achieve better results. Earlier, we documented the failure of that approach with regard to APs, but what about ADs? In one review of this strategy,[6] the authors cited a number of small studies in which SSRIs were supplemented with various ADs, but with mixed results. In the STAR★D study,[7] augmentation of citalopram with bupropion was no more effective than augmentation with buspirone, an antianxiety agent. Remission rates were only 30% with either drug.

Despite these mixed but unimpressive results, the search for effective drug combinations has been intensive, as witnessed by a meta-analytic study[8] that found over 3,000 articles published between 1996 and 2010. However, the authors included *only* RCTs that examined results when ADS were combined at study start (rather than as augmentation), where there were quantifiable outcomes, and where the combination was compared with a single AD. These simple inclusion criteria left *only* five studies with 250 patients for an analysis of efficacy and 284 patients for an analysis of dropout rates! Keeping in mind the limits just noted, the *overall remission rates doubled for the combination* while mirtazapine plus an SSRI yielded an 88% increase in the remission rate vs a single agent. This was not true for response, which is odd indeed, since response rates are usually higher than remission rates.

Before the reader returns to the office and doubles the prescriptions for ADs, the caveats voiced by the authors need emphasis, particularly the scarcity of placebo-controlled trials. In addition, there was little data on adverse events, except for weight gain in the mirtazapine groups. No study lasted longer than eight weeks, and, as noted previously, the population was small, and other potential combinations were not investigated. With regard to the TCA plus SSRI outcome, Spijker and his group[6] found the evidence for that combination doubtful. Similarly, the Canadian Network for Mood and Anxiety Treatments Clinical Guidelines found the evidence for combination treatments considerably weaker than for augmentation strategies.[9, p. 36]

A later study by Rush et al.[10] was not included in the preceding review and meta-analysis, but did correct some of the methodologic problems, including the use of an acute-phase 12-week duration with single-blinding at various points, followed by randomization to three treatments: escitalopram plus placebo, bupropion plus escitalopram, or mirtazapine plus bupropion. *Remission rates at 12 weeks did not differ among the three groups (37% to 39%), nor did response rates (51% to 52%).* Although the mirtazapine plus bupropion group had a greater risk of adverse events, the dropout rates were similar. Note that clinicians were not blinded to treatment, and diagnoses were not based on structured interviews, so this study was more representative of what one finds in the clinic—and it didn't work! Yet in the Blier et al. study of 105 people with major depression,[11] the authors found that the remission rate doubled with combination therapy (46% to 52%) compared with fluoxetine alone (25%). There were no significant differences in dropout rates, but people in the combination groups gained significant weight. There was no placebo arm. The NNTs were impressively low at 3 to 5.

What are we to make of this? First, the evidence suggests poor results with ADs generally, and virtually every study acknowledges the need for better treatment. Second, the combination studies suffer from low numbers and a paucity of RCTs. Third, despite the impressive results found by several groups, Michael Thase concluded[12] that the evidence for combination treatment has not been well validated, a conclusion similar to that of Cowen[13] in 2017.

Switching Antidepressants

This is often the first strategy, with an ongoing debate over switching to a drug from a different class (SSRI to SNRI) or within a class (SSRI to SSRI). In the STAR*D studies, several switch strategies were employed, but they seemed to make little difference,[14] although people with treatment-resistant depression (TRD) were not targeted. Of interest, remission rates dropped to about 15% if the first two trials failed! In a meta-analysis[15] of SSRI-resistant depression, switching to another SSRI yielded a remission rate of 23%; if the patient was switched to a non-SSRI (bupropion, mirtazapine), the response rate was 28%, with a 28% increase in remission. However, the NNT was 22, far higher than the clinically useful NNT of 10.

Yet the authors noted that this increase might be important, given the numbers of people with TRD. In addition, the NNT with venlafaxine (an SNRI) was 13, making this a more reasonable choice. In a meta-analysis[16] of 93 trials comparing SSRIs with SNRIs (venlafaxine, mirtazapine, duloxetine, mianserin, moclobemide) for MDD, SNRIs did show a "modest advantage," but note an *NNT of 24*. A reminder: An NNT of 24 means that one would have to treat 24 additional patients to get a response beyond that obtained with an SSRI. Whether this would be cost effective is not at all clear.

In 2017, Cowen[13] summed up other psychotropics thought to be effective in TRD, including TCAs and MOAIs, but TCAs have a high rate of side effects, and the MAOIs require dietary restrictions in order to avoid hypertensive crises. I have been hesitant indeed to prescribe either group of drugs, given their adverse events and possible fatalities with overdoses. Nevertheless, we have reviewed evidence in previous chapters pointing to undertreatment of many chronically depressed patients.[2, 17]

Augmentation Strategies

Another approach to TRD involves supplementing an antidepressant with a non-antidepressant drug. Indeed, there are many such options.[7, 9, 13] For example:

- Add lithium to the AD, with meta-analytic studies showing this to be superior to placebo, whether added to TCAs or SSRIs.
- Add triiodothronine (Cytomel) to the AD, but the evidence is weaker. On the other hand, side effects are fewer, and, if there is no response in three to six weeks, it can be stopped without tapering.
- Add buspirone, pindolol, or stimulants, but these steps have even weaker evidence, so should be avoided.
- Add psychotherapy, a move we shall consider later.
- Add an antipsychotic, an increasingly popular move that deserves more examination.

However, a 2019 meta-analysis[18] of augmentation therapies found an overall effect size of only 1.19 for pharmacological treatments and 1.43 for psychological treatments. The highest ES (1.48) for medication was found in NMDA-targeting drugs, including ketamine, D-cycloserine, and minocycline. Note that the ES for APs was only 1.12, although aripiprazole was better, at 1.33. The authors concluded that the evidence was "sparse." Controlled trials of psychological interventions were comparatively few, unfortunately.

Adjunctive Use of Antipsychotics

As of this writing, the only FDA-approved strategies for *adjunctive* use of APs in major depression are aripiprazole, extended-release quetiapine, and brexipiprazole, while ketamine and a combination of fluoxetine and olanzapine (Symbyax) have been approved for TRD. Symbyax has also been approved for bipolar depression.[18] *Caution*: Symbyax is clearly a marketing ploy since one could easily give fluoxetine and olanzapine (both are generic) as separate drugs, but Symbyax is packaged in odd doses not available in the separate drugs. For example, 3 mg of olanzapine/25 mg of fluoxetine, 6 mg of olanzapine/25 mg of fluoxetine, etc. I have not seen any evidence showing that the 6 mg/25 mg capsule is superior to 10 mg of olanzapine plus 20 mg of fluoxetine.

Antipsychotics as Antidepressants

One comparatively easy and less expensive route toward the better treatment of depression would be to find new uses for an already FDA-approved drug class, which is precisely what has happened in the rush to market APs as ADs. The reader may recall that FDA approval for a new indication of a previously approved drug *requires only one RCT, a low standard indeed.*

Although some might see the dual role of APs as something novel in the field, that is not historically accurate. Earlier in this volume, we cited Winkelman's large outpatient study[19] of chlorpromazine, in which 41% of depressed patients showed at least "moderate" improvement. However, the focus was not on depression itself. Paradoxically, Heinz Lehmann stressed in a classic paper[20, p. 229] that the *primary goal* of chlorpromazine was to produce motor retardation, sedation, and emotional indifference, all of which can be found in major depression. Regardless, interest in the antidepressant properties of APs continued, although dampened historically by growing concerns over TD, parkinsonian side effects,[21] and, more recently, the metabolic syndrome.

In a meta-analysis of AP augmentation in the treatment of major depression,[21] the authors noted that the first report of atypical antipsychotic augmentation for depression came out in 1999, but it had very few patients. However, this study included 16 trials involving 3,480 patients with TRD.

There was a substantial difference in the response rates, with 44% of those taking an SGA responding vs 30% with placebo, yielding an odds ratio of 1.69, a highly significant result. The odds ratio for remission was impressive, at 2.00, while 30% remitted in the atypical group vs 17% with placebo. The NNT was 9 for both remission and response. Interestingly, there were *no differences between and among the four SGAs*, which itself is odd, given the differences in FDA approval of these agents for depression and the endless TV commercials touting aripiprazole.

I must say that the results are impressive, in that almost half of those who had failed treatment responded, and almost one third remitted. The authors correctly noted that the number of patients in this trial was far larger than in comparable trials of adjunctive agents (lithium, thyroid hormone), but there were problems, including a lack of data on adverse events and prior treatment. In addition, a careful reader will have noted that Dr. Nelson was a speaker and consultant for some 20 pharmaceutical companies, raising the question of bias. It appeared that an independent review was needed. In 2010, the Cochrane Collaboration[22] reviewed and analyzed 28 RCTs of SGAs as adjunctive agents and found less optimism. For example, risperidone had limited benefit, accompanied by weight gain and parkinsonism, while olanzapine was no more effective than add-on placebo. Quetiapine resulted in more symptom reduction than placebo, but sedation was common.

In 2013, another meta-analysis[23] incorporated ratings of remission, quality of life, and safety, with significant advantages found for aripiprazole, quetiapine, and risperidone. Olanzapine was also effective, but the NNT was elevated at 19. A summary recommendation of this study by Cowan[13] failed to mention that the meta-analysis lacked evidence for any improvement in quality of life or the presence of adverse events, including weight gain, with all four drugs; abnormal metabolic changes; and aripiprazole-induced akathisia.

Clinical Notes

1. It seems fair to conclude that SGAs may have some limited usefulness in treatment-resistant MDD, but the *primary problem is the paucity of data on metabolic side effects, especially when the drugs are used over a period of five years or longer.* In Chapter 4, we stressed that SGAs can significantly increase body fat and induce metabolic changes within weeks, so careful monitoring is a must.

2. Clinicians must document in writing that a full discussion of the risks vs benefits has occurred. These discussions should take place at least yearly, with a full discussion and documentation of any metabolic changes.

3. Monitoring for neurological side effects is necessary, regardless of the class of AP.

4. Do not neglect the benefits of psychotherapy! We shall discuss this in detail later, but there is significant evidence for the use of cognitive

behavioral therapy (CBT) and other approaches, either as monotherapy or in combination with medication.

Neurotherapeutics and Depression

The burgeoning interest in a variety of procedures aimed at directly stimulating the brain seems to reflect not only the never-ending effort at expanding the medicalization of depression and the growing clout of the medical device companies[24] but also an acknowledgment that 60 years of drug development have failed to produce any real gains in the pharmacological treatment of depression. We have already reviewed the poor outcomes of many studies earlier in the volume, a view reinforced by Holtzheimer and Mayberg,[25] who noted that about 65% of patients fail to respond to a first antidepressant, and one third fail to achieve remission after four trials of an FDA-approved AD. In primary care settings, where a great deal of treatment takes place, non-response has ranged from 10% to 51% while a partial response has been found in 11% to 45% and remission in 25% to 65%.[26]

Vagus Nerve Stimulation

Once again, we find an approach that initially seemed to hold some promise, but serious questions arose after the FDA approved vagus nerve stimulation (VNS) as an adjunctive treatment for MDD in July of 2005—only one year after the agency had rejected it! What happened?

Before proceeding, let's note that the procedure involves implantation of a pulse generator in the left chest wall, the insertion of a steel shaft through a channel under the skin through which wire leads are threaded. The wires are wrapped around the vagus nerve, which is close to the carotid artery. The pulse generator is programmable. Note that the VN is closely connected with areas thought to be important in mood, including the serotonergic system and the hypothalamus, while stimulation of the VN leads to increased blood flow in the amygdala and the cingulate gyrus.[27] During VSN treatment of convulsive disorders, some observed improvement in mood, leading to the initial studies.

In 2000, Rush et al. published an open-label trial[28] of 30 patients with TRD, in which VNS led to a 40% response rate, a very good result considering that this group had failed two to five trials of ADs and psychotherapy. This led Cyberonics, the manufacturer, to develop a 21-site RCT involving 235 patients with MDD or bipolar depression.[29] The patients were highly treatment resistant, having failed treatment with ADs in at least four episodes of major depression. They had also failed at least six weeks of psychotherapy in any depressive episode. The baseline Hamilton Depression Rating scale was 20 or greater. Medications were left unchanged. Patients were randomized to active or sham treatment; even those in sham treatment had the device implanted. The raters were blind, but programmers of the device could not be blinded, for obvious reasons. So far, so good . . . but what were the results at ten weeks?

Sadly for Cyberonics—and the patients—*only 15.2% of the active treatment group responded on the Hamilton Rating Scale for Depression, compared with 10% of the sham group*, a non–statistically significant difference. On a global rating of change, 13.9% of the active treatment group responded vs 11.8% of the sham group, another non-significant result. Several other ratings, with one exception, also failed to show meaningful improvement. These results were not close to those required of a drug, but the authors concluded that the study did not "yield definitive evidence of short-term efficacy," a statement remarkable for its optimism. In addition, it wasn't clear if study procedures had insured adequate blinding, an important issue given the many side effects of VNS. In addition, there was one suicide in the active group and one infection. Depression became worse in 11 patients (4 in the active group), while 2 in the active group became manic or hypomanic. Other adverse events included voice changes in 68%, cough and shortness of breath in 23% to 29%, and wound infection in 8%.

Not to be deterred, Cyberonics then did a 12-month follow-up *open-label* study[30] in which those on sham treatment could have active treatment at a certain level of depression. Raters were blinded to settings, but the treating physicians were a mixed group of study personnel and others. In this uncontrolled study, 27% responded, and almost 16% remitted. Another definition of benefit was added, ranging from worse to extraordinary benefit, with 57% of the evaluable sample receiving at least meaningful benefit. *However, an intent-to-treat analysis by the FDA[31] found that only 38% had a meaningful benefit!*

Cyberonics then sponsored another study[32] with the goal of comparing VNS with treatment as usual (TAU). Results were again superior to those found in the RCT, with 27% of the VNS patients responding vs 13% of the TAU group, a significant difference. However, this study was *badly flawed* by *switching the primary outcome measure* from the Hamilton scale to the Inventory of Depressive Symptomatology Self-Report. With regard to adverse events, 1 patient committed suicide, 6 attempted suicide, and 30 of 177 had to be hospitalized for worsening depression, while 3 developed hypomania. Two other deaths occurred, one from unknown causes after 10 weeks of VNS, and one person died due to a pre-existing malignancy. (If the patient was that ill, why was he/she enrolled in the study?)

A Blue Cross/Blue Shield Technology Evaluation Summary[33] in 2005 found *no substantial evidence* that VNS improved net health outcomes, nor was VNS as effective as alternative treatments. We must note that the studies noted here were sponsored by the manufacturer, and the investigators were predominantly employees of and/or consultants to Cyberonics, with obvious financial stakes in the outcome. Given such poor results, we must also stress that the cost of the system is not trivial: about $15,00 to $18,000, while the surgical procedure can run to some $15,000 as of 2005. The company, however, favorably compared the VNS system to the cost of dealing with treatment-resistant depression.

So why did the FDA choose to approve VNS in August of 2005? It appears this was done on the basis of testimony by patients and relatives who understandably were seeking help for depression—but the decision was not evidence-based. Indeed, the Public Citizen Health Research Group[34] stated that the FDA decision was among the worst regulatory decisions in recent memory and predicted that thousands of depressed patients would be implanted, regardless of the data.

Subsequent studies of VNS[35, 36, 37] demonstrated response rates of 43% to 53% but with significant side effects, including worsening depression, suicides, a switch into mania, coughing, and voice changes. A systematic review of VNS in TRD was done by Daban et al.,[38] in which all studies save the original RCT were uncontrolled. Some predictors of a positive response included a previous response to ECT and the output current of the device, although one group did not find that significant. It's difficult to know what to make of these findings, given the seriously flawed methodology and the desperate search for results. In addition, VNS is a long-term process involving daily stimulation of the vagus nerve with noticeable side effects, and it is both expensive and invasive. Moreover, several case reports have surfaced in which the authors found an increase in sleep apnea with VNS,[39] and another in which mild neck trauma led to vocal cord paralysis and injury to the vagus nerve itself during surgery.[40]

In the meantime, the problems with TRD led to the creation in 2006 of a treatment-resistant registry in the United States, with 61 sites representing a mix of academic, private clinics, and institutions.[41] One of the motivations for this was the FDA's insistence on a post-marketing surveillance study after granting approval for VNS in TRD. This naturalistic study,[41] carried out over five years, included 795 patients with MMD or bipolar depression who were also receiving treatment as usual (TAU). The adjunctive VNS clearly outperformed the TAU-only group, with a response rate of 67% vs 40% and a remission rate of 43% vs 25%. The VNS group also had more reduction in suicidality and all-cause mortality.

Despite these impressive results, a systematic review[42] of VNS in 2019 found a limited number of RCTs. A qualitative analysis found no significant differences between VNS and sham VNS on a number of standard rating scales used to gauge depressive symptoms. On the brighter side, adjunctive VNS *combined* with TAU led to a significant decrease in depressive symptoms and improved quality of life.[43] These mixed results have led some to develop transcranial auricular VNS, in which the lower half of the back ear is stimulated, with modulatory effects similar to invasive VNS. A meta-analysis[44] of this approach in 2018 found statistically significant improvements in MDD in four studies.

Clinical Notes

1. All in all, I would not refer any patient for VNS, absent positive results in at least two well-done, long-term RCTs sponsored by the NIMH or other independent agency with investigators not tied to the manufacturers.
2. The side effects have been serious, with worsening depression, suicidality, obvious voice changes, site infections, and technological problems with the wires and pulse generator requiring corrective surgery.
3. Other, safer alternatives are available for treatment-resistant depression and, in most instances, are not invasive.

Transcranial Magnetic Stimulation (TMS)

Repetitive TMS (rTMS) employs the passage of an alternating current through a metal coil, which is placed over the patient's scalp, a procedure that induces a magnetic field over brain areas and depolarizes neurons to a depth of about 2 cm. Repetitive TMS was first used to map neurons in the motor cortex, with the goal of delineating neurons involved in memory, vision, and muscle control.[45] When treating depression, the coil usually placed over the left dorsolateral prefrontal cortex (DLPC), an area involved in regulation of mood, but also in the proposed pathology of schizophrenia. The first devices emitted only a single pulse but later emitted a rapid succession of pulses, leading to the term *rTMS*. Similarly, frequencies have increased from 1 Hz or less to 5 to 20 Hz. Treatment can be affected by coil placement, stimulus intensity, frequency of treatment, and other variables. Repetitive TMS is often given in 20 sessions. *In contrast to ECT, no anesthesia is needed, and, in contrast to VNS and deep brain stimulation, it is non-invasive.* TMS was FDA approved for the treatment of depression in October of 2008, with the proviso that the patient have failed one trial of an AD, rather than two.

Proposed mechanisms of action include many of the same effects produced by ADs and ECT, including an increase in BDNF, increased turnover of DA and NE, and normalization[45] of the hypothalamic-pituitary-adrenal axis (HPA), which is in overdrive in depression. Stimulation of the prefrontal cortex (PFC) may help restore the putative imbalance between the PFC and the limbic system found in some depressed patients. Yet several studies[46, 47] have shown that rTMS induces ipsilateral release of subcortical DA. And, in contrast to ADs, experiments with adult male rats found that rTMS did not increase neurogenesis in the hippocampus but down-regulated the HPA axis.[48] One group found that a well-known polymorphism (the Val66Met, in which valine is substituted for methionine) in the gene coding for BDNF modified the motor response to rTMS, perhaps as a result of effects on synaptic plasticity.[49]

The relatively benign nature of rTMS led to a much larger pool of randomized, controlled trials than we found with VNS. That being the case,

Couturier[50] performed a meta-analysis of 6 RCTS that had met strict inclusion criteria, although 19 RCTS had been located—but most were methodologically compromised. Sadly, *rTMS was no better than sham treatment*, perhaps because of a small sample size. The authors compared their results with another meta-analysis of 14 trials by Martin et al.,[51] who found a statistically significant effect of rTMS at two weeks of active treatment, but this was *not significant at four weeks*. Once again, sample sizes were small, and the trials were felt to be methodologically poor due to small sample sizes, failures to do intent-to treat analyses—despite dropouts in half the studies—and inconsistencies in allowing medications during treatment. The authors concluded that the evidence *did not* support the use of rTMS for depression.

One of the larger and frequently cited studies[52] was a multi-site RCT of daily rTMS in 301 medication-free patients. This study deserves a detailed review, given its size and attention to detail. After 20 sessions over four weeks, active rTMS was *not superior to sham on the primary outcome measure*; the effect size was 0.26. In contrast to many of the VNS studies, the patients were not highly treatment resistant; they had failed, on average, only 1.6 ADs in the episode prior to study entry. On the other hand, they had been depressed for an average of 13 months, and half had failed to benefit from two or more treatments. Consistent with what we observed in the RCT of VNS, the authors found a way around the results—but, in fairness, we should note that the sham group actually was more severely depressed at baseline, but *only* by 1.1 points, a difference which is not recognizable clinically. At any rate, the authors did a supplementary analysis that resulted in a statistically significant improvement with active treatment at week four, *despite* the failure of the first analysis to find an effect of active treatment on the primary outcome measure. Rates of remission did not differ at four weeks: 7% to 9%, depending on the scale, vs 6% to 8% with sham. The response rate at four weeks was 18% vs 11% with sham, with very similar rates on the Hamilton depression scale. After a number of adjustments, the authors concluded that the efficacy of rTMS is "comparable to that of standard pharmacotherapy."[52, p. 1214] They also noted several shortcomings, including the usual lack of data on prior treatment resistance and failure to assess the adequacy of the blind.

My major concern, however, mirrors what we found in studies of VNS: namely, the fact that *every investigator* was closely tied to either Cyberonics or Neuronetics, not to mention the usual ties to multiple pharmaceutical companies. Virtually all authors had been recipients of grants from Neuronetics, the study sponsor, and were often consultants to the company, as well as members of company speaker bureaus, positions that can be quite lucrative. Clearly, the possibility of bias in this study cannot be discounted. *One can only wonder why the principal investigators did not find at least one independent collaborator, given the rampant conflicts of interest.*

More clinical trials soon followed, as did multiple meta-analytic studies with response rates hovering around 43% to 53%.[53–55] A more inclusive meta-analysis of treatment-resistant depression, negative symptoms of schiz-ophrenia, auditory-visual hallucinations, and obsessive-compulsive disorder found an mean weighted effect size of 0.55 (moderate) in depression, of 0.39 in negative symptoms of schizophrenia, but of only 0.15 for OCD. In addition, ECT was superior to rTMS.[56] In a study of veterans with TRD, PTSD, and a history of substance abuse, rTMS as adjunctive therapy pro-duced an overall response remission rate of 39%, but remission rates did *not* differ between the active and sham groups.[57] Clearly, these results were at least in part secondary to careful monitoring of medications and more staff interaction.

Finally, a 2014 meta-analysis of high-frequency (at least 5 Hz) rTMS found 29 RCTs of this form of rTMS. Almost 30% responded, and 18.6% remitted, with NNTs of 6 and 8, respectively. Dropout rates were no differ-ent in the active vs sham groups, which is encouraging.[58]

rTMS in Bipolar Disorder

We should note that studies of bipolar disorder have been compromised by the concomitant use of a mélange of medications, making analysis difficult.[59] Early but uncontrolled results were promising, with a decline in a stand-ard rating scale of 71% with right prefrontal cortex rTMS compared with a 29% improvement when stimulating the left side, but a later controlled study found *no* difference between sham and active treatment.[60] However, a large study found that active treatment was superior,[61] with 100% of 41 patients achieving remission. Interestingly, *65% of the sham-treated patients also achieved remission*, but all the patients were receiving APs, 53% were receiving lithium, and 31% were receiving carbamazepine, leaving the results open to question.

In a retrospective review[62] of 100 consecutive patients with bipolar depres-sion or major depression, the primary outcome was the aforementioned CGI-1, a simple scale of clinical assessment. Patients had failed an average of 3.4 AD trials. In addition, 31 of the final sample of 85 patients had failed ECT or found it intolerable, by self-report. Treatment was flexibly dosed, with up to 30 sessions. *There was no placebo arm.* The CGI-1 response rate at six weeks was 50.6%, while the remission rate was 24.7%. These are impres-sive figures, but several problems should be noted. First, the patients were taking a very large number of concomitant medications from virtually every class of drug, but there was *no data* on polypharmacy and no review of phar-macy or medication records. In addition, one third had undescribed medi-cation changes during rTMS. In an interesting comparative study, Gross et al.[63] compared the results of a meta-analysis published in 2003[51] with a newer meta-analysis[63] involving another five trials and found that the effect size had increased significantly, but the authors admitted that the quality of the newer studies was still "variable" and that patient expectations might well have increased over time, given the publicity surrounding rTMS.

Clinical Notes

1. In summary, rTMS is much better tolerated than VNS and has considerably higher response rates in depression, with generally acceptable NNTs. Note, however, that a number of studies failed to show superiority over sham treatment.
2. There appear to be much lower rates of treatment-induced depression and/or suicidality.
3. It is non-invasive, does not require anesthesia, and the costs are no doubt much lower.
4. Obviously, one avoids any risk of infections or other operative complications, and the patient doesn't have to worry about battery failure and replacement. Some studies were compromised by potential conflicts of interest and bias.
5. Theta-burst stimulation was also approved in 2018 for TRD and employs 600 pulses in three minutes, with the possibility of shorter treatment sessions.

Transcranial Direct Current Stimulation

This approach utilizes a different technique than rTMS,[59] in that an anode is placed over the left dorsolateral prefrontal cortex, and a cathode over the right lateral orbit. Saline-soaked rubber electrodes are held in place by a band. The idea is to use direct current instead of an alternating current and to ramp up the current intensity from less than 1 mA to 1 to 2 mAs. Neurons under the positively charged anode are more excitable while neurons under the negatively charged cathode are inhibited. Treatment is given for 20 minutes in about 15 to 20 daily sessions,[64] but some of the early studies used alternate days and different numbers of sessions. It appears to modify cortical excitability, neural plasticity, and long-term potentiation, a process involved with memory.

In a double-blind, sham-controlled trial of tDCS, Loo et al. reported[64] clinically meaningful improvement with ten treatment sessions in 40 patients, but at the end of the five-day sham-controlled period, there was *no statistically significant improvement.* They then extended this work[65] in a three-week randomized, sham-controlled trial involving 64 people with MDD. Treatment was given every weekday for three weeks. Fifty-eight patients completed the three-week blinded trial in which there was only a *13% response rate in each group; no one remitted.* The NNT was 16, considerably higher than the standard of 10.

Despite these poor results, the authors insisted that the study confirmed the efficacy of tDCS while lamenting the fact that several earlier studies (see their discussion for a review and citations) had found response rates of 43% to 60% after two weeks or less. There was no decline in neuropsychological functioning after three to six weeks of treatment. Side effects included skin redness, burning, itching, headache, and dizziness, as well as other, very infrequent experiences of watery eyes, feeling spaced out, etc. In contrast to the many studies described earlier, this effort was independently funded by a national agency in Australia.

In another RCT of tDCS,[66] Loo et al. found no differences between active and sham treatment in the unipolar or bipolar depressed groups, although mood improved significantly in both. They also found that the BDNF genotype played no role, but this sample was badly underpowered for a genetic study. Yet a systematic review and meta-analysis[67] of studies in bipolar depression in 2017 found a significant decrease in depressive symptoms, although the treatment parameters were heterogeneous. Note, too, that in six cases, a switch to hypomania occurred.

Clinical Notes

1. In a lengthy review, Loo et al.[59] concluded that the evidence for rTMS in bipolar disorder was not definitive. They also concluded that ECT is the treatment of choice for severe bipolar depression, mania, and mixed mood episodes. With regard to non-bipolar MDD, the FDA has approved rTMS for adults who have failed to respond to at least one treatment episode with an AD used at or above the minimal dosage and duration. However, there is still ongoing debate about coil placement, number of rTMS stimulations, and whether rTMS should be used as maintenance therapy.
2. With regard to tDCS, the data is skimpy, with even less evidence of efficacy.
3. Evidence suggests that in cases of very serious depression, ECT is preferable to rTMS or tDCS but carries the risks of anesthesia and more side effects, including stigma. Cost-benefit data obtained from a single-blind, "pragmatic" trial[68] 46 patients who volunteered to be randomized to rTMS or ECT found that 59% achieved remission with ECT compared with 17% in rTMS, yet the Hamilton scores were no different at six-month follow-up! There was no difference in quality of life. Cost of treatment favored ECT, but other work has shown the reverse, with tDCS costing some $5,000 to $12,000 per course of treatment vs at least $20,000 for ECT.
4. In a review of Medline papers on tDCS, I found references to tDCS in alleviating post-stroke aphasia, enhancing motor recovery after stroke, enhancing cognitive abilities in a variety of conditions, in treating autistic disorder, and many other conditions. The majority of these papers involved small case series or single case reports, so I shall not cite references.

Deep Brain Stimulation (DBS)

Research into DBS treatment of psychiatric disorders has become much more popular in recent years, a remarkable and, indeed, curious development in view of the history of psychiatry and its early focus on lobotomy, insulin coma, ECT, and the other intrusive "therapies" described in Chapter 1. An even more extreme approach involved treating hallucinations by cutting out portions of the cerebral cortex (Burckhardt, 1891, cited in Holtzheimer and Mayberg).[25]

Despite the lack of solid evidence for lobotomies, tens of thousands of were performed in the U.S. over a 25-year period starting in the late 1930s.[69] (This was the era of forced sterilizations as well.) During the same period, another 10,000 were performed in Great Britain.[70] The results of lobotomy: indifference to symptoms, profoundly regressive behavior, passivity, and late-onset seizures.[70] As cited by Whitaker, the California Department of Mental Hygiene wrote in 1949 that lobotomy had been used primarily to pacify uncooperative and belligerent patients,[71, p. 135] exactly as shown in *One Flew Over the Cuckoo's Nest*. Ironically, the pioneer of prefrontal lobotomy, Egas Moniz, suffered paralysis after being shot by a patient he lobotomized and later was fatally assaulted by another lobotomized patient not happy with the results.[72]

In a lengthy 2008 editorial[70] in the *American Journal of Psychiatry*, Yudofsky took note of the historical course of lobotomy in the U.S. and how psychosurgery had become synonymous with the exploitation of psychiatric patients by callous, unethical, and unchecked professionals. Despite this history, Yudofsky's editorial was aimed at smoothing the path back to psychosurgery, in part by recommending that we do away with the term *psychosurgery* and replace it with the term *neurosurgical intervention*, but others questioned the wisdom of this strategy.[72] It is my intention to review representative studies in this area and to examine the data on efficacy and safety.

Let's begin with DBS, which is a reversible procedure involving placement of electrodes bilaterally in various brain areas, accompanied by the subcutaneous implantation of a programmable neurostimulator that sends an electrical current to the electrodes. There appears to be disagreement with regard to whether the current produces brain lesions.[73, 74]

In 1997, the FDA approved DBS for the treatment of Parkinson's disease, but it soon came to be used for the treatment of tremor, dystonias, chronic pain, and cluster headaches.[73] By 2007, some 35,000 patients with movement disorders had been treated with DBS.[75] With additional time, psychiatric disorders came to be treated with DBS, including major depression, OCD, Tourette's syndrome, and addiction.[76] In 2009, the FDA approved a Medtronic DBS device for chronic and severe obsessive-compulsive disorder under a humanitarian device exemption.[77]

The expanding list of psychiatric disorders began to cause some discomfort in the field, such that enthusiasts began to ask if DBS should be considered psychosurgery. For example, Sachdev[74] argued in 2007 that DBS should be considered distinct from psychosurgery since no lesion is being created, a debatable conclusion.[73] Sachdev further added that there are no obvious structural deficits in psychiatric disorders—an interesting statement, given the hundreds of papers showing a variety of structural brain changes in multiple disorders.

One of the remarkable findings in these studies is the variety of brain sites that have been stimulated, with generally similar results. As of 2010, 17 different brain areas had been targeted with DBS![76] We will review a representative study in detail, but first, here is a summary of the more important sites and response rates as described by Holtzheimer and Mayberg.[25]

> Ventral anterior accumbens, 6 months, response rate of 50%.
> Inferior internal capsule/ventral striatum, 6 months, response rate of 53%.
> Nucleus thalamic peduncle in one patient, 24 months, "dramatic improvement, but relapsed.
> Lateral habenula, one patient, 60 weeks, poor response until high stimulation, then 4 months to remission.

While the response rates are impressive, *these studies were all uncontrolled, open-label studies with very small numbers of patients,* thus leaving considerable doubt about placebo effects and efficacy. Granted, these patients were highly resistant to standard therapies—including ECT in some cases—which certainly makes the response rates more impressive. Yet there is no doubt that the ethics of DBS and other invasive techniques needs serious consideration, given the risks of these procedures, even with contemporary neurosurgical techniques. In addition, this deeply flawed methodology would never result in FDA approval of a new drug.

Fortunately, at least from a scientific viewpoint, we now have several studies with larger numbers and longer follow-ups. The first report by Mayberg et al.[78] included only *six patients* with TRD who had failed at least four treatment efforts, including ECT in five of the six. All patients had undergone cognitive behavioral therapy with poor results. Persons with active suicidality were not accepted. I want to describe these early studies in detail, since they illustrate the problems with this approach.

The procedure involved implanting four electrodes in the subgenual cingulate gyrus white matter on each side of the brain (Brodmann area 25). Electrodes were inserted through burr holes in the skull. Electrode locations were guided by MRI and confirmed by MRI scans. A pulse generator was implanted in the chest wall. Voltage was increased as tolerated every 30 seconds, with monitoring of changes in visual perception, verbal expression, and mood. Patients were blinded as to which electrode was stimulated over the five-day post-operative period, during which refinements were made to the stimuli according to symptoms experienced by the patient, including heightened sensations, sharper visual details, increased attention, and rather mystical experiences. Changes in rate and volume of speech were also noted, but *sham stimuli failed to result in such changes.* The patients were then discharged home with no stimulation for one week, after which the stimuli were programmed and generally remained constant for six months. Stimulus parameters on average were 4.0 volts, 60s pulse width, with a frequency of 60 Hz.

As with AD studies, response was defined as a 50% drop on the HAM-D and remission as a HAM-D score of less than 8. Medications given before surgery were not changed. *The response rate was 66% (n = 4) at four months.* The authors then tried to rule out a placebo response by blinded discontinuation of the stimuli in a single patient who had shown a robust response. After two weeks, the patient gradually worsened, so stimulation was resumed, with normalization of symptoms at 48 hours. This is interesting, but it doesn't merit serious scientific consideration as a blinded methodology. We shall discuss mechanisms of action later, but we should note that two of the six patients developed infections around the connector cable in the chest and were treated with IV antibiotics. The devices were taken out at six months without worsening of depression. (How long were they subsequently followed?) Another patient developed erosion of the skin over the hardware and was also treated with antibiotics. Note that all patients were given prophylactic antibiotics hours after each procedure, pointing to obvious concerns over the possibility of infection. Comprehensive neuropsychological testing revealed no adverse effects on IQ, language, or visual-spatial functions.

PET scans were done in the first five patients and compared with normal controls, with the depressed patients showing elevated subgenual cingulate blood flow at baseline, a finding not previously found in non-TRD patients. Decreases in cerebral blood flow were found pre-frontally and elsewhere, *but similar patterns were seen in responders and non-responders.* However, the magnitude of the prefrontal decrease after treatment was greater in responders. The scans were repeated at three and six months and showed normalization of blood flow in the subgenual cingulate and prefrontal cortices as well as the hypothalamus, consistent with changes associated with AD treatment. Note that the subgenual hyperactivity found at baseline was different from previous studies in bipolar and unipolar depression, where hypoactivity was common.

This group of 6 patients was later expanded to 20. The response rate at 12 months was 60%; the remission rate was 30%.[79] However, 2 patients underwent explantation due to lack of efficacy, and 2 more were lost to follow-up, although 1 eventually returned. By the start of year three,[80] 14 patients remained, but one committed suicide 35 months post implantation. Using an intent-to-treat analysis, 55% responded, and 20% remitted at one year; 60% responded, and 40% remitted at three years; and 55% responded, and 35% remitted at the last follow-up visit. Interestingly, there was *no difference between responders and non-responders in quality of life* as measured by the SF-36. However, *90% of those who responded returned to work vs 33% of those who did not, a significant difference.*

Adverse Events in the Mayberg,[78] Lozano,[79] and Kennedy[80] Studies

There were no additional adverse device-related events after the first year. However, eight patients required surgery for battery replacement at a mean of 43 months. Eight patients were hospitalized on 12 occasions, with *half experiencing worsening depression or suicidality.* Two patients committed suicide. The patient with confirmed suicide had a strong family history of suicide. Two other patients attempted suicide, both in the first year after surgery. The use of ADs decreased in nine patients; only one began an AD. Five of fourteen taking an SGA discontinued it. Outcome was not predicted by stimulus parameters or variation in electrode placement.

The suicide rate was 10%. The authors cited data indicating that suicide occurs in 2% of severely depressed outpatients and 6% to 15% of inpatients suffering melancholic depression, so whether the suicide rate in this small group is excessive is difficult to determine. Yet we need to remember that potential candidates for this study (starting with Mayberg et al.[78]) *were not accepted if they had active thoughts of suicide,* nor could they be included if suffering from schizophrenia, bipolar disorder, or current substance abuse, including use of alcohol in the previous three months.[78, p. 657] We have no knowledge of the subsequent course of these patients. Did they continue DBS, and will they continue it indefinitely?

Despite repeated calls for controlled studies, a larger and primarily uncontrolled study[81] came out in 2012 but with an interesting ethical twist we shall describe in a moment. The study was sponsored by Emory University and sought to enroll adults with failure to respond to at least four treatment episodes with ADs, failure to respond to ECT, or intolerance or inability to receive ECT. As we found earlier, patients with significant psychiatric co-morbidities were excluded, as were patients with substance abuse in the previous 12 months, those currently suicidal, and those with personality disorders. Psychotherapy was not only permitted, but patients were encouraged to continue therapy if they had started it six months prior to study enrollment. Current psychotropics were allowed if doses had been stable for four weeks prior to surgery. In the later observational phase, meds/therapy could be altered. Details of the surgery and electrode placement were similar to those found in Mayberg et al.[78]

All patients were told that they would be randomized to active or sham stimulation, *but, in fact, all patients received sham stimulation.* Although this was approved by the Emory University Institutional Review Board, *I maintain that this maneuver, in fact, was unethical.* Subsequent reviews of DBS,[82] which included this study, failed to mention the ethical lapse, as did two papers specifically examining the ethics of DBS.[83, 84] In a single-blind discontinuation phase, patients were told that they were being randomized to active or sham treatment, *but all received sham.* Sadly, the first 3 patients to have treatment discontinued developed suicidality. This resulted in elimination of this phase. An observational follow-up phase was next, in which the 17 patients continued to receive open-label stimulation, with evaluations monthly for three months, then every three months for nine months, then every six months. *During this phase, there were no restrictions on changes in medications and psychotherapy if they were approved by the study team or the primary care doctor.*

Results: 14 patients completed one year of stimulation, 11 completed two years, with response rates of 36% to 92%, and remission rates of 18% to 58%. But keep in mind the length of time needed for response and remission. These are complex neurosurgical procedures! No patient experienced a spontaneous relapse in the presence of active stimulation, and there was no difference in response rates in unipolar vs bipolar patients, although the numbers were quite small. *Neuropsychological testing scores did not worsen* with during the study, and several improved.

Adverse Events

Adverse events occurred in 65% of the cases and serious events in 24%. (75% of those occurred in one bipolar patient.) No manic or hypomanic episodes occurred. Two episodes of infection occurred in one patient; these required explantation. One patient developed two episodes of suicidality, and two made attempts in conjunction with undescribed stressors. Two patients developed five episodes of anxiety; *53% had surgery to replace the battery* after 72 weeks of active stimulation.

One group did a meta-analytic study of adverse events with DBS[73] and found 2,095 unique articles published after 1996. Interestingly, only 30 were published in 1996, but this rose to 338 by 2008, an astonishing increase. Not surprisingly, 65% of the procedures were aimed at Parkinson's disease, with only 3% of the studies aimed at psychiatric conditions. In general, mood improved in these studies, and there was little evidence of cognitive deterioration, but about 10% gained weight. *The primary finding was an increase in completed suicides*, although there were problems in interpretation since the mean time to suicide was two years after surgery. Kennedy et al.[80] cited a number of studies employing DBS for movement disorders in which 4.3% of patients committed suicide about three years after the procedure. As we mentioned earlier, the authors had compared this data with several reports showing that some 2% of depressed outpatients commit suicide, but in TRD, the rate is said to be about 15%. All-cause mortality in TRD is said to be 13% at four to eight years and as high as 32% at seven years.

Clinical Notes and Issues

1. Given the severity of TRD in these studies, the results in DBS seem impressive, with response rates hovering around 50%. The results improved over time, *but*, with longer study periods, the rate at which

confounders come into play also increases, as witnessed by the freedom to alter medications and/or therapy in some studies.

2. In addition, some have commented on the very high motivation to enroll, which in some instances involved moving to a different city in order to obtain treatment,[83, p. 77] raising the issue of bias.

3. The response rates are further compromised by the absence of sham studies and the very small number of patients in each study. While some investigators used the word "sham," this usually meant observations of very brief periods during which batteries failed, the stimulus dose was lowered, or the patient stopped treatment. These appear to be "accidental" controls. Truly blinded studies involving such an invasive procedure are unlikely.

4. Infections, while uncommon, are not rare and require treatment.

5. In 2012,[85] one group reported electrical short circuits in almost 9% of cases at routine follow-up examination, with symptoms such as dysarthria, difficulties controlling eyelid movements, and a fall-off in efficacy in patients with movement disorders.

6. Battery failure requires a brief surgical procedure to replace it, leaving another opportunity for infection, although this appears to be unusual.

7. The question re the true suicide rate remains open, but remember that patients with baseline significant suicidality were excluded.

8. To what extent do these studies apply to the general population of patients with TRD? Patients with significant co-morbid psychiatric disorders have been excluded, no doubt due in part to safety concerns, but in part due to a legitimate wish for homogeneity of the population in order to examine the science behind DBS. However, this gives us a very limited view of the usefulness of DBS in the clinic.

9. The lack of independently funded studies is worrisome, as are the very close ties of the principal players in the field, many of whom are funded by the device makers and receive licensing fees from St. Jude Medical Neuromodulation, Boston Scientific, Medtronic, and other companies. The field is rife with conflicts of interest, which may have been justified as the field began to develop but not a decade later.

10. I could find only one report[86] (from Germany) in which an outside expert was called in to review the study prior to the inclusion of patients. These investigators also required informed consent from the closest caregiver and a two-week interval before consent could be signed. *These steps should be required in every study!*

11. While the focus of DBS in psychiatry has been on depression and OCD, its application is broadening steadily. Additional studies are underway on the use of DBS in treating various addictions.[87] It appears that the effects of DBS are non-specific and involve normalizing pathological activity and oscillations within a basal ganglia and thalamocortical network.[88]

12. Finally, what are the limits of DBS in depression? Since major depression is often chronic, will DBS continue for years? If so, what are the

risks? What happened to patients in these studies after study completion? Have autopsy studies been carried out on long-term participants with psychiatric disorders in order to assess tissue damage?

Irreversible Brain Surgery

We now enter a more worrisome arena, wherein neurosurgeons either resect brain tissue or insert probes, which are heated to a temperature that destroys cells. Gamma knife radiation is another technique, but it does not involve burr-hole placement or insertion of electrodes. It does, however, irreversibly damage brain cells. Each technique results in irreversible brain lesions, in contrast to VNS and tCMS.

We have already reviewed the early work by Moniz and Freeman on prefrontal lobotomies, so let us proceed to the next chapter in this story, although historically, there is overlap, since surgery on the cingulate gyrus began 1948 at Oxford, where neurosurgeons performed open, bilateral resections of the gyrus.[89] In 1949, Spiegel and Wycis[90] were the first to use a stereotactic technique, which allowed for more precise positioning of instruments and the approach to the target area, which in this paper was the dorsomedial thalamic nucleus. At the same time, however, lobotomies were still in vogue. For example, 232 patients were lobotomized at the Stockton State Hospital in California during the years 1947 through 1954.[91] Nevertheless, stereotactic neurosurgical procedures gained popularity, with 400 operations performed between 1971 and 1973.[92]

Not surprisingly, the controversy over brain surgery continued, especially with the widespread publicity given to Mark and Ervin's book *Violence and the Brain*, published in 1970.[93] The authors proposed that the United States begin widespread screening for a social dyscontrol syndrome, emphasizing the high rate of brain pathology in those who committed violent acts. The real debate, however, grew out of their suggestion that violence could be prevented and controlled by various forms of psychosurgery. As documented by Elliot Valenstein in his book *Brain Control*,[94] many other physicians embraced this concept, and the NIMH supported Mark and Ervin with grant money. Massachusetts General Hospital (MGH) continued to play a pivotal role in these debates, with MGH physicians Mark, Ervin, and Sweet suggesting in a letter[95] to the American Medical Association that brain disease was playing a role in race riots and that proper screening for brain pathology might be helpful in prevention.

However, with the advent of chlorpromazine and ADs in the mid-1950s, interest in both lobotomy and the more precise neurosurgical interventions began to decline. A 2001 overview by MGH staff[92] estimated that fewer than 25 patients are operated on yearly in Great Britain and the United States and perhaps several each year in Australia. However, the U.S. number seems low, given the studies to be reviewed and the current interest in neurosurgical procedures for an expanding list of conditions.

Cingulotomy

In 1962, Thomas Ballentine and his group at Massachusetts General Hospital (MGH) began what would be a long-term study of bilateral stereotaxic anterior cingulotomy in treatment-refractory psychiatric patients.[96, 97] Indeed, MGH spearheaded this approach, such that some 800 cingulotomies were performed by MGH staff between 1962 and 1968.[98] The initial paper[96] from this group reported on 57 patients, but only 40 psychiatric patients, of whom 26 were diagnosed with manic-depressive illness and 10 with schizophrenia. A few had OCD, and others had a mixed bag of difficulties including alcoholism, anorexia, and "sexual aberrations." They had been ill for an average of ten years. How these 40 were selected from the patient population of 2500—of whom 800 had been given intensive shock therapy—was not evident. *No diagnostic testing was reported,* except IQ testing in a few, and there were no data whatever on medications or co-morbid medical conditions. The authors reported that 95 cingulotomies were performed on this group, but how they were distributed was not clear. *There was no mention of informed consent or the use of an institutional review board (IRB).*

The authors reported that "useful improvement" was found in 30 of the 40 psychiatric patients in follow-ups ranging from three months to four years, with 23 functioning effectively in society.[96, p. 495] The best results (77% to 80% improvement) were found in manic-depressives and women with manic-depressive illness. They also emphasized that the patients, relatives, and doctors had not observed any serious physical or psychological complications and therefore judged the risk of cingulotomy as negligible. However, two patients with a seizure history had one seizure each, and one patient with no seizure history had a seizure. There were four late deaths, including a suicide; a pulmonary embolus seven months post operatively; a case of emphysema at age 82 some six months after surgery; and a young woman was found dead in her bathroom three months after surgery, possibly of myocarditis.

The authors concluded that this was an interim study, and they could not know if recurrence would take place, or why the surgery is successful, if indeed it is,[96, p. 494] a refreshingly candid statement. However, I must stress that the gaps in data are so profound that it's impossible to assess the results by today's standards, including the ethical issues. This prompted an essay by Alan Stone in 2008,[98] severely criticizing MGH for its rejection of his proposal that an outside consultant review each case, a proposal made when he chaired a committee charged with developing regulations for psychosurgery in Massachusetts. *Why did MGH veto the idea of an independent review?* The IRB at MGH consisted of a psychiatrist, a neurologist, and an operating surgeon, all appointed by MGH. This would not be allowed today, give the obvious conflicts of interest.

Given the need to focus on current treatment approaches, I will describe the results of a 2010 summary[99] of the procedures and results instead of attempting a more detailed examination of each paper. The authors relied on the Proceedings of the World Congress of Psychiatric Surgery and articles found on a Medline database. Only 29 reports of 470 met their inclusion criteria. Given the variations in reporting methods and scales, the authors attempted to standardize the data using a five-point scale: Minus 1= worse; 0 = no change; 1 = minimal improvement; 2 = significant improvement; 3 = symptom free. Results:

Generalized Anxiety Disorder, n = 177 with anterior capsulotomies, yielding a mean score of 2.4. Most were in the 2 to 3 range, but with cingulotomy, the scores were more widely distributed.

Obsessive-Compulsive Disorder, n = 303 with anterior capsulotomies, resulting in a mean score of 2.1, but this procedure was not significantly different from cingulotomy, frontal leucotomy, frontal leucotomy plus cingulotomy, or subcaudate tractotomy.

Bipolar Disorder, n = 42 with cingulotomy, yielding a mean score of 2.8, higher than any other disorder. More patients fell into the 3 category than with any other disorder. Cingulotomy was significantly more effective than frontal leucotomy.

Depressive Disorder, n = 413, mean score of 2.3 with cingulotomy, which was significantly better than other procedures.

Schizoaffective Disorder, total not reported. Mean score of 2.3 with cingulotomy, which was superior to anterior callostomy.

Schizophrenia, total not reported. Cingulotomy had the best outcome of all procedures, but the results were poor at 1.6. Outcomes were similarly poor in addictive disorders. The cumulative mean score was 2.1, indicating significant improvement at the low end of this informal and non-validated rating scale.

Limbic leukotomy is yet another form of psychosurgery, dating to 1973. This involves combining anterior cingulotomy and subcaudate tractotomy, with reports of improvement in 89% of patients with obsessive-compulsive disorder, 66% of patients with anxiety disorders, and 78% of patients with major depression. However, the studies were short term and did not use validated rating scales.[100] That being the case, Cho et al. carried out testing for seven years post limbic leukotomy for intractable major affective disorders, utilizing well-validated scales.[100] They claimed no significant side effects and a reduction in depression, anxiety, and negative symptoms but did not utilize neuropsychological testing. Why not?

Clinical Notes and Issues in Neurotherapeutics

1. One obvious question: Why is it that many of the same brain areas are targeted by DBS and lesional (ablative) surgery? One would think stimulating the cingulate gyrus might have an entirely different effect from

destroying cells in the same area. I am not alone in noticing that these radically different procedures targeted different areas but with similar efficacy. An overview at MGH stressed the same issue.[92] The usual explanation is that both DBS and brain lesions correct a malfunctioning corticostriatal-thalamocortical circuitry involving frontal associative and limbic areas of the basal ganglia and thalamus.[76, p. 478] The authors note that much of the same circuitry is involved not only in depression but also in OCD. Other targets in this wide-ranging circuitry are the nucleus accumbens and the subthalmic nucleus, areas have that have been targeted with DBS in studies aimed at treating alcoholism, cocaine addiction (in rats), anxiety, and Tourette's syndrome.

2. Helen Mayberg, a pioneer in the area, emphasizes the same systemic circuits but with a focus on the subgenual cingulate, which appears to be metabolically overactive in depression, but with normalization by with a variety of treatments, including ADs, ECT, TMS, DBS, and lesional surgery. (See Mayberg et al.[78] for a detailed review.) In addition, DBS increases blood flow in the prefrontal cortex, thus correcting pretreatment hypofrontality. However, *Mayberg does not explain why a lesion in the same area has comparable efficacy.* In any event, Holtzheimer and Mayberg have rejected the notion of discrete biological subtypes of depression—an explanation often used to explain the variation in response to treatment of whatever sort—and instead have proposed that depression is not an abnormal state in and of itself, but an "inability to regulate the state appropriately."[20, p. 6]

3. *It seems not to matter whether we stimulate or destroy brain cells; the results appear to be similar.* Note that the MGH staff stated that *the scientific rationale for psychiatric neurosurgery is not evident.*[93, p. 2]

4. Given the number of sites and techniques, a scientific approach demands head-to-head comparisons, but none have been done. While the results appear similar, we still don't know if one approach is better than another. Krack et al.[76, p. 480] stated plainly that there has been no real breakthrough in terms of reliability and magnitude of benefit. This group also pointed out that while DBS for Parkinson's disease has benefited from relevant animal models, this has not been case for mental disorders.

5. *We should add that the lack of relevant biochemical laboratory data in the clinical studies is shocking. The absence of studies on potentially relevant neurotransmitters, metabolites, and proteins such as BDNF is difficult to understand.*

6. Similarly, the data is either missing or skimpy regarding pharmacologic treatment pre- and post-operatively. Investigators typically minimize such data, noting that patients have failed to respond to standard treatment, with the inference being that continued drug or other therapies are more or less irrelevant. But how do we know? Isn't it possible that DBS might somehow set the stage for a better response to pharmacotherapy or behavioral therapy?

7. We have mentioned a number of times the lack of controls, but the problem persists. Again, one can understand the ethical concerns surrounding sham brain surgery, but the combination of small numbers and no controls is a serious problem. In some studies, a brief period of sham stimulation was employed, but patients knew that they would later receive active stimulation, thus maintaining a set of expectations. Observation of patients who have suffered battery failure is interesting but is not a valid means of estimating placebo effects. And even should a sham lesioning trial be done, one would have to wonder about the profile of volunteers, but careful screening could resolve that issue. Such a trial would require a very expensive *national or international* effort in order to recruit sufficient numbers.

8. *A large-scale trial should be independently funded in order to have credibility.* As we have seen, the majority of studies have been funded wholly or in part by the relevant companies and staffed by personnel employed by or with financial connections to the device manufacturers. Ample research has consistently found bias in favor of company-sponsored drugs or devices, as we discussed earlier. Research staff have every reason to maximize benefit and minimize adverse effects, despite their best intentions. Unfortunately, potential bias has continued to be an issue, as was noted in a 2018 meta-analysis of nine studies on DBS for depression.[101] We should note that DBS, as opposed to sham, did produce an odds ratio of 5.50, but the effects were attenuated in subgroup and sensitivity analyses, and there were 131 serious adverse events.

9. Given the recent news that some $7 billion is being devoted to the Human Brain Initiative and similar projects (see the final chapter), we have every reason to believe that *neurotherapeutics* will continue to expand. Indeed, the FDA approved the Brainsway Deep TMS system for OCD in 2018,[102] after a large study reported 38% of actively treated patients had a greater than 30% reduction of symptoms vs 11% with sham treatment.

10. In addition, the commercial market for non-invasive devices is rapidly expanding. The website[103] Total tDCS, recently listed the five best tDCS devices for 2019, while another[104] noted availability of vagus nerve stimulation devices but questioned their efficacy and safety. The marketing of these devices may soon become an issue in the clinic and may complicate research into depression.

11. Investigators are always looking for a different method to establish the usefulness of tDCS and other devices. Brunoni and his group did a meta-analysis[105] of individual patient data, rather than simply aggregating the results. In MDD, the overall response favored active treatment, 34% vs 19%, with an NNT of 7; for remission, active treatment results were 23% vs 12.7%, with an NNT of 9.

12. I would be very reluctant to refer anyone for *irreversible* brain surgery. While the response rates in a few studies have been impressive, we have

to stress that repeated operations have been necessary in a number of cases, and almost all studies have lacked substantial data on previous treatment and long-term follow-up. Further, the range and availability of pharmacological, psychological, and non-invasive brain stimulation devices would seem to argue against these procedures.

13. In the meantime, studies in 2019 continue to confirm that genetics offers nothing in the way of biomarkers that might help identify those with a greater risk for TRD or guide treatment.[106] A meta-analysis[107] of three independent samples examining TRD failed to identify any gene or polymorphism associated with TRD, although suggestive signals were found in genes associated with calcium signaling, regulation of the cytoskeleton, and transcription modulation. Several gene sets were identified that could be eventually used as biomarkers, but it seemed clear that their clinical usefulness is distant at best.

References

1. Cole J. Depression. *American Journal of Psychiatry* 1974;131:204–205.
2. Keller MB, Bell WH, Endicott J, et al. Findings from the collaborative depression study. In: *Clinical Guide to Depression and Bipolar Disorder*. American Psychiatric Publishing, Washington DC and London, 2013.
3. Ormel J, Spinhoven P, de Vries YA, et al. The antidepressive standoff: why it continues and what to do about it. *Psychological Medicine* 2019. https://doi.org/10.1017//S003329171003295.
4. Leichsenring F, Steinert C, Ioannidis JPA. Toward a paradigm shift in treatment and research of mental disorders. *Psychological Medicine* 2019;49:2111–2117.
5. Joyner ML, Paneth N, Ioannidis JPA. What happens when underperforming big ideas in research become entrenched? *JAMA* 2016;316:1355–1356.
6. Spijker J, Nolen WA. An algorithm for the pharmacological treatment of depression. *Acta Psychiatrica Scandinavaca* 2010;121:180–189.
7. Trivedi MH, Fava M, Wisniewski SR, et al. STAR*D Study Team. Medication augmentation after the failure of SSRIs for depression. *New England Journal of Medicine* 2006;354:1243–1252.
8. Rocha FL, Fuzikawa C, Riera C, et al. Combination of antidepressants in the treatment of major depressive disorder. A systematic review and meta-analysis. *Journal of Clinical Psychopharmacology* 2012;32:278–281.
9. Lam RW, Kennedy SH, Grigoriadis S, et al. Canadian network for mood and anxiety treatments (CANMAT) Clinical guidelines for the management of major depressive disorder in adults. III. Pharmacotherapy. *Journal of Affective Disorders* 2009;117:S26–S43.
10. Rush AJ, Trivedi MH, Stewart JW, et al. Combining medications to enhance depression outcomes (CO-MED): acute and long-term outcomes of a single-blind randomized study. *American Journal of Psychiatry* 2011. Doi:10.1176/appi.ajp.2011.10111645.
11. Blier P, Ward HE, Tremblay P, et al. Combination of antidepressant medications from treatment initiation for major depressive disorder: a double-blind randomized study. *American Journal of Psychiatry* 2010;167:281–288.

12. Thase ME. Antidepressant combinations: widely used, but far from empirically validated. *The Canadian Journal of Psychiatry* 2011;56:317–323.

13. Cowen PJ. Backing into the future: pharmacological approaches in the management of depression. *Psychological Medicine* 2017;47:2569–2577.

14. Rush AJ, Trivedi MH, Wisniewski SR, et al. Acute and longer-term outcomes in depressed outpatients requiring one or several steps: a STAR*D report. *American Journal of Psychiatry* 2006;163:1905–1917.

15. Papakostos GI, Fava M, Thase ME. Treatment of SSRI-resistant depression: a meta-analysis comparing within-versus across-class switches. *Biological Psychiatry* 2008;63:699–704.

16. Papakostos GI, Thase ME, Fava M, et al. Are antidepressant drugs that combine serotonergic and noradrenergic mechanisms of action more effective than selective serotonin reuptake inhibitors in treating major depressive disorder? A meta-analysis of studies of newer agents. *Biological Psychiatry* 2007;62:1217–1227.

17. Kocsis JH, Gelenberg AJ, Rothbaum B, et al, Chronic forms of major depression are still undertreated in the 21st century: systematic assessment of 801 patients presenting for treatment. *Journal of Affective Disorders* 2008;110:55–61.

18. Stawbridge R, Carter B, Marwood L, et al. Augmentation strategies for treatment-resistant depression: systematic review and meta-analysis. *The British Journal of Psychiatry* 2019;214:42–51. Doi:10.1192/bjp.2018.233.

19. Winkelmann, Jr NW. Chlorpromazine in the treatment of neuropsychiatric disorders. *JAMA* 1954;155:18–21.

20. Lehmann HE, Hanrahan GE. Chlorpromazine: new inhibiting agent for psychomotor excitement and manic states. *Archives of Neurology and Psychiatry* 1955;72:91–98.

21. Nelson JC, Papakostas GI. Atypical augmentation in major depressive disorders: a meta-analysis of placebo-controlled randomized trials. *American Journal of Psychiatry* 2009;166:980–991.

22. Komossa K, Depping AM, Gaudcha A, et al. Second-generation antipsychotics for major depression and dysthymia (review). *Cochrane Data Base of Systematic Reviews* 2010;(12):CD008121.

23. Spielmans GI, Berman MI, Linardatos E, et al. Adjunctive atypical antipsychotic treatment for major depressive disorder: a meta-analysis of depression, quality of life, and safety outcomes. *Public Library of Science* 2013;10:e1001403.

24. Carlat D. Unhinged. In: *The Trouble with Psychiatry—A Doctor's Revelations about a Profession in Crisis.* Free Press, New York, London, Toronto and Sydney, 2010.

25. Holtzheimer PE, Mayberg HS. Stuck in a rut: rethinking depression. *Trends in Neuroscience* 2011;34:1–5.

26. Mauskopf JA, Simon GE, Kalsekar A, et al. Nonresponse, partial responses, and failure to achieve remission: humanistic and cost burden in major depressive disorders. *Depression and Anxiety* 2009;26:83–97.

27. George MS, Sackeim HA, Rush AJ, et al. Vagus nerve stimulation: a new tool for brain research and therapy. *Biological Psychiatry* 2000;47:287–295.

28. Rush AJ, George MS, Sackheim HA, et al. Vagus nerve stimulation (VNS) for treatment-resistant depression: a multicenter study. *Biological Psychiatry* 2000;47:276–286.

29. Rush AJ, Marengell LB, Sackheim HA, et al. Vagus nerve stimulation for treatment-resistant depression: a randomized, controlled acute phase trial. *Biological Psychiatry* 2005;58:347–354.

30. Rush AJ, Sackheim HA, Marangell LB, et al. Effects of 12 months of vagus nerve stimulation in treatment-resistant depression: a naturalistic study. *Biological Psychiatry* 2005;58:355–363.

31. *FDA Summary of Safety and Effectiveness (SSE) for Cyberonic's VNS Therapy System^TM for TRD.* www.fda/gov/cdrh/PDF/P970003S050.html.

32. George MS, Rush AJ, Marangell LB, et al. A one-year comparison of vagus nerve stimulation with treatment as usual for treatment-resistant depression. *Biological Psychiatry* 2005;58:364–373.

33. Kucia K, Merk W, Zapalowicz K, Medrala T. Vagus nerve stimulation for treatment-resistant depression. *Blue Cross and Blue Shield Assessment Program* 2005;20:1–20.

34. Lurie P. FDA approves depression device without proof of effectiveness. *The Public Citizen Health Research Group Health Letter,* August 2005, p. 9.

35. Schlaepfer TE, Frick C, Zobel A, et al. Vagus nerve stimulation for depression: efficacy and safety in a European study. *Psychological Medicine* 2008;38:651–661.

36. Najas Z, Marangell LB, Husain MM, et al. Two-year outcome of vagus nerve stimulation (VNS) for treatment of major depressive episodes. *Journal of Clinical Psychiatry* 2005;66:1097–1104.

37. Cristancho P, Cristancho MA, Baltuch GH, et al. Effectiveness and safety of vagus nerve stimulation for severe treatment-resistant depression in clinical practice after FDA approval: outcomes at one year. *Journal of Clinical Psychiatry* 2011;72:1376–1382.

38. Daban C, Martinez-Aran A, Cruz A, et al. Safety and efficacy of vagus nerve stimulation in treatment-resistant depression: a systematic review. *Journal of Affective Disorders* 2008;110:1–15.

39. Parhizgar F, Nugent K, Raj R. Obstructive sleep apnea and respiratory complications associated with nerve stimulators. *Journal of Clinical Sleep Medicine* 2011;7:401–407.

40. Tran Y, Shah AK, Mittal S. Lead breakage and vocal cord paralysis following blunt neck trauma in a patient with a vagal nerve stimulator. *Journal of the Neurological Sciences* 2011;304:132–135.

41. Aaronson ST, Sears P, Ruvuna F, et al. A 5-year observational study of patients with treatment-resistant depression treated with vagus nerve stimulation or treatment as usual: comparison of response, remission, and suicidality. *American Journal of Psychiatry* 2017;174:640–648.

42. Lv H, Zhao Y-H, Chen J-G, et al. Vagus nerve stimulation for depression: a systematic review. *Frontiers in Psychology* 2019;10. Article Number 64.

43. Conway CR, Kumar A, Xiong W, et al. Chronic vagus nerve stimulation significantly improves quality of life in treatment-resistant depression. *Journal of Clinical Psychiatry* 2018;79:18m12178.

44. Wu C, Liu P, Fu H, et al. Transcutaneous auricular vagus nerve stimulation in treating major depressive disorder: a systematic review and meta-analysis. *Medicine* 2018;97:52, e13845.

45. George MS, Post RM. Daily left prefrontal repetitive transcranial magnetic stimulation for acute treatment of medication-resistant depression. *American Journal of Psychiatry* 2011;168:356–364.

46. Strafella AP, Paus T, Barrett J, et al. Repetitive transcranial magnetic stimulation of the human prefrontal cortex induces dopamine release in the caudate nucleus. *The Journal of Neuroscience* 2001;21:RC 157.

47. Strafella AP, Paus T, Fraraccio M, et al. Striatal dopamine release induced by repetitive transcranial magnetic stimulation of the human motor cortex. *Brain* 2003;126:2609–2615.

48. Czeh B, Welt T, Fischer AK, et al. Chronic psychosocial stress and concomitant repetitive transcranial magnetic stimulation: effects on stress hormone levels and adult hippocampal neurogenesis. *Biological Psychiatry* 2002;52:1057–1065.

49. Cheeran B, Talelli P, Mori F, et al. A common polymorphism in the brain-derived neurotrophic factor gene (BDNF) modulates human cortical plasticity and the response to rTMS. *Journal of Physiology* 2008;586:5717–5725.

50. Couturier JL. Efficacy of rapid-rate repetitive transcranial magnetic stimulation in the treatment of depression: a systematic review and meta-analysis. *Journal of Psychiatry and Neuroscience* 2005;30:83–90.

51. Martin JL, Barbanoj J, Schlaepfer TD, et al. Repetitive transcranial magnetic stimulation for the treatment of depression: systematic review and meta-analysis. *The British Journal of Psychiatry* 2003;182:480–491.

52. O'Reardon JP, Solvason HB, Janicak PG, et al. Efficacy and safety of transcranial magnetic stimulation in the acute treatment of major depression: a multisite randomized controlled trial. *Biological Psychiatry* 2007;62:1208–1216.

53. Lam RW, Chan P, Wilkins-Ho M, et al. Repetitive transcranial magnetic stimulation for treatment-resistant depression: a systematic review and meta-analysis. *The Canadian Journal of Psychiatry* 2008;53:621–631.

54. Schutter DJLG. Antidepressant efficacy of high-frequency transcranial magnetic stimulation over the left dorsolateral prefrontal cortex in double-blind sham-controlled designs: a meta-analysis. *Psychological Medicine* 2009;39:65–75.

55. Gaynes BN, Lloyd SW, Gartlehner G, et al. Repetitive transcranial magnetic stimulation for treatment-resistant major depression. A systematic review and meta-analysis. *Journal of Clinical Psychiatry* 2014;75:477–489.

56. Slotema CW, Dirk Blom J, Hoek HW, et al. Should we expand the toolbox of psychiatric treatment methods to include repetitive transcranial magnetic stimulation (rTMS)? A meta-analysis of the efficacy of rTMS in psychiatric disorders. *Journal of Clinical Psychiatry* 2009;71:873–884.

57. Yesavage JA, Fairchild K, Zhibao M, et al. Effect of repetitive transcranial magnetic stimulation on treatment-resistant depression in US veterans. A randomized trial. *JAMA Psychiatry* 2018;75:884–893.

58. Berlim MT, van den Eynde F, Tovar-Perdomo S, et al. Response, remission and drop-outs following high-frequency repetitive transcranial magnetic stimulation (rTMS) for treating major depression: a systematic review and meta-analysis of randomized, double-blind and sham-controlled trials. *Psychological Medicine* 2014;44:225.

59. Loo C, Katalinic N, Mitchell P, et al. Physical treatments for bipolar disorder: a review of electroconvulsive therapy, stereotactic surgery and other brain stimulation techniques. *Journal of Affective Disorders* 2011;132:1–13.

60. Kapstan A, Yaroslavsky Y, Applebaum J, et al. Right prefrontal TMS vs sham treatment of mania: a controlled study. *Bipolar Disorders* 2003;5:36–39.

61. Praharaj S, Ram D, Arora M. Efficacy of high frequency (rapid) suprathreshold repetitive transcranial magnetic SK stimulation of right prefrontal cortex in bipolar mania: a randomized sham-controlled study. *Journal of Affective Disorders* 2009;117:146–150.

62. Connolly KR, Helmer A, Cristancho MA, et al. Effectiveness of transcranial magnetic stimulation in clinical practice post-FDA approval in the United States: results observed with the first 100 consecutive cases an academic medical center. *Journal of Clinical Psychiatry* 2012;73:e567–e573.

63. Gross M, Nakamura L, Pascaul-Leone A, et al. Has repetitive transcranial magnetic stimulation (rTMS) treatment for depression improved? A systematic review and meta-analysis comparing the recent vs. the earlier rTMS studies. *Acta Psychiatrica Scandinavica* 2007;116:165–173.

64. Loo CK, Sachdev P, Martin D, et al. A double-blind, sham-controlled trial of transcranial direct stimulation for the treatment of depression. *International Journal of Neuropsychopharmacology* 2010;13:61–69.

65. Loo CK, Alonzo A, Martin D, et al. Transcranial direct current stimulation for depression: 3 week, randomized, sham-controlled trial. *The British Journal of Psychiatry* 2012;200:52–59.

66. Loo CK, Katalinic N, Mitchell P, et al. Physical treatments for bipolar disorder: a review of electroconvulsive therapy, stereotactic surgery, and other brain stimulation techniques. *Journal of Affective Disorders* 2011;132:1–13.

67. Donde C, Amad A, Nieto I. Transcranial direct-current stimulation for bipolar depression: a systematic review and meta-analysis. *Progress in Neuro-Psychopharmacology & Biological Psychiatry* 2017;78:121–131.

68. McLoughlin DM, Mogg A, Eranti S, et al. The clinical effectiveness and cost of repetitive transcranial magnetic stimulation vs electroconvulsive therapy in severe depression: a mulicentre pragmatic randomized controlled trial and economic analysis. *Health and Technology Assessment* 2007;11:1–54.

69. Valenstein ES. *Great and Desperate Cures. The Rise and Decline of Psychosurgery and Other Radical Treatments for Mental Illness.* Basic Books, New York, 1986.

70. Yudofsky SC. Changing tides in neurosurgical interventions for treatment-resistant depression. *American Journal of Psychiatry* 2008;165:671–674.

71. Whitaker R. *Mad in America. Bad Science, Bad Medicine, and the Enduring Mistreatment of the Mentally Ill.* Perseus Publishing, Cambridge MA, 2002.

72. A come back for psychosurgery? Alliance for Human Research Protection (AHRP). www.namiscc.org/News/2003/Summer/Psychosurgery.htm. Accessed June 23, 2008.

73. Appleby BS, Duggan PS, Regenberg A, et al. Psychiatric and neuropsychiatric adverse events associated with deep brain stimulation: a meta-analysis of ten years' experience. *Movement Disorders* 2007;22:1722–1728.

74. Sachdev P. Is deep brain stimulation a form of psychosurgery? *Australasian Psychiatry* 2007;15:97–99.

75. Kringelbach ML, Jenkinson N, Owen SLF, et al. Translational principles of deep brain stimulation. *Nature Reviews Neuroscience* 2007;8:623–635.

76. Krack P, Hariz MI, Baunez C, et al. Deep brain stimulation: from neurology to psychiatry? *Trends in Neurosciences* 2010;33:474–484.

77. US Food and Drug Administration (2009). New humanitarian device approval. www.fda.gov/cdrh/mda/docs/HO50003.html. Accessed May 26, 2009.

78. Mayberg HS, Lozano AM, Voon V, et al. Deep brain stimulation for treatment-resistant depression. *Neuron* 2005;45:651–660.

79. Lozano AM, Mayberg HS, Giacobbe P, et al. Subcallosal cingulate gyrus deep brain stimulation for treatment-resistant depression. *Biological Psychiatry* 2008;64:461–467.

80. Kennedy SH, Giacobbe P, Rizvi SJ, et al. Deep brain stimulation for treatment-resistant depression: follow-up after 3 to 6 years. *American Journal of Psychiatry* 2011;168:502–510.

81. Holtzheimer PE, Kelley ME, Gross RE, et al. Subcallosal cingulate deep brain stimulation for treatment-resistant unipolar and bipolar depression. *Archives of General Psychiatry* 2012;69:150–158.

82. Anderson RJ, Frye MA, Abulseod OA, et al. Deep brain stimulation for treatment-resistant depression: efficacy, safety, and mechanisms of action. *Neuroscience and Biobehavioral Reviews* 2012;36:1920–1933.

83. Fisher CE, Dunn LB, Christopher PP, et al. The ethics of research on deep brain stimulation for depression: decisional capacity and therapeutic misconception. *Annals of the New York Academy of Sciences* 2012;1265:69–79.

84. Fins JJ, Dorfman GS, Pancrazio JJ. Challenges to deep brain stimulation: a pragmatic response to ethical, fiscal, and regulatory concerns. *Annals of the New York Academy of Sciences* 2012;1265:80–90.

85. Samura K, Miyagi Y, Okamoto T, et al. Short circuit in deep brain stimulation. *Journal of Neurosurgery* 2012;117:955–961.

86. Bewernick BH, Hurlemann R, Matusch A, et al. Nucleus accumbens deep brain stimulation decreases ratings of depression and anxiety in treatment-resistant depression. *Biological Psychiatry* 2010;67:110–116.

87. Wing VC, Barr MS, Wass CE, et al. Brain stimulation methods to treat tobacco addiction. *Brain Stimulation* 2012. http://dx.doi.org/10.1016/j.brs.2012.06.008.

88. Miocinovic S, Somayajula S, Chitnis S, et al. History, applications and mechanisms of deep brain stimulation. *JAMA Neurology* 2013;70:163–171.

89. Whitty CWM, Duffield JE, Tow PM, et al. Anterior cingulectomy in the treatment of mental disease. *Lancet* 1952;262:475–481.

90. Spiegel EA, Wycis HT, Freed H. Thalamotomy: neuropsychiatric aspects. *New York State Medical Journal* 1949;49:2273–2274.

91. Starks SL, Braslow JT. The making of contemporary American Psychiatry, Part I: patients, treatments, and therapeutic rationales before and after World War II. *History of Psychology* 2005;8:176–193.

92. Eskandar EN, Cosgrove GR, Rauch SL. Psychiatric neurosurgery overview. *Massachusetts General Hospital Web Site: Functional and Stereotactic Neurosurgery.* http://mgh.harvard.edu/functional/Psychosurgery2001.htm. Accessed January 24, 2013.

93. Mark VH, Irvin FR. *Violence and the Brain.* Harper and Row, New York, 1970.

94. Valenstein ES. *Brain Control. A Critical Examination of Brain Stimulation and Psychosurgery.* A Wiley-Interscience Publication. John Wiley & Son, New York, London, Sydney and Toronto, 1973.

95. Mark VH, Sweet WH, Ervin FR. Role of brain disease in riots and urban violence. *American Medical Association* 1967;201:895.

96. Ballantine HT, Cassidy WL, Flanagan NB, et al. Stereotactic anterior cingulotomy for neuropsychiatric illness and intractable pain. *Journal of Neurosurgery* 1967;26:488–495.

97. Ballantine HT, Bouckoms AJ, Thomas EK, et al. Treatment of psychiatric Illness by stereotactic cingulotomy. *Biological Psychiatry* 1987;22:807–819.

98. Stone AA. Psychosurgery—old and new. *Psychiatric Times*, June 2008, pp. 30–34.

99. Leiphart JW, Valone III FH. Stereotactic lesions for the treatment of psychiatric disorders. *Journal of Neurosurgery* 2010;113:1204–1211.

100. Cho D-Y, Lee W-Y, Chen C-C. Limbic leukotomy for major affective disorders: a 7-year follow-up study using nine comprehensive psychiatric test evaluations. *Journal of Clinical Neuroscience* 2008;15:138–142.

101. Kisely S, Li A, Warren N, Siskind D. A systematic review and meta-analysis of deep brain stimulation for depression. *Depression and Anxiety* 2018;35:468–480.

102. FDA permits marketing of transcranial magnetic stimulation for treatment of obsessive compulsive disorder [press release]. Silver Spring MD. www.fda.gov/News Events/Newsroom/PressAnnouncements/ucm617244.htm.

103. Total tDCS. 5 best tDCS devices of 2019. https://totaltdc.com. Accessed December 15, 2019.

104. BrainFacts. Org. Are commercial vagus nerve stimulation devices safe and effective? https://brainfacts.org. Accessed December 15, 2019.

105. Brunoni AR, Moffa AH, Fregni F, et al. Transcranial direct current stimulation for acute major depressive episodes: meta-analysis of individual patient data. *The British Journal of Psychiatry* 2016;208:522–531.

106. Fabbri C, Souery FCD, Kasper S, et al. The genetics of treatment-resistant depression: critical review and future perspectives. *International Journal of Neuropsychopharmacology* 2019;22:93–104.

107. Fabbri C, Kasper S, Kautzky A, et al. Genome-wide association study of treatment-resistance in depression and meta-analysis of three independent samples. *The British Journal of Psychiatry* 2019;214:36–41. Doi:10.1192/bjp.2018.256.

12 Desperately Treating Depression

On Psychotogenic and Hallucinogenic Drugs, Anti-Inflammatories, Antidiabetics, Hyperthermia, and Opioids

Introduction

In the past several chapters, we have noted the failure of psychiatry to significantly advance the treatment of major depression, despite decades of research and the development of an ever-larger array of ADs, a variety of psychotherapeutic approaches, multiple forms of non-invasive brain stimulation, and invasive and irreversible neurosurgical approaches. Yet we have been faced with an epidemic of depression, increasing rates of suicidality, and an epidemic of opioid abuse and deaths from overdoses. Given these realities, psychiatry has chosen to embrace approaches that were popular from the 1950s to the 1970s, including the use of LSD and other hallucinogenic and psychotogenic agents. In addition, positive results have been found for so-called "novel" therapies, including nitrous oxide, anti-inflammatory agents, oral antidiabetic drugs, botulinum toxin, and whole-body hyperthermia, once popular in the asylums. We shall explore the benefits and risks of these strategies, starting with ketamine and ending with the enthusiastic embrace of opioids for depression, despite the opioid epidemic. I propose that socioeconomic problems are dampening the results of our therapeutic adventures, whether old or new.

Ketamine

Ketamine has become extremely popular in recent years, with private and academic ketamine clinics opening up across the country, despite a number of concerns. For example, a 2018 editorial in the *American Journal of Psychiatry*[1] warned that some people are shopping for infusion clinics to obtain ketamine, while others are diverting the drug from its intended use in pediatric and veterinary anesthesia. A consensus statement[2] on the use of ketamine in 2017 emphasized the potential for abuse and noted that clinical trials have focused only on efficacy and short-term safety, not the long-term effects. Others[3] have called for the establishment of a registry of patients receiving ketamine in order to better balance the risks and benefits, but, to my knowledge, this has not been accomplished.

Ketamine Basics

In 1963, Parke-Davis synthesized ketamine for use as a dissociative anesthetic. Seven years later, the FDA approved it for anesthesia in cases where muscle relaxation was not required, for the induction of anesthesia prior to the use of other agents, and as a supplement for low-potency anesthetics. With regard to ketamine and psychiatry, we should note first that ketamine is a derivative of phencyclidine (PCP) and, in fact, binds to the PCP-binding site in the ion channel of the N-methyl-d-aspartate (NMDA) receptor,[4] an ionotropic glutamate receptor. The NMDA receptor itself is very complex,[5, 6] with two protein subunits, one of which has multiple variants, while the other is coded by four different genes! It also interacts strongly with a number of membrane and cytoplasmic proteins, making research into its actions quite difficult. In addition, ketamine may act as a low-potency opioid agonist and antagonist, with the highest affinity for the μ receptor. Like antidepressants, it inhibits the transporters for NE, DA, and 5-HTA,[4] giving it a wide range of actions. We should note as well its short half-life of 2 to 2.5 hours, which comes into play when evaluating the prolonged effects of ketamine infusions—although the half-life of esketamine is 7 to 12 hours. Note, too, that a metabolite, hydroxynorketamine, may have antidepressant properties *independently of ketamine*, but more on this later. A 2019 review[7] has summarized multiple pathways pointing to the effects of ketamine on synaptic plasticity and the relevant neurocircuitry.

Making matters even more complex, ketamine comes in two isomers, S and R, with esketamine being the S-enantiomer. Esketamine, about which we will say more shortly, binds to the NMDA receptor with triple the potency of the R-isomer but induces fewer psychotomimetic symptoms. As we shall see, the FDA approved esketamine nasal spray for TRD on March 6, 2019.[8] However, it is available *only* through a risk evaluation and mitigation strategy (REMS), a requirement clearly reflecting concerns over the possibility of adverse outcomes.[1, 2, 8]

A significant issue in the therapeutic development of ketamine and PCP has been their involvement in schizophrenia research, in which both were used to stimulate and model the production of psychotic symptoms.[9, 10] As recently as 2012, Domino et al.[11] continued to stress the importance of ketamine and PCP in modeling schizophrenia. However, the adverse effects of PCP (abuse liability, prolongation of psychotic episodes, neuropathologic changes in the rat brain) soon led to a greater focus on ketamine, with its shorter half-life and fewer side effects. Nevertheless, similar concerns soon surfaced with regard to the ethics of ketamine challenge studies in schizophrenia, as documented by Carpenter[12] in 1999. In his essay, Carpenter defended the use of challenge studies in general and ketamine in particular, claiming that the media reports had been inflammatory.

However, he did not acknowledge the specific problems at the Maryland Psychiatric Research Center, where Robert Whitaker[13, p. 245] had found that the consent forms for the experimental use of ketamine were misleading at best! The investigators fully expected that ketamine would worsen symptoms, but the consent form indicated that ketamine would be used as a medication that might offer symptom relief! Yet ketamine had been tested in normal volunteers, in whom it produced psychotic symptoms, as Krystal et al. noted in 1994.[14] The volunteers complained of paranoid ideation, ideas of reference, excitement, and thought disorder—all classic symptoms of schizophrenia. In addition, they exhibited perseverative errors and delayed verbal recall, indicating an adverse effect on cognition. In a similar study,[15] the investigators found disruptions in immediate recall and long-term retention, as well as thought disorder, increased anxiety, and depression. Multiple other studies found similar results. In addition, ketamine also produced an exacerbation of symptoms in antipsychotic-free patients with schizophrenia.[16] These and similar studies reinforced the idea that deficits in NMDA receptors could play a significant role in the pathogenesis of schizophrenia,[11] a model that was reinforced by an imaging study showing that ketamine induced a *reduction of NMDA receptors* in the human brain, a reduction that correlated with a higher rate of negative symptoms.[17]

The burning question: Through what feat of alchemy did a psychotogenic, memory-impairing drug of abuse become transformed into a reputedly safe antidepressant?

Ketamine and Depression

While that work was in progress, ketamine was becoming known as a club drug (vitamin K, super K), along with GHB (Xyrem) and rohypnol, a benzodiazepine. Reports began to surface of people binging on ketamine and developing signs of tolerance and cravings.[18] The emphasis was on ketamine-induced dissociative states and out-of-body experiences, although some found these experiences pleasant, or even euphoric, resulting in compulsive use.[19] Indeed, in another study, healthy volunteers did not report psychotic symptoms but instead described euphoria and disinhibition.[20] No doubt these reports helped to stir interest in ketamine as an antidepressant, but other factors were at work as well, including abnormalities in concentrations of excitatory neurotransmitters (glutamate, glutamine) in MDD, with more severe abnormalities in TRD.[4] Studies also found that stress leads to excessive production of glucocorticoids and increased activation of glutamate receptors, which, in turn, leads to neurotoxicity, as found in studies of depression.[7] Given this data, interest grew in the idea that NMDA receptor blockade might be effective in stress-associated conditions, including depression.

Clinical Studies

In 2000, Berman et al. published a study[21] comparing a single infusion of ketamine, dosed at 0.5 mg/kg, and sham treatment in eight patients with

TRD. They reported a significant drop in the Hamilton Depression Rating Scale at 4 hours, with further reductions at 24 and 48 hours, followed by a 14-point drop at 72 hours. (Keep in mind ketamine's 2 to 3 hour-half-life.) Zarate et al.,[22] using the same dose in 17 patients, reported a 71% response rate and a 29% remission rate at 24 hours in people with TRD, while 35% maintained their response at one week. Others[23] found a significant decrease in suicidality in TRD, using the same single-dose strategy. Even patients who had failed ECT responded to a single 0.5 mg/kg dose at almost 4 hours post infusion,[24] although this was an open-label study.

By 2015, enough studies had been done to warrant four meta-analyses of ketamine. For example, Coyle et al.[25] reviewed 21 studies of patients who received ketamine. Single infusions were significant at 4 hours, 24 hours, and seven days, but effect sizes were even larger with multiple infusions. *Only a few studies examined responses at 12 to 14 days; the results were not statistically significant. Effect sizes for open-label studies were not significant at any point.* With regard to adverse events, many studies found dissociative effects and mild psychomimetic effects, as well as transient headaches, dizziness, and nausea.

In a second meta-analysis, McGirr et al[26] examined seven RCTs involving patients with MDD and bipolar depression, with outcomes similar to those mentioned earlier, but adding the NNT, which at 24 hours was 5, and at seven days was 6, well within the clinically significant range. The third, by Newport et al.,[27] also reported on seven controlled trials and found an odds ratio of 9.87 for response and 14.47 for remission, accompanied by brief dissociative and psychomimetic effects. However, D-cycloserine and raspinel, *partial agonists at the NMDA co-agonist site, also significantly reduced depressive symptoms* but without inducing dissociative or psychotomimetic effects. The agonistic effects of these two drugs raised more doubts about the viability of NMDA-receptor blockade as the primary action behind ketamine's antidepressant effects. (We shall note other possibilities shortly.)

But first, the obvious problem: What comes next? How many people relapse after the infusions? In a summary of studies examining relapse rates, Coyle et al.[25] noted that the median time to relapse was 18 days in one study and 19 days in another. In an open-label follow-up of ten patients, eight of nine had responded well to a first infusion, then had an additional five infusions, after which eight of the nine relapsed at a mean of 30 days following the last infusion.[28] Indeed, a study of the natural history[29] of *untreated* depressive episodes noted that 52% recover by three months while another 15% recover during the next three months, so the relapse rates with ketamine are of concern.

Clearly, additional work is needed on the long-term effects of ketamine, the appropriate doses, modes of administration, rates of addictive behaviors following treatment, and, if possible, studies of brain tissue in patients who have been repeatedly exposed to the drug. More attention should be given to the cognitive effects of ketamine, especially after long-term and/or repeated use.[7] We should also ask: *What are the legal implications of the outpatient use of ketamine?* Who bears responsibility if the patient becomes addicted or shops ketamine clinics for additional treatments, diverts the drug, becomes psychotic, or develops serious cognitive deficits?

Esketamine and FDA Approval of the Nasal Spray

As this data indicate, we need better strategies to prevent relapse into depressive symptoms, especially in those with TRD. To that end, Daly et al.[30] began a multi-site RCT of esketamine nasal spray *plus* assignment to a new AD after tapering of the previous drug. Esketamine was started at a dose of 56 mg or 84 mg twice weekly. Patients with suicidal ideation or suicidal behavior in the previous year were excluded, as were those with psychotic features, substance abuse, or alcohol abuse disorders. The study design was quite complex, with five phases.

The combination of esketamine and a new AD significantly delayed relapse in those patients who had achieved stable remission or a stable response after 16 weeks of treatment. The NNT was 6, which is quite good. When compared with those taking an AD and placebo, relapse rates in the combination were *reduced* by 51% in patients with a stable remission and by 70% in those who achieved a stable response. Adverse events were judged mild to moderate, with dizziness, somnolence, vertigo, and dissociation. No fatalities occurred, nor were there any cases of interstitial cystitis (infection of the bladder), a problem described in a number of case reports. There were no significant EKG changes and only transient hypertension. These were impressive results, but we should ask the degree to which the results can *generalize* to the usual clinic population, who suffer from multiple co-morbidities, including suicidality and substance use disorders.

Of considerable interest is a 2018 double-blind proof-of-concept study[31] that utilized intranasal ketamine plus standard of care to assess its potential for rapidly reducing not only depressive symptoms, but also suicidality, over a four-week period. In contrast to other studies in which suicidality blocked study enrollment, patients had to present with an *imminent risk of suicide* but could *not* have a moderate substance use disorder or a psychotic disorder. Esketamine was dosed at 84 mg (reduced to 56 mg if necessary) and given twice weekly for four weeks. The most commonly used AD was sertraline. Significant improvement in the esketamine group was found in depressive symptoms at 4 hours after the first dose, at 24 hours, and at day 11, but not at day 25. Similarly, significant improvement of suicidality post first dose with esketamine occurred at 4 hours, but *not* at 24 hours or at day 25. *Indeed, there were no group differences at the end of double-blind treatment or at post-treatment follow-up.*

The authors stressed that esketamine might be a helpful bridge on the path to improvement with an AD, but, if ADs take three to four weeks to act, that bridge needs to be much longer. The authors did not explain why twice-weekly dosing of esketamine failed to differentiate from placebo at day 25, but this is a significant question. *They did note that the results should not be viewed as evidence of effectiveness in the clinical population.* On the bright side, only transient elevations in blood pressure occurred, and there was *no* evidence of misuse, diversion, or withdrawal and *no* evidence of such behaviors in past clinical trials. However, it was not at all clear how these problems were assessed during the studies. We should say as well that this trial was sponsored by the manufacturer, and nine of the authors were company employees while another was a patent holder on the technology. In addition, medical writing assistance was provided by a communications company, and editorial advice was provided by the manufacturer. *One must be cautious when this degree of manufacturer involvement is present.* (Similar problems occurred in a 2019 study[32] of esketamine nasal spray combined with an AD, with heavy involvement of company personnel.)

Yet the 2019 study[32] is interesting in that it also switched patients with TRD from an ineffective AD to flexibly dosed esketamine nasal spray dosed twice weekly plus a new AD, vs a placebo nasal spray and a new AD. These were given during the 28-day double-blind treatment phase involving 197 patients. An impressive 86% of patients completed the treatment phase, far greater than in many studies of ADs and APs. *In contrast* to the previous study,[31] esketamine nasal spray plus AD was significantly superior to AD plus placebo at day 28. Significant differences were found at 24 hours after dosing and at days 8 through 28. In a post-hoc analysis, 69% of the active esketamine plus AD group were responders at day 28 vs 52% in the AD plus placebo arm, NNT = 6. *However, the effect size at day 28 was only 0.3, a small effect size.* Adverse events ranged from 20% to 26%, with dizziness, dissociation, vertigo, nausea, and a bad taste being the most common; 7% in the esketamine active arm had to discontinue the drug due to anxiety, panic, headache, etc. There were no psychotic symptoms.

The effect size of only 0.3 prompted a commentary[33] that questioned *whether efficacy had actually been demonstrated and emphasized that two previous pivotal trials of the nasal spray had not achieved statistical significance.* Nevertheless, the FDA approved the nasal spray with restrictions, as noted earlier. Other difficulties with esketamine were noted by *The Medical Letter* in 2019,[34] which warned of neurotoxicity in the breast-fed offspring of animals given NMDA antagonists, including ketamine. *The Medical Letter* further stated that esketamine should not be used in pregnancy or in patients with a history of cerebral aneurysms, AV malformations, or intracerebral hemorrhage, given its hypertensive effects.

In the meantime, research into the pathophysiology of ketamine and its actions continued, with some finding that ketamine stimulates release of endogenous opioids as part of its pain relief effectiveness, while naloxone, a mu receptor antagonist, blocks pain relief in animal studies.[33] How this fits with our recent enthusiasm for using opioids as antidepressants is a matter I will discuss shortly. The NMDA receptor blockade hypothesis regarding the actions of ketamine continues to fall from favor, since a metabolite, norhydroxyketamine, stimulates the AMPA receptor and appears to be a step necessary for its efficacy. The relationship between ketamine and BDNF is marked by inconsistent results, with studies showing that ketamine increases BDNF levels, or results in no change, or increases concentrations in dendrites. Importantly, other NMDA blocking agents are *not* effective as ADs, another argument against the NMDA hypothesis.[7]

Hallucinogens and Depression: Psilocybin, LSD, and the Trip Treatment

Psilocybin is one of the psychedelic drugs known to induce hallucinations and feelings of depersonalization, loss of reality, altered sense of time, and various psychotic symptoms. The history of psychedelics is long and in some respects infamous, not only because of their abuse potential but also because of their use by the CIA and government scientists eager to find ways of breaking down resistance and disorienting individuals, as noted by Whitaker.[13] There have also been concerns about the ethics of experimentally induced psychosis.[12, 35, 36] The following history leans heavily on the accounts by Whitaker,[13] Hoch,[35] and Healy.[36]

Briefly, the history of LSD (lysergic acid diethylamide) dates to 1938 with the synthesis of ergot alkaloids by Albert Hoffman and his collaborators. Ergot compounds had long been suspected of causing serious behavioral changes, including St. Vitus's Dance. In 1943, Albert Hoffman accidentally ingested LSD-25 and developed intense perceptual changes, which were repeated when he gave himself another dose under supervision. Investigators found it remarkable that such profound changes could result from such minute doses of LSD. Some began using LSD in psychotherapy, in order to break down defenses and, in an oft-used phrase, "open an avenue to the unconscious." Indeed, by 1965, LSD had become the subject of some 2,000 publications focused on the treatment of alcoholism, neuroses, and personality disorders.[37] However, Paul Hoch in New York began using LSD and mescaline to investigate the chemistry of psychosis and, in an echo of the work with ketamine, reported that the drugs led to serious disorganization, delusions, and hallucinations in patients with schizophrenia—experiments that were ethically dubious. He even gave mescaline to patients who had been lobotomized![35]

By the late 1960s, social and governmental concerns over LSD, mescaline, and similar drugs led to strict controls on their use. Nevertheless, these experiments laid the groundwork for later work *designed to exacerbate symptoms in patients with schizophrenia* by giving them dopaminergic drugs such as amphetamines, apomorphine, and ketamine.[35, 37] Hallucinogens were also used in the 1950s to 1970s to treat patients with metastatic cancers, who reportedly had significant improvements in their mood, a general sense of well-being, and improvement in pain.[38] Despite the apparent advantages of these agents, the political and moral climate of that era soon put an end to such research.

Psilocybin, the Magic Mushroom

The formal name of this hallucinogen is daunting: 4-phosphoryloxy-N, N-dimethyltrypramine, a compound found in some mushrooms. Psilocybin is quickly metabolized to psilocin, a powerful agonist at multiple 5-HTA receptors. *Indeed, psilocybin-induced activation of the 5-HT2a receptor correlates with the onset of hallucinations,*[38, 39] although work we shall describe later has cast doubt on this process. Nonetheless, we should note that antagonists (ketanserin) at the 5-HT2a receptor block the effects of psilocybin, as does deletion of the relevant gene.[40]

In a widely cited study,[41] psilocybin, in doses of 30 mg/70 kg, was given to 36 healthy volunteers and compared with a stimulant, methylphenidate. Interestingly, subsequent citations of this work never acknowledge that the volunteers were very well educated, with 97% being college graduates while 83% were working full time. (*I daresay that these demographics have been unmatched in any study of APs and ADs.*) In addition, the study was skewed toward people already affiliated with various religious and/or community groups. The volunteers denied prior involvement with hallucinogenic agents (verified by urine toxicology screens) but had responded to recruitment flyers describing the use of a psychoactive agent that had been used "sacramentally in some cultures." The stated goal of the study was to investigate states of consciousness.

Two monitors were with the subjects at all times. The study setting was like a comfortable living room, where subjects could listen to classical music using headphones. Two or three eight-hour sessions were conducted at two-month intervals. Twenty-two of 36 subjects described a complete mystical experience after using psilocybin vs 4 of 36 after taking methylphenidate.

While the authors stated that this dose of psilocybin can be given safely, 22% reported periods of anxiety and dysphoria, 31% reported significant fear, and some developed transient ideas of reference. However, symptoms were managed by reassurance from the monitors; no rescue drugs were needed, but the authors noted that the risks of hallucinogens should not be underestimated. After all, psilocybin is a Schedule I controlled drug, although in animal studies, it has not produced the kind of compulsive drug-seeking behaviors found with cocaine, heroin, and alcohol.[41]

Another study in 2006 of nine patients with OCD found that psilocybin was not only safe and well-tolerated but also effective in reducing symptoms[42] These studies and others led Grob et al. to proceed with a pilot study[38] of psilocybin for the treatment of anxiety in patients with advanced-stage cancer, the first to do so in three decades. This was a double-blind, placebo-controlled study. Patients were excluded if they had any psychotic disorder or a history of anxiety or mood disorders in the year prior to the study. They could not be enrolled if taking insulin, chemotherapy, or psychotropics in the previous two weeks. Four subjects were hallucinogenic naïve, but the rest were not. There were two experimental sessions, two weeks apart. Sessions took place in a hospital research unit decorated with flowers and wall hangings. The subjects wore eye shades and used headphones. They were told they would receive either psilocybin or niacin as a placebo. Standard rating scales were administered at intervals for six months. Results?

Subjective psychological effects included significant increases in depersonalization, derealization, hallucinations, visual pseudo-hallucinations, mania-like feelings, facilitation of imagination, and auditory changes not further described. "Oceanic boundlessness" was especially remarkable. In plain English, they were high! However, they did not have more thought disorder or fear of loss of control. Interestingly, the scale ratings of psychotic symptoms were similar after placebo and psilocybin, a finding *not consistent* with the reported symptoms. Mood was significantly improved at one month after the second treatment session. Anxiety ratings fell at one and three months but were elevated at six months, perhaps because of worsening physical status. There was no significant decrease in pain perception or the use of pain medication.

Patients and investigators were aware of whether drug or placebo had been given. The authors admitted that the placebo effect was important and that the setting and attention given to the subjects influenced outcomes. Nonetheless, the authors felt that this study provided a model for dealing with the profound existential anxiety and despair often found in patients with advanced cancer.

While no one begrudges these severely ill patients a respite from their struggle, the fact is that psilocybin, even at this minimal dose, clearly resulted in very significant changes in the psychological states of this group, despite the lack of change in the Brief Psychiatric Rating Scale—but note that this scale was used only at the end of the experimental sessions and not during the lengthy follow-up period. *Why not?* Did the authors have no interest in the longer-term effects of psilocybin on symptoms and behavior? Nor do we have any data on the safety of this agent with longer-term dosing. In addition, the majority of these patients had had prior experience with hallucinogens, so this was a biased population from the outset, and the study settings were far different from the usual research setting.

The contrast between this study and one done earlier by Vollenweider et al.[40] could not be more striking. Those authors recruited 25 healthy volunteers from a university staff and *excluded* previous users of illicit drugs. A slightly higher dose of psilocybin was used (0.25 mg/kg), with a placebo control. In addition, subjects were pretreated with 0.02 mg/kg of haloperidol, 1 mg orally of risperidone, or 20 mg or 40 mg of ketanserin, a drug that strongly blocks serotonin 5-HT2a receptors. Two experimental formats were used, during which comparisons were made in order to assess differences in working memory, psychotic symptoms, and mood between psilocybin, placebo, and pretreatment with the antipsychotic drugs.

The authors did not mince words, writing that psilocybin produced a psychotic syndrome that lasted one to two hours. Symptoms included grandiosity, euphoria, loss of reality testing, thought disorder, and paranoid ideation. They drew attention to the similarity of these symptoms to those of acute schizophrenia and, in some instances, chronic schizophrenia. This "model psychosis" was largely prevented by the two atypical APs and almost completely so by 40 mg of ketanserin, thus validating the hypothesis that activation of 5-HT2a receptors is a key to the psychotogenic action of psilocybin. Spatial working memory was clearly worsened by psilocybin, boosting the argument for the similarity between the drug-induced state and schizophrenia.

Back and forth we go: In a 2011 pooled analysis[43] of eight RCTS of psilocybin involving 110 subjects, doses ranged from 2 to 28 mg. Assessment scales focused on changes in perception and mood. The authors found "profound changes" in perception, mood, and thought, but "most" subjects found these to be satisfying and pleasurable. Only a few, given high doses, experienced more severe dysphoria and/or panic. No rescue drug therapy was needed, and subjects did not report drug abuse/dependence or psychotic symptoms at follow-up. To the authors' credit,[43] they admitted that generalization with regard to the safety of psilocybin in the larger population is risky, since subjects were carefully screened with a variety of tests. We should note, too, that 40% of the subjects had used at least one hallucinogen prior to the study. In addition, the very favorable stance regarding the safety of psilocybin stands in contrast to the Vollenweider et al. study[40] described earlier, although Vollenweider helped write both studies. (Apparently another 12 years had altered his perceptions!)

In an open-label pilot study[44] of TRD involving twelve patients, eight of twelve achieved remission at one week after receiving two oral doses of psilocybin one week apart. As is usually found in these psychedelic studies, treatment occurred in a supportive treatment setting with medical supervision. Seven of the eight responded at three months, with five in remission. No serious adverse events were reported.

Note that the lead author Carhart-Harris has been among the most prolific writers and supporters of psychedelic therapy. However, he has also been involved in a number of studies examining brain changes with use of psilocybin. For example, in a 2017 study[45] of psilocybin in TRD, he and his associates examined changes in cerebral blood flow and blood oxygen–level dependent (BOLD) resting state functional connectivity using fMRI before and after treatment with psilocybin; 47% met criteria for response at five weeks. Interestingly, decreased blood flow in the amygdala correlated with a decrease in depressive symptoms. Decreased blood flow was found in the temporal cortex as well, and increased resting state functional connectivity was found in the default mode network post treatment. However, the most important finding, according to the authors, was a decrease in resting-state functional connectivity between the bilateral para-hippocampus and the prefrontal cortex that correlated with the peak level of mystical experience.

In another study of functional connectivity, Carhart-Harris et al.[46] proposed an increase in coupling between the default-mode and task-positive network (found in psychotic states) along with preservation of thalamocortical connectivity, resulting in preservation of arousal but blurring of the separation of inner thought and external foci. *However, there was no control group in either study.*

LSD

A 2016 systematic review by Rucker et al.[47] of psychedelics in the treatment of mood disorders found 19 studies involving 423 people, but the majority of investigations focused on LSD. The overall improvement rate was 79.2%, a remarkable finding but one that came with a number of caveats I will mention shortly. Rucker et al. also noted a meta-analysis of LSD in the treatment of alcoholism, in which LSD achieved an odd ratio of 1.96 vs placebo. Other studies have focused on advanced cancer, obsessive-compulsive disorder, addiction, cluster headaches, and neuroses, a term not found in DSM-5. In depression, improvement rates varied from 80% to 91%, far exceeding rates found with ADs, with doses ranging from 20 to 1,500 µg. Unfortunately, the many studies done between 1949 and 1973 were marked by significant methodological problems, despite the four million dollars spent by federal agencies to fund over 100 studies of LSD.[48] *Indeed, only four of the studies reviewed by Rucker et al.[47] had control groups.*

Outcomes were vague, and positive outcomes varied between 40% and 95%. The therapeutic effects are closely tied to the setting, an issue that remains today. Blinding is difficult since it is obvious if the subject is experiencing a psychedelic effect. On the other hand, Rucker et al. cited a number of studies indicating that psychedelic use has been associated with a lower relative risk of suicide, less need for psychotropics, decreased recidivism, and very low rates of psychotic symptoms. However, distinguishing psychotic symptoms from the primary effects of psychedelics is difficult and clearly depends on the setting and experimental goals. In the clinic setting, for example, a patient exhibiting derealization, depersonalization, and perceptual disturbances would be considered psychotic but, in the psychedelic world, would be rated as having a profound mystical experience.

In a 2014 study[49] of LSD-assisted psychotherapy for anxiety associated with life-threatening illnesses in 12 patients, 200 µof LSD was the experimental dose, while 20 µg was used as a control dose. Subjects were required to taper off psychotropic drugs. LSD was given in two full-day sessions two to three weeks apart, with the setting being a comfortable office with a co-therapist and music. Reduction in anxiety occurred at the two-month follow-up but *only at a trend level, with an effect size of 1.1 to 1.2, which is quite low.* However, the authors took an optimistic view. Nevertheless, we must note that LSD impairs inhibitory performance,[49] as measured by fMRI imaging in a go/no-go task. LSD also impairs working memory, executive functions, and cognitive flexibility but not risk-based decision-making.[50] However, pretreatment with ketanserin, a 5-HT2a antagonist, normalized the cognitive deficits.

Despite these problems, the use of psychedelics in psychiatry is blooming, and the public seems enthusiastic. Witness the publication in *The New Yorker* of an essay, "The Trip Treatment," by Michael Pollan in 2015,[48] followed by his book *How to Change Your Mind* in 2018.[52] One year later, the FDA[53] granted the Ursona Institute in Madison a breakthrough designation for psilocybin in the treatment of MDD, resulting in a phase-two trial of psilocybin for MDD at seven study sites in the U.S., with a targeted enrollment of 70 patients. The field gained additional legitimacy in 2019, when Johns Hopkins announced the first U.S. Center for Psychedelic and Conscious Research, funded by a private foundation and several philanthropists.[54]

MDMA

In August of 2017, the FDA announced yet another breakthrough designation, this for the treatment of PTSD with 3,4-methylenedioxymethamphetamine (MDMA, commonly known as ecstasy or molly). Evidence supporting the designation had come from the Multidisciplinary Association for Psychedelic Drug Studies (MAPS), a group that reported more improvement with a combination of MDMA and integrated psychotherapy than antidepressants. This resulted in an agreement with the FDA to work jointly on the design of three phase-three studies. The $25 million cost is significant, but, by 2017, MAPS had raised half the funding[55] and has continued to expand its access to MDMA-assisted psychotherapy.

MDMA Basics

This is an amphetamine analog, first synthesized in 1912, but it received little interest until the U.S. Army Chemical Center funded a series of studies in animals and humans as part of the work aimed examining the toxicity and lethal doses of a number of chemicals. In the 1960s, it gained fame as a drug that enhanced well-being and connectedness, thereby winning use as an adjunct in psychotherapy, as did LSD. In 1985, its use became illegal, but it found popularity as a drug in the rave party scene. We should note that MDMA is closely related structurally to methamphetamine, and *both are toxic to serotonergic neurons*. Readers at times may be confused by the nomenclature of the four related compounds: amphetamine, methamphetamine, 3,4-methlene dioxyamphetamine (MDA), and 3,4-methylenedioxymethamphetamine (MDMA).[56]

MDMA acts by stimulating production of 5-HTA (serotonin), DA, and NE, and, like ADs, MDMA blocks the transporter for each, resulting in increased levels of these transmitters at the synapse. Like ketamine, it has two isomers, with the R (-) form being the most active at 5-HTA receptors. The half-life is six to nine hours. Doses in humans range from 75 to 150 mg. It also has sympathomimetic effects, so it can increase blood pressure, heart rate, and pupillary constriction and elevate body temperature to the point that malignant hyperthermia can develop.[56]

Unfortunately, many studies have shown that MDMA can deplete stores of 5-HT, its metabolite, and the 5-HT transporter. *MDMA can also induce structural changes in 5-HT neurons.* In other words, it can be neurotoxic. The margin for safety in this regard is low. Abstinent MDMA users have been shown to have reductions in the transporter and the primary metabolite of 5-HT. The longer-term effects include impairment in immediate and delayed memory and verbal learning. The threshold for pain may be lowered. In addition, MDA, the MDMA metabolite, appears to be a factor in the development of valvular heart disease.[57]

However, debate continues over the extent of 5-HT neurotoxicity in humans. Yet Gerra et al., in a study[58] of 15 male users (8 to 25 months) done three weeks after the last dose found an impaired response to a 5-HT agonist (fenfluramine), with decreased release of cortisol and prolactin. However, release of cortisol improved after 12 months of abstinence. Indices of hostility also improved at 12 months. However, problems with this study included the lack of a control group and the use of other substances during the study.

Despite these concerns, studies have continued. For example, in a 2018 study[59] of MDMA and psychotherapy in service personnel afflicted with PTSD of at least six months, MDMA was dosed at 30 mg (active control), 75 mg, or 125 mg in two eight-hour sessions. At one month, the 75 mg and 125 mg groups had a very significant reduction in PTSD symptom severity, with an effect size of 2.8, which is quite large. In a subsequent open-label crossover, a significant reduction in symptoms was found in the 75 mg and 125 mg groups. Only five subjects had a serious adverse event, with four related to the study drug.

Finally, psychiatry continues its enthusiasm for MDMA and psychedelics, as witnessed by a long review in 2019 by David Nutt,[60] who writes that these efforts portend a new era in psychiatry, and a 2018 editorial[61] in *JAMA Psychiatry* that notes with favor the FDA approval of MDMA and its potential for use in pediatric patients! Ben Sessa,[62] while making the case for the use of MDMA in addictions and the treatment of trauma, also insists that the drug has very low rates of morbidity and mortality, citing a coroner's report of deaths in the UK. This report found 81 deaths in the years 1997 through 2000, but only 7% involved the use of MDMA alone, indicating 6 deaths in three years occurring among 120 million doses of MDMA in more than 100 million users. In his view, the media, public, and health professionals have badly misjudged the safety of MDMA. However, Sessa seems to have minimized the possibility of long-term use damaging the serotonergic system.

"Novel" Treatment Alternatives for Depression

Anti-Inflammatories

The use of anti-inflammatory agents, including NSAIDs (celecoxib, ibuprofen), statins, and cytokine inhibitors, rests on evidence pointing to an inflammatory process in depression, as witnessed by an increase in biomarkers of inflammation during depressive episodes,[63] an increased frequency of depression in infections and autoimmune diseases,[64] and evidence of greater symptom severity in the presence of inflammatory biomarkers.[65] Pro-inflammatory cytokines have been found in the prefrontal cortexes of adolescent victims of suicide[66] while low levels of IL-8 have been associated with anxiety in suicidal patients.[67] (As a reminder: Biomarkers of inflammation include tumor necrosis factor, interleukin (IL-1ß, IL-6), and c-reactive protein (CRP), perhaps the most commonly studied.)

In a 2019 meta-analysis of this work,[68] the authors included 15 agents investigated in 36 RCTs involving 10,891 patients. Anti-inflammatory agents as add-ons to antidepressants were significantly superior to placebo, with a risk ratio of *1.76 for response and 2.14 for remission.* NSAIDs as monotherapy were also superior to placebo, but the effect size was low. Statins were superior to placebo as add-on agents but not as monotherapy. The authors admitted that, in many instances, the effect sizes fell into the medium category, but the studies were highly heterogeneous. Worse, *all* trials showed a high risk of bias stemming from publication bias, concealment, sequence generation, and for-profit bias. Importantly, the risk of adverse events could not be fully assessed, due to the absence of reports in 17 of the 36 studies, an omission difficult to explain. However, there was no increase in the risk of gastrointestinal symptoms or cardiovascular events compared with placebo. *Inexplicably, only five trials examined the influence of baseline inflammatory markers!*

Other Novel Strategies

A number of other novel but less-well studied approaches have been found effective, but the database is sparse. For example, oral scopolamine, a cholinergic receptor antagonist, delivered in a 4 μg/kg infusion, achieved a remission rate in TRD of 56% at three days.[69] Pioglitazone, an oral antidiabetic drug, has demonstrated success in three RCTs of major depression.[70] Nitrous oxide, an inhibitor of NMDA receptors, had significant antidepressant effects at 2 hours and 24 hours, with no psychedelic effects,[71] but only 20% improved. In 2014, Magid et al. noted that one injection of botulinum toxin A yielded a 33% to 55% response rate, but patients could simultaneously take up to three psychotropics.[72] In an RCT of whole-body hyperthermia,[73] elevation of the body temperature to 101.3° in one session led to more improvement in depressive symptoms than did sham treatment. Note that the induction of hyperthermia was common in the asylum. It was championed in the 1920s by Wagner-Jauregg, who first injected patients with a variety of vaccines and then found success with injections of blood from malaria patients into patients with syphilis. He claimed success rates of 80% in stemming the progression of the disease and, in 1927, was awarded the Nobel Prize in medicine.[74, pp. 30-31]

For a detailed review of "novel" approaches, see a 2017 review by Henter et al.[75] Given the rapidly increasing numbers of studies, these strategies may not be novel in the near future. This includes the use of opioids, an approach that deserves a separate critique.

Opioids in Depression

The rationale for opioids rests in part on the history of these drugs and their therapeutic use, dating to at least the third millennium BC. The record shows that opioids were used to treat suffering secondary to melancholia, pain, agitation, and crying babies,[76] with Sumerians calling poppy the plant of joy. At the turn of the last century, Kraepelin recommended opium for the treatment of agitated depression. Indeed, it was considered a specific treatment for melancholia even prior to Kraepelin's endorsement.[77] The rise of organic chemistry made the synthesis of cocaine and morphine possible in the 1800s, while the advent of the hypodermic syringe in the mid-1800s marked a turning point in the widespread use of opiates.[78]

Despite the centuries-old use of opioids, the enthusiasm of many in psychiatry for using opioids in the treatment of mental disorders appears *illogical* in view of the opioid epidemic and the epidemic of deaths by overdose. Indeed, the overall mortality rate for unintentional drug poisoning in the U.S. has grown exponentially since 1979,[79] although this has varied with individual drugs. In 2005 and 2006, cocaine was the leading cause of death, mostly among those ages 40 to 50. Death rates increased with prescription opioids and then with synthetic opioids, especially fentanyl, while the age range dropped to 20 to 40 years. Geography matters,[79] with deaths from fentanyl and heroin dominating in the Northeastern U.S. while deaths from methamphetamine were common in the Southwestern U.S. *In 2017, 67% of the 70,327 overdose deaths involved opioids, with a 45% increase from 2016 to 2017.*[80] There is no doubt that excessive prescribing by physicians played a major role in the epidemic, with sales of opioids rising 300% over the past two decades, in part due to the campaign that designated pain as the fifth vital sign[80] and the willingness of manufacturers to flood certain areas of the country with opioids.[81, 82] *Unfortunately, the chronic use of opioids results in more depressive symptoms than found in non-users—independent of pain—and a 25% increase in the risk of developing TRD.*[83, 84]

Background

Briefly, opioid receptor subtypes modulate regulation of 5-HT in the midbrain, forebrain, and raphe and activate DA systems, reflecting a significant interplay between the endogenous opioid systems and monoaminergic systems, although some have found that the rewarding effects of opioids may be independent of DA systems. There is little question but that the opioid receptors, kappa (KORs), delta (DORs), and mu (MORs), have a significant impact on reward processing and mood control. These receptors are linked to the endogenous opioid peptides (ß-endorphins, enkephalins, dynorphins) and are found in high density in the limbic system.[85, 86] A deficiency in the endogenous opioid system has been proposed as a model for depression, similar to the concept of a monoaminergic deficit. MOR and DOR agonists increase extracellular concentration of DA in the nucleus accumbens while KOR agonists decrease DA levels. If one accepts a mono-aminergic theory of depression, which emphasizes low levels of DA and other monoamines, it seems reasonable to propose that antagonists of the KORs might be useful for depression and KOR agonists for mania.[85] However, things aren't that simple since dose size make a considerable difference. This brings us to buprenorphine.

Clinical Studies of Opioids in Psychiatry

Buprenorphine, a Schedule 3 drug, is a partial MOR agonist, but, at doses below 2 mg, buprenorphine acts as a KOR antagonist, with *increased release of DA. At that dose or below, it has been widely abused.* It received FDA approval in 2002 for treatment of opioid abuse, with dose ranges from 8 mg to 24 mg sublingually, and acts as a MOR antagonist, thus *blocking* the release of DA and its rewarding effects. At that dose, it relieves cravings and withdrawal while blocking the effects of other opioids.[87]

In an RCT of TRD,[88] Fava et al. took this a step further, by comb-ing buprenorphine with samidorphin, a potent MOR antagonist, in order to block the MOR agonist effects of buprenorphine. Previous studies had shown that this combination to be effective in blocking euphoria and crav-ing. The combination was given in a single, sublingual tablet, dosed in ratio of 2 mg/2 mg, 8 mg/8 mg, or placebo, with all patients continuing the same AD. The 2 mg/2 mg group showed a significantly greater improvement vs placebo, while the 8 mg/8 mg group improved, but not significantly, a sur-prising finding. The effect size was 0.50, with a 47% response rate for the 2 mg/2 mg group vs 26% with placebo and 36% for the 8 mg/8 mg group. The most common adverse events were gastrointestinal symptoms, dizzi-ness, and headache. There was no opiate withdrawal. The authors noted that the better response in the 2 mg/2 mg group may have been secondary to higher rates of nausea and vomiting in the higher dose group, thus skew-ing the response.

In a 2016 commentary, Kosten[87] emphasized the abuse potential of buprenorphine and stressed that the development of a mucosal film and depot implant containing buprenorphine was itself problematic, since the implant requires surgery and replacement in a few months. Importantly, the implant contains some 300 mg of the drug, making it attractive for potential abusers. On the other hand, such strategies carry the possibility of reducing abuse and diversion.

The dosing issue was also explored in a study[89] of ultra-low-dose buprenorphine (0.1 mg daily, up to 0.44 mg daily) for patients who were severely suicidal as an adjunctive treatment over a four-week period. This included use at home. Buprenorphine was clearly superior to placebo in reducing suicidality, with the principal side effects being fatigue, nausea, constipation, and dry mouth. At the end of four weeks, the medication was stopped, but there were no withdrawal symptoms. A systematic review[86] of buprenorphine in MDD in 2018 found over 2,000 potentially relevant studies, *but only 10 met the inclusion criteria!* The authors concluded that buprenorphine is effective, well tolerated, and safe, but the relative contributions of various combinations and doses need to be established.

Nevertheless, psychiatry's enthusiasm for opioids continues, with a long review in 2019 of their promising potential for treating TRD.[90] In an extraordinary statement, the authors insist that concerns over opioid dependency and overdoses are badly out of balance when compared with the importance of opioids as treatments for mood and anxiety disorders! But they offer no data on or discussion of the possibility of opioid-treated patients becoming addicted, dying from an overdose, or becoming involved in selling or otherwise misusing the drugs. Nor do they explore the legal consequences of such behaviors and events. Who will bear responsibility in these cases? Have we learned nothing from our role in fostering the opioid epidemic?

In addition, one author has been working with the manufacturer of buprenorphine for use in TRD, with funds provided for his laboratory and other work, but at least this obvious conflict of interest was acknowledged.[90] Similarly, a 2020 review[91] in the *American Journal of Psychiatry* notes evidence-based support for the use of MDMA for the treatment of PTSD and psilocybin for the treatment of depression and anxiety in patients with cancer, but again, there was no discussion of the clinical and legal consequences of prescribing psychotogenic drugs.

Clinical Notes

1. The rapid development of private and university ketamine clinics in the U.S. has already resulted in patients shopping for infusion clinics in order to obtain additional drug. I strongly advise against such behavior. Ketamine is an addictive and potentially psychotogenic agent.
2. Healthy people have developed psychotic symptoms with the use of ketamine.
3. Short-term use of ketamine has produced impressive results in depression, but relapse rates are high, although use of the esketamine nasal spray has significantly delayed relapse.

4. While the FDA has approved the nasal spray, there are significant restrictions on its use. It must be given in a certified clinic, and a two-hour post-dose observation period is required before discharge.

5. Psychiatry has returned to practices dating to the 1950s and 1960s in its enthusiasm for use of LSD and psilocybin, often as adjunctive agents in psychotherapy, but also for relief of depression. I caution that the risks of hallucinogens should not be underestimated. Psilocybin clearly can produce a psychotic state, but, in tightly controlled, rather elegant experimental settings, with intensive monitoring and support, patients can experience intense mystical feelings with mood-elevating effects. How these results could be developed in the context of the usual clinic settings isn't at all clear, nor is it clear how psilocybin could be used therapeutically in schizophrenia or bipolar disorder. As we noted earlier, psilocybin has been used in challenge studies aimed at studying the impact of more psychotic symptoms.

6. A long review published in 2020 emphasized studies showing that psychedelics are low on the list of social harms, especially compared with alcohol, and noted that some, including PCP, are potentially addictive but do not lead to uncontrollable drug-seeking behaviors.[91]

7. Both LSD and PCP have been used in cancer patients to alleviate depression and anxiety with positive results. Older and newer studies have found LSD helpful in treating alcohol use disorders, but the studies are biased by the settings, which are far different from those in the usual clinic, with intense supervision, music, and mentors.

8. LSD has been shown to impair working memory and other cognitive functions.

9. Research in psychedelic agents is booming, with breakthrough designations by the FDA for psilocybin and MDMA (ecstasy) and the establishment of a research center at Johns Hopkins.

10. Please note that the data does not support the use of any psychedelic drug outside the confines of a research setting.[91]

11. MDMA may deplete serotonin and indeed cause neurotoxicity with cognitive impairment. Its use in PTSD is a subject of active research, with one study showing a significant reduction in PTSD symptoms.

12. Research into depression has been advanced by a focus on inflammation, but the same can be said for many other disorders. Elevated markers of inflammation (C-reactive protein) have been found in depression, suicidality, completed suicide, and COVID-19.[92] Anti-inflammatory agents have shown superior results in MDD vs placebo, as have statins, but they have the potential for significant adverse events, including gastrointestinal bleeding. Anti-inflammatories have also shown positive results in schizophrenia.[93]

13. Even in the face of the opioid epidemic and an extraordinary rise in overdose deaths from opioids and fentanyl, psychiatry has become enthused about opioids as antidepressants, with a number of studies finding

significant response rates in TRD. A systematic review of buprenorphine found it efficacious, tolerable, and safe. However, it is clearly an addictive drug, as emphasized by a number of authors.

14. Regarding the therapeutic use of opioids in psychiatric disorders, serious questions have yet to be answered, as I noted earlier. Who is responsible if the patient becomes addicted? Who is responsible if the patient or doctor misuses the drug and attempts to sell it or gives it to friends? Who is responsible if the patient overdoses and perhaps dies? What should the clinician do if the patient has had a good response but later relapses and insists on resuming an opioid—which I guarantee will happen. The same can be said for the use of ketamine and hallucinogenic agents such as psilocybin and MDMA.

15. By embracing these agents, is psychiatry helping legitimize the drug culture and enhance the drug-saturated society that is the United States? Are we helping blur the line between recreational and therapeutic use of psychotogenic drugs? *Have we forgotten our role in abetting the opioid epidemic?* While the COVID-19 crisis has overshadowed the opioid epidemic, the latter has not disappeared. Indeed, concerns have been raised about the stress of COVID-19 worsening the abuse of opioids and other drugs, not to mention its effect on depression and suicidality.

16. The studies just reviewed seldom dive into the socioeconomic status of the patient, despite work that demonstrates the significant impact of the environment and unemployment on depression. A study in 2019,[94] for example, noted that unemployment, the death of a friend, and disability were indicators of outcome in MDD. Case and Deaton[95] stressed the association between the lack of a BA degree and the rising rates of depression, alcoholism, alcoholic liver disease, pain, and "deaths of despair" in non-Hispanic white males, ages 45 to 54, a development seen only in the United States. Perhaps these problems constitute a major block to the effectiveness of our current crop of 32 antidepressants, 23 antipsychotics, and the many adjunctive agents and strategies we have reviewed.

References

1. Freedman R, Brown AS, Cannon TD, et al. Can a framework be established for the safe use of ketamine? *America Journal of Psychiatry* 2018;175:587–589.

2. Sanacora G, Frye MA, McDonald W, et al. A consensus statement on the use of ketamine the treatment of mood disorders. *JAMA Psychiatry* 2017;74:399–405.

3. Sanacora G, Heimer H, Hartman D, et al. Balancing the risks of ketamine for mood disorders. *Neuropsychopharmacology* 2017;42:1179–1181.

4. Mathew SJ, Shah A, Lapidus K, et al. Ketamine for treatment-resistant unipolar depression: current evidence. *Central Nervous System Drugs* 2012;26:189–204.

5. Iversen LL, Iversen SD, Bloom FE, Roth RH. *Introduction to Neuropsychopharmacology*. Oxford University Press, Oxford, 2009.

6. Hass D, Harper D. Ketamine: a review of its pharmacologic properties and use in ambulatory anesthesia. *Anesthesiology Progress* 1992;39:61–68.

7. Mischel NA, Kritzer MD, Paktar AA, et al. Updates on preclinical and translational neuroscience of mood disorders. A brief historical focus on ketamine for the clinician. *Journal of Clinical Psychopharmacology* 2019;39:665–672.

8. US Food and Drug Administration. FDA approves new nasal spray medication for treatment-resistant depression: available only a certified doctor's office or clinic. www.fda.gov/news-events/press-announcements/fda-approves-new-nasal-spray-medication-treatment-resistant-depression-available-only-certified. Accessed December 16, 2019.

9. Luby ED, Cohen BD, Rosenbaum G, et al. Study of a new schizophrenicmimetic drug: sernyl. *American Medical Association Archives of Neurology and Psychiatry* 1959;81:363–369. Note: sernyl is PCP, or phencyclidine.

10. Javitt DC, Zukin SR. Recent advances in the phencyclidine model of schizophrenia. *American Journal of Psychiatry* 1991;148:1301–1308.

11. Domino EF, Luby ED. Phencyclidinine/Schizophrenia: one view towards the past, the other to the future. *Schizophrenia Bulletin* 2012;38:914–919.

12. Carpenter WT Jr. The schizophrenia ketamine challenge debate. *Biological Psychiatry* 1999;46:1081–1091.

13. Whitaker R. *Mad in America. Bad Science, Bad Medicine, and the Enduring Mistreatment of the Mentally* Ill. Perseus Publishing, Cambridge MA, 2002.

14. Krystal JH, Karper LP, Seibyl JP, et al. Subanesthetic effects of the noncompetitive NMDA antagonist, ketamine, in humans. *Archives of General Psychiatry* 1994;51:199–214.

15. Malhotra AK, Pinals DA, Weingartner H, et al. NMDA receptor function and human cognition: the effects of ketamine in healthy volunteers. *Neuropsychopharmacology* 1996;14:301–307.

16. Malhotra AK, Pinals DA, Adler CM, et al. Ketamine-induced exacerbation of psychotic symptoms and cognitive impairment in neuroleptic-free schizophrenics. *Neuropsychopharmacology* 1977;17:141–150.

17. Stone JM, Erlandsson K, Arstad E, et al. Relationship between ketamine-induced psychotic symptoms and NMDA receptor occupancy: a [^{123} I]CNS-1261 SPET study, *Psychopharmacology* (Berlin) 2008;197:401–408.

18. National Institute on Drug Abuse. Drug Facts: club drugs (GHB, Ketamine, Ropypnol). Revised July 2010. www.drugabuse.gov/publications/drugfacts/club-drugs-ghb-ketamine-rohypol.

19. Jansen KR. Non-medical use of ketamine. Dissociative states in unprotected settings may be harmful. *British Medical Journal* 1993;306:601–602.

20. Harborne G, Watson FL, Healy DT, et al. The effects of sub-anesthetic doses of ketamine in memory, cognitive performance, and subjective experience in healthy volunteers. *Journal of Psychopharmacology* 1996;10:134–140.

21. Berman RM, Cappiello A, Anand A, et al. Antidepressant effects of ketamine in depressed patients. *Biological Psychiatry* 2000;47:351–354.

22. Zarate, Jr CA, Singh JB, Carlson PJ, et al. A randomized trial of an N-methyl-D-aspartate antagonist in treatment-resistant major depression. *Archives of General Psychiatry* 2006;63:856–864.

23. Diaz Granados N, Ibrahim LA, Brusche NE, et al. Rapid resolution of suicidal ideation after a single infusion of an N-methyl-D-aspartate antagonist in patients

with treatment-resistant major depressive disorder. *Journal of Clinical Psychiatry* 2010;71:1605–1611.

24. Ibrahim L, Diazgrandos N, Luckenbaugh DA, et al. Rapid decrease in depressive symptoms with an N-methyl-D-aspartate antagonist in ECT-resistant major depression. *Progress in Neuropsychopharmacology & Biological Psychiatry* 2011;35:1155–1159.

25. Coyle CM, Laws KR. The use of ketamine as an antidepressant: a systematic review and meta-analysis. *Human Psychopharmacology* 2015;30;152–163.

26. McGirr A, Berlim MT, Bond DJ, et al. A systematic review and meta-analysis of randomized, double-blind, placebo-controlled trials of ketamine in the rapid treatment of major depressive episodes. *Psychological Medicine* 2015;45:693–704.

27. Newport DJ, Carpenter LL, McDonald WM, et al. Ketamine and other NMDA antagonists: early clinical trials and possible mechanisms in depression. *American Journal of Psychiatry* 2015;172:950–966.

28. aan het Rot M, Collins KA, Murrough JW, et al. Safety and efficacy of repeated-dose intravenous ketamine for treatment-resistant depression. *Biological Psychiatry* 2010;67:139–145.

29. Posternak MA, Solomon DA, Leon A, et al. The natural history of unipolar major depression in the absence of somatic therapy. *The Journal of Nervous and Mental Disease* 2006;194:324–329.

30. Daly EJ, Trivedi MH, Janik A, et al. Efficacy of esketamine nasal spray plus oral antidepressant treatment for relapse prevention in patients with treatment-resistant depression. A randomized clinical trial. *JAMA Psychiatry* 2019;76:893–903.

31. Canuso CM, Singh JB, Fedgchin M, et al. Efficacy and safety of intranasal esketamine for the rapid reduction of symptoms of depression and suicidality in patients at imminent risk for suicide: results of a double-blind, randomized, placebo-controlled study. *American Journal of Psychiatry* 2018;175:620–630.

32. Popova V, Daly EJ, Trivedi M, et al. Efficacy and safety of flexibly dose esketamine nasal spray combined with newly initiated oral antidepressant in treatment-resistant depression; a randomized double-blind active-controlled study. *AJP in Advance*. Doi:10.1176/appi.ajp.2019.1902172.

33. Schatzberg A. A word to the wise about intranasal esketamine. *Ajp.Psychiatryonline. org*. https:doi.org/10.1176/appi.ajp.2014.13101434.

34. The Medical Letter on Drugs and Therapeutics. Esketamine nasal spray (Spravoto) for treatment-resistant depression. *The Medical Letter on Drugs and Therapeutics* April 8, 2019;61(1569);54–56.

35. Hoch P. Experimentally-induced psychosis. *American Journal of Psychiatry* 1952;107:607–611.

36. Healy D. *The Creation of Psychopharmacology*. University Press, London, 2002.

37. Sessa B. Can psychedelics have a role in psychiatry once again? *The British Journal of Psychiatry* 2005;186:457–458.

38. Grob CS, Danforth AL, Chopra GS, et al. Pilot study of psilocybin treatment for anxiety in patients with advanced-stage cancer. *Archives of General Psychiatry* 2011;68:71–78.

39. Glennon RA, Titeler M, McKenney JD. Evidence for 5-HT2 involvement in the mechanism of action of hallucinogenic agents. *Life Sciences* 1984;35:2505–2511.

40. Vollenweider FX, Vollenweider-Scherpenhuyzen MF, Andreas B, et al. Psilocybin induces schizophrenia-like psychosis in humans via a serotonin-2 agonist action. *NeuroReport* 1998;9:3897–3902.

41. Griffiths RR, Richards WA, McCann U, et al. Psilocybin can occasion mystical-type experiences having substantial and sustained personal meaning and spiritual significance. *Psychopharmacology* 2006;187:268–283.

42. Moreno FA, Weisand CB, Taitino EK, et al. Safety, tolerability, and efficacy of psilocybin in 9 patients with obsessive-compulsive disorder. *Journal of Clinical Psychiatry* 2006;67:1735–1740.

43. Studerus E, Kometer M, Hasler F, Vollenweider FX. Acute, subacute and long-term subjective effects of psilocybin in healthy humans: a pooled analysis of experimental studies. *Journal of Psychopharmacology* 2011;25:1434–1452.

44. Carhart-Harris RL, Bolstridge M, Rucker J, et al. Psilocybin with psychological support for treatment-resistant depression: an open-label feasibility study. *The Lancet* 2016;3:619–627.

45. Carhart-Harris R, Roseman L, Bolstridge M, et al. Psilocybin for treatment-resistant depression: fMRI-measured brain mechanisms. *Nature Scientific Reports* 2017. Doi:10.1038/s41598-107-13282-7.

46. Carhart-Harris RL, Leech R, Errizoe D, et al. Functional connectivity measures after psilocybin inform a novel hypothesis of early psychosis. *Schizophrenia Bulletin* 2012;39:1343–1351.

47. Rucker JJH, Jelen LA, Flynn S, et al. Psychedelics in the treatment of unipolar mood disorders: a systematic review. *Journal of Psychopharmacology* 2016;30:1220–1229.

48. Pollan M. The trip treatment. *Annals of Medicine, The New Yorker*, February 9, 2015.

49. Gasser P, Holstein D, Michel Y, et al. Safety and efficacy of lysergic acid diethylamide-assisted psychotherapy of anxiety associated with life-threatening diseases. *The Journal of Nervous and Mental Disease* 2014;202:513–520.

50. Schmidt A, Müller F, Lenz C, et al. Acute LSD effects on response inhibition neural networks. *Psychological Medicine*. Published online 2017:1464–1473.

51. Pokorny T, Duerler P, Seifritz E, et al. LSD impairs working memory, executive functions, and cognitive flexibility, but not risk-based decision-making. *Psychological Medicine*. Published online 10 September 2019:1–10.

52. Pollan M. *How to Change Your Mind. What the New Science of Psychedelics Teaches Us About Consciousness, Dying, Addiction, Depression, and Transcendence*. Penguin Press, New York, 2018.

53. FDA grants Breakthrough Therapy Designation to Ursona Institute's psilocybin program for major depressive disorder [press release]. Ursona Institute, Madison WI, November 22, 2019. www.businesswire.com/news/home/20191122005452/en/FDA-grants-Breakthrough-Therapy-Designation-Usona-Institutes.

54. Rubin R. Philanthropists fund Johns Hopkins center for study of psychedelics. *JAMA* 2019;322:1849–1851.

55. Press release: FDA grants breakthrough therapy designation for MDMA-assisted psychotherapy for PTSD, agrees on special protocol assessment for phase 3 trials. https://maps.org. Accessed August 26, 2017.

56. McCann UD, Ricaurte GA. Effects of MDMA on the human nervous system. Chapter 15. *The Effects of Drug Abuse on the Human Nervous System*. https://dx.doi.org/10.1016/B978-0-12-418679-8-8.00015-0.

57. Baumann MH, Rothman RB. Neural and cardiac toxicities associated with 3,4-methylenedioxymethamphetamine (MDMA). *International Review of Neurobiology* 88. Doi:10.1016/S0074-7742(09)88010-0.

58. Gerra G, Zaimovic A, Ferri M, et al. Long-lasting effects of (±)3,4-methylenedioxymethanphetamine (Ecstasy) on serotonin system function in humans. *Biological Psychiatry* 2000;47:127–136.

59. Mithoefer MC, Mithoefer AT, Feduccia AA, et al. 3–4-methylenedioxymethanphetamine (MDMA)-assisted psychotherapy for post-traumatic stress disorder in military veterans, firefighters, and police officers: a randomized, double-blind, dose-response, phase 2 clinical trial. *The Lancet Psychiatry* 2018;5:486–497.

60. Nutt D. Psychedelic drugs—a new era in psychiatry? *Dialogues in Clinical Neuroscience* 2019;21:139–147.

61. Bedi G. 3,4-methylenedioxymethamphetamine as a psychiatric treatment. *JAMA Psychiatry* 2018;75:419–420.

62. Sessa B. Why psychiatry needs 3,4-methylenedioxymethamphetamine: a child psychiatrist's perspective. *Neurotherapeutics* 2017;14:741–749.

63. Howren MB, Lamkin DM, Suls J. Associations of depression with C-reactive protein, IL-1, and IL-6. A meta-analysis. *Psychosomatic Medicine* 2009;71:171–186.

64. Benros ME, Waltoft BL, Nordentoft M, et al. Autoimmune diseases and severe infections as risk factors for mood disorders. A nationwide study. *JAMA Psychiatry* 2013;70:812–820.

65. Postal M, Lapa AT, Sinicato NA, et al. Depressive symptoms are associated with tumor necrosis factor alpha in systemic lupus erythematosus. *Journal of Neuroinflammation* 2016;13:5. https://doi.org/10.1186/s12974-015-0471-9.

66. Pandey GN, Rizavi HS, Ren X, et al. Proinflammatory cytokines in the prefrontal cortex of teenage suicide victims. *Journal of Psychiatric Research* 2012;46:57–63.

67. Janelidze S, Suchankova P, Elman A, et al. Low IL-8 is associated with anxiety in suicidal patients: genetic variation and decreased protein levels. *Acta Psychiatrica Scandinavica* 2015;131:269–278.

68. Köhler-Forsberg O, Nicolaisen Lydholm C, Hjorthøj C, et al. Efficacy of anti-inflammatory treatment on major depressive disorder or depressive symptoms: meta-analysis of clinical trials. *Acta Psychiatrica Scandinavica* 2019;139:404–419.

69. Drevets WC, Zarate CAJ, Furey ML. Antidepressant effects of the muscarinic cholinergic receptor antagonist scopolamine: a review. *Biological Psychiatry* 2013;73:1156–1113.

70. Colle R, de Laminat D, Rotenberg S, et al. PPAR-γ agonists for the treatment of major depression: a review. *Pharmacopsychiatry* 2017;50:49–55.

71. Nagele P, Duma A, Kopec M, et al. Nitrous oxide for treatment-resistant major depressive depression: a proof of concept trial. *Biological Psychiatry* 2015;78:10–18.

72. Magid M, Finzi E, Kruger TH, et al. Treating depression using botulinum toxin A: a pooled analysis of randomized controlled trials. *Pharmacopsychiatry* 2015;48:205–210. Note: the 2nd author has patents on the use of botulinum toxin for depression.

73. Janssen CW, Lowry CA, Mehl MR, et al. Whole-body hyperthermia for the treatment of major depressive disorder. *JAMA Psychiatry* 2016;73:789–795.

74. Valenstein ES. *Great and Desperate Cures. The Rise and Decline of Psychosurgery and Other Radical Treatments for Mental Illness.* Basic Books, New York, 1986.

75. Henter ID, de Sousa RT, Gold PW, et al. Mood therapeutics: novel pharmacological approaches for treating depression. *Expert Reviews in Clinical Pharmacology* 2017;10:153–166.

76. Saxena PP, Bodkin JA. Opioidergic agents as antidepressants: rationale and promise. *CNS Drugs* 2019;33:9–16.

77. Bodkin JA, Zornberg GL, Lukas SE, et al. Buprenorphine treatment of refractory depression. *Journal of Clinical Psychopharmacology* 1995;15:49–57.

78. Musto DF. Opium, cocaine, and marijuana in American history. *Scientific American*, July 1991, pp. 20–27.

79. Jalal H, Buchanich JM, Roberts MS, et al. Changing dynamics of the drug overdose epidemic in the United States from 1979 through 2016. Science 2018;361:1218.

80. Garcia MC, Heilig CM, Lee SH, et al. Opioid prescribing rates in nonmetropolitan and metropolitan counties among primary care providers using and electronic health record system—United States, 2014–2017. *MMWR Morbidity and Mortality Weekly Report* 2019;68:25–30.

81. Madras BK. The surge of opioid use, addiction, and overdoses. Responsibility and response of the US health care system. *JAMA Psychiatry*, published online March 29, 2017. jamapsychiatry.com.

82. Quinones S. *Dreamland. The True Tale of America's Opiate Epidemic.* Bloomsbury Press, New York, London, New Delhi and Sydney, 2015.

83. Scheerer JF, Salas J, Schneider FD, et al. Characteristics of new depression diagnoses with and without prior chronic opioid use. *Journal of Affective Disorders* 2017;210:125–129.

84. Scheerer JF, Salas J, Sullivan MD, et al. The influence of prescription opioid use duration and dose on the development of treatment-resistant depression. *Preventive Medicine* 2016;91:110–116.

85. Carlezon, Jr WA, Béguin C, Knoll A, et al. Kappa-opioid ligands in the study and treatment of mood disorders. *Pharmacology & Therapeutics* 2009;123:334–343.

86. Serafini G, Adavasto G, Canepa G, et al. The efficacy of buprenorphine in major depression, treatment-resistant depression, and suicidal behavior: a systematic review. *International Journal of Molecular Sciences* 2018;19:2410. Doi:10.3390/ijms19082410.

87. Kosten TR. An opioid for depression? *American Journal of Psychiatry* May 2016;173:5. Ajp.psychiatryonline.org.

88. Fava M, Memisoglu A, Thase M, et al. Opioid modulation with buprenorphinie/samedorphan as adjunctive treatment for inadequate response to antidepressants: a randomized double-blind placebo-controlled trial. *American Journal of Psychiatry* 2016;173:499–508.

89. Yovell Y, Bar G, Mashiah M, et al. Ultra-low-dose buprenorphine as a time-limited treatment for severe suicidal ideation: a randomized controlled trial. *American Journal of Psychiatry* 2016;173:491–498.

90. Saxena PP, Bodkin JA. Opioidergic agents as antidepressants: rationale and promise. *CNS Drugs* 2019;33:9–16.

91. Reiff CM, Richman EE, Nemeroff CB, et al. Psychedelics and psychedelic-assisted psychotherapy. *American Journal of Psychiatry*, published online 26 February 2010. https://doi.org/10.1176/appi.ajp.2019.190910035.

92. Matheson NJ, Lehner PJ. How does SARS-Cov-2 cause COVID-19? The viral receptor on human cells plays a critical role in disease progression. *Science* 2020;369:510–511.

93. Çakici N, van Beveren NJM, Judge-Hundai G, et al. An update on the efficacy of anti-inflammatory agents in patients with schizophrenia: a meta-analysis. *Psychological Medicine* 2019;49:2307–2319.

94. Zisook S, Johnson GR, Tal I, et al. General predictors and moderators of depression remission: a VAST-D report. *American Journal of Psychiatry* May 2019;176:5. ajppsychiatryonline.org.

95. Case A, Deaton A. *Deaths of Despair and the Future of Capitalism.* Princeton University Press, Princeton NJ, 2020.

13 Psychiatric Diagnoses

The DSM and the Roots of Failure

Introduction

In Faulkner's novel *As I Lay Dying*, Cash muses on whether Darl might be crazy but wonders who has the right to make the judgment. He then asks if anyone is completely crazy or sane.[1, p. 157] Faulkner wrote this in 1930, but we struggle with the same questions today. What are the boundaries between illness and normality? Who is the final arbiter in the mental health and judicial systems? Have we made any progress in how we diagnose mental illness and how we validate the diagnosis? The problems presented by diagnostic systems in psychiatry can be illustrated by the following clinical sketch. The narrative is substantially accurate, but with changes designed to conceal the patient's identity.

About eight years ago, a 27-year-old veteran came to my office in Minneapolis after discharge several weeks earlier from a prominent medical center on the West Coast. He was admitted after his family had become concerned over his increasingly odd ideas and behaviors, including hearing voices from Satan, some of which commanded him to destroy the family bible. He finally set up candles around the basement, lit them, and set several curtains on fire. The family called the fire department and the police, who took Bob to an emergency room, where he was admitted to a psychiatry ward. Copies of the hospital records confirmed the history and added a rather complete family and social history. There was no family history of mental illness, no history of child abuse, and no evidence of perinatal trauma. Bob's academic history was impressive, but he admitted to a few episodes of disciplinary problems in high school and several instances when he had used cannabis. Routine laboratory studies, a CT scan of the head, and an EEG were normal. An MMPI indicated a psychotic disorder coupled with depression; the working diagnosis was schizoaffective disorder. Bob was treated with risperidone and citalopram. Within ten days, he appeared well enough to travel. A family member flew to the coast and escorted him back to Minneapolis. In my interview, he was quite pleasant, spoke well, and denied current psychotic symptoms and depression.

In reviewing the medical records, I found that the attending psychiatrist was a well-known investigator who had published multiple articles on schizophrenia. He had interviewed Bob on three occasions and had dictated the discharge summary using the DSM-IV diagnostic system.[2] The discharge recommendations included the usual concerns about consistency of medications, close follow-up, monitoring for metabolic and neurologic side effects, and avoiding use of illicit drugs. So what's not to like? Bob had been treated well and had avoided commitment and long-term hospitalization, and his family was pleased with the results. He planned to live at home for a time and begin the process of applying to college and obtaining a degree in computer science.

Problem: Old Wine in Old Bottles

The process by which Bob's diagnosis and treatment plan had been developed was virtually identical to the process I had used as a resident at the University of Cincinnati General Hospital in the mid-1960s! Bob's attending psychiatrist was surrounded by the latest technology, but he still used the clinical history and observation as the foundation for his diagnosis and treatment. Should any of us—whether mental health professionals, families, patients, or taxpayers—be content with this state of affairs? After all, we have invested billions in research on mental illness and have, without question, learned a great deal about brain function, *but we still can't independently validate the presence of any psychiatric disorder with a biomarker*—although claims pop up with some frequency, only to break up on the shores of replication, specificity, and the lack of a relevant database.[3, 4] In response to this obvious failure, we continue to develop ever more elaborate statistical methods, various forms of brain scans, and fiendishly clever neuropsychological tests, not to mention an impressive array of psychotropic drugs, non-invasive and invasive brain stimulation, and validated forms of psychotherapy.

We are now entering the era of complete brain mapping, as evidenced by former President Obama's proposals, with additional funding by a number of philanthropists, the European Union, and entities worldwide, with costs of at least $10 billion.[5, 6] (I will describe these in more detail in the final chapter.) While one hopes for success with brain mapping, I have described in the foreword decades of work aimed at clarifying the pathophysiology of mental disorders, but the practical payoff for the clinician has been slim. With regard to forging a complete map of the brain, concerns have already been raised over the massive amounts of data that would emerge and how to store it, much less interpret it.[7, 8] The human brain has about 100 billion neurons, each of which has at least several thousand connections with other neurons, giving us a system that would generate around 300,000 petabytes of data annually. In addition, research on neural circuitry has often uncovered common patterns of disruptions across diagnostic categories,[9, 10] results that appear incompatible with our current categorical diagnostic system. Unfortunately, the current categories are well entrenched and have taken on a life of their own.[11]

Indeed, a large and growing body of work has shown us that these diagnostic boundaries are largely illusory. If so, we are badly in need of a different diagnostic system. One alternative model is a dimensional system,[12] in which the clinical focus is on a range of symptoms, rather than a specific DSM diagnosis. This would ameliorate the growing and somewhat embarrassing shift to the use of the NOS (not otherwise specified) diagnosis,[11] a maneuver that essentially admits to the presence of symptoms and behaviors outside the DSM criteria lists. A dimensional system would also largely eliminate the vexing problem of co-morbidity: that is, the presence of symptoms and behaviors that qualify the patient for a second or even three or more simultaneous diagnoses. (Perhaps the Research Domain Criteria, or RDoC,[13] will help, but more on this later.) Co-morbidity is not a new problem, as witnessed by a study[14] in 1984 of DSM-III, showing that the presence of a major depressive episode increased the odds ratio for a diagnosis of schizophrenia to 28.5, of simple phobia to 9.0, and of OCD to 10.8!

Query: To what degree will the newer models advance the diagnosis and treatment of mental disorders? Can a computerized brain map actually model the multiple inputs to the living human brain from both the interior and the exterior? After all, the brain is constantly bombarded with stimuli, is criss-crossed with blood vessels carrying many kinds of neurochemicals, and is subject to epigenetic changes induced by medications, stress, exercise, and a host of other experiences. In addition, the brain has a built-in system of spontaneous rhythms and patterns and incorporates a host of individual genetic influences on the structure and functions of receptors. That being the case, will a computerized brain map provide clinicians with better tools and patients with better outcomes? Other recent investigations include gathering real-time data from cell phones and other mobile devices,[15] using data from electronic health records,[8] and exploring deep neural networks with machine learning.[16] Before we attempt answers, we should reverse course and describe how psychiatry arrived at its present dysfunctional and outdated diagnostic system.

A Brief History of Psychiatric Diagnoses

Our present problems with diagnoses don't stem from a lack of effort, as summarized by Karl Menninger in his book *The Vital Balance*.[17] What follows leans heavily on his historical review of diagnostic systems, as well as Edward Shorter's *A History of Psychiatry*.[18] Menninger cites historical work[17, pp. 419–489] showing that descriptions of melancholia and hysteria date to 2,600 BCE. By 460 BCE, mania had been added to the list, while melancholia and hysteria continued to be discussed by Hippocrates and Plato. In the first century CE, Aretaus began to subdivide mania into three different types while adding senility and secondary dementia to the diagnostic list. The humoral theory of mental illness made an appearance in the fourth century CE. By 700 CE, at least 20 forms of mental illness were listed.

Along the way, various writers began to incorporate religious themes, with possession by evil spirits becoming a popular explanation for various symptoms. Melancholia continued its run, with the focus on black and yellow bile, phlegm, and changes in circulation of the blood. By the 18th century, one writer claimed that there were 14 different types of melancholia. However, Phillipe Pinel rebelled against the growing number of categories, and in 1801, he wrote that only four types were clinically useful: melancholia, mania, idiocy, and dementia. Carrying this even further, Benjamin Rush claimed that only one mental illness existed, as did Heinrich Neumann— who named it insanity. At the other pole, Thomas Sydenham insisted that there were multiple and specific diseases and that classification should follow the pattern developed by botanists, with detailed descriptions of species of illness. But the move toward simplification of diagnoses was not compatible with the growing emphasis on collecting statistics in the asylums,[19] reinforcing the urge to subdivide. By 1863, the diagnostic list had grown to five major classes, with some 29 subdivisions. Clearly, the splitters were beating the lumpers!

With regard to the etiology of mental illness, one can find dramatically opposing ideas, ranging from Heinroth's notion that sin was the causal factor, to the humoral theory, to Esquirol and Morel's notion of hereditary insanity, to moral degeneracy, and to Griesinger, who famously stated in 1845 and 1861 that mental diseases are brain diseases.[18] Variations on the theme of brain disease soon followed, with Meynert proposing an oppositional tension between the cerebral cortex and brain stem. We shouldn't leave off this list Kraepelin and Freud, both of whom felt that mental disorders were "organic" in nature. Others were certain that changes in the brain vasculature or brain chemistry were critical.

Diagnoses and Statistics

With the development of asylums across Europe and the United States in the 19th century, superintendents began to call for better data aimed at demonstrating the positive effects of asylum care. Beyond the pragmatics, some noted that such data could provide better estimates of recovery rates and help clarify the pathophysiology of mental disorders.[20, p. 422] However, much of the data was demographic. Diagnoses themselves seemed of little statistical or clinical consequence. Indeed, many of the prominent "alienists" had a dim view of diagnoses, with many voicing opinions identical to those found today.[17, 20] For example, in 1838, Isaac Ray wrote that no classification could be correct since the subdivisions did not originate in nature, while in 1843, Amariah Brigham noted that diagnoses had little practical utility. In 1850, Samuel Woodward observed that therapy is independent of any diagnostic system. I invite the reader to revisit the foreword to this volume for quotations from TR Insel, Steven Hyman, and Eric Nestler, all of whom have made similar comments—in the 20th century! As we shall see a bit later, Woodward's statement could be made in 2020, given the widespread use of APs and ADs without regard to diagnoses.[21]

But let's get back to our earlier struggles and recognize several sentinel events that seemed to promise advances in diagnoses. One was the discovery by Robert Koch of the tubercle bacillus in 1882, as well as the bacterial causes of anthrax and cholera. *Here we finally had definitive evidence of specific causal factors in the development of diseases.* This was reinforced in 1913 by the discovery of treponema pallidum in the brains of people with tertiary syphilis, a disease that had begun to draw a great deal of attention in the asylums, due to its profound neurologic and psychiatric consequences. The concept of disease specificity got more boosts with the awarding of the Nobel Prize in Medicine to Robert Koch in 1905 and then to Wagner von Jauregg in 1927 for his work on malarial therapy for syphilis. As Healy pointed out, this work marked a paradigm shift for psychiatry and medicine.[22]

By 1918, psychiatry had its first standardized diagnostic manual, the *Statistical Manual for the Use of Institutions for the Insane*, which described 22 principal groups of mental disorders. The manual went through ten editions between 1918 and 1942[20, p. 426] but had only marginal significance in the everyday lives of patients and psychiatrists. This is not to say that less emphasis was being placed on mental illness, given the advent of Freud, the seminal work by Kraepelin on manic-depressive insanity (MDI), and Eugen Bleuler's work on dementia praecox—which he renamed schizophrenia in 1908. Other diagnoses had come to the forefront in the late 1800s, including hebephrenia in 1863, an illness thought by Kahlbaum to be one of a number of specific and distinct psychotic disorders.[18, p. 104] Eleven years later, Kahlbaum also described catatonia.

In 1899, Kraepelin described 13 groups of mental disorders but then became a lumper, deciding that all affective or mood disorders should be included under the rubric of manic-depressive insanity (MDI) while non-affective psychoses could be lumped under dementia praecox. He went on to characterize MDI as a cyclical process with good inter-episode functioning, as opposed to dementia praecox.[17, 21] This is worth emphasizing since the alleged division between these disorders haunts psychiatry to this day, with literally thousands of studies aimed at finding the genetic/biologic/clinical differences between the two. As we shall see, recent genetic studies have, in fact, affirmed similarities, not differences.

Crosscurrents: Biologically Based Treatment and the Rise of Psychoanalysis/Psychodynamics

The 1930s and 1940s marked another transition in psychiatry—the era[22, 23] of great and desperate cures—with the development of insulin coma, electroconvulsive therapy (ECT), and prefrontal lobotomies, all of which were applied with little regard for specific diagnoses, although some claimed that insulin coma was specific for schizophrenia and ECT for melancholia.[24]

Similarly, ideas began to float around with regard to more specific biologic abnormalities in MDI and schizophrenia, but these were largely vague and non-specific.[24] The population of the asylums had grown rapidly, but medical staff was in short supply and desperate for better methods of treatment. As Valenstein described in detail, many in the medical establishment and the community at large were supportive of these often bizarre and punitive treatments.[23]

The onset of WWII was another sentinel event, since it led to (a) an influx of psychoanalysts in the U.S. who were fleeing the Nazi regime; (b) increasing concerns over the mental health of the those in the armed services and, by extension, the population as a whole; and (c) the need for effective treatment of the so-called "war neuroses." By 1944, psychiatry, which had been held in low esteem, was deemed important enough to be elevated to an organizational level equal to medicine and surgery by the Office of the Surgeon General.[20, p. 427] The emphasis began to switch to the general population and away from psychotic disorders, thus giving more legitimacy to the psychodynamic and psychoanalytic approach espoused by the incoming wave of psychoanalysts, a development that further diminished interest in specific diagnostic categories. These shifts led to a doubling of psychiatric residencies, from 155 in 1946 to 294 a decade later; an official stamp of approval by the American Board of Psychiatry for a psychodynamic approach to therapy; and a marked increase in the hours devoted to training. However, by 1950, it was apparent that these shifts had resulted in even more diagnostic confusion, leading to recommendations that the nomenclature be substantially revised. Within two years, the DSM-I had been published,[25] a remarkably fast turnaround time when compared with more recent editions. The term "reaction" came into vogue, with diagnostic labels of schizophrenic reaction, antisocial reaction, depressive reaction, etc. The alleged boundaries between illness and normality were blurred, a significant change, but a spokesperson for DSM-I[26] still insisted that accurate diagnosis remained the foundation of appropriate treatment and the prediction of outcome.

Nevertheless, the psychosocial model continued to expand. By 1955, the Group for the Advancement of Psychiatry[27] noted that its goal was to examine "Man in Transaction with the Universe," a lofty goal indeed. However, it elicited considerable criticism in 1965 from Roy Grinker,[28] who decried the ever-increasing reach of psychiatry into social and cultural issues at the expense of research and scientific training. Grinker went on to describe psychiatry as a field riding madly in all directions.[29] By way of confirmation, John Reusch[30] noted in 1957 that virtually all recent advances in psychiatric theory and knowledge had originated in Europe, citing work on phenothiazines, ECT, and Pavlovian reflex theory, to which we could add John Cade's work in Australia on lithium, the advent of psychodrama, and community-oriented home treatment. Adding to the debate over the goals of psychiatry were economic problems, including a decrease in funding by the NIMH from 1965 to 1972, and decisions by the major insurance companies to limit reimbursement for the treatment of mental illnesses.[31]

Despite the criticism, Gaskill and Norton[32] emphasized in 1968 that the *basic science of psychiatry consisted of the knowledge and understanding of the unconscious and its role in the origin of psychological conflicts*. Not surprisingly, psychiatrists in large numbers decided to enter private practice, for both economic reasons and the emphasis on psychotherapy, which was largely aimed at those suitable for psychodynamic therapy. Clearly, private practice and psychotherapy had become the dominant models in psychiatry. As a corollary, there was little interest in diagnostic systems. Robert Spitzer, who was to become the principal developer of DSM-III, recalled that no one would attend the sessions on diagnoses at the APA annual meetings in the 1960s.[31, p. 403]

Yet criticism continued to mount. In 1961, Thomas Szasz published his famous book *The Myth of Mental Illness: Foundations for a Theory of Personal Conduct*,[33] which stimulated an intense debate only to be outdone in 1973 by David Rosenhan's paper[34] in *Science*, with the wonderful title "On being sane in insane places." Although his work has recently been discredited, it stimulated additional interest in diagnosis and whether any psychiatric diagnosis had a valid basis. The tension between those who would seek a more scientific foundation for psychiatry and those who wished to broaden our involvement with social issues continued apace.

The Neo-Kraepelinian School of Washington University and the Rise of DSM-III

Along the way, DSM-II was published in 1968,[35] listing 83 separate mental disorders in nine major groups in a volume of 134 pages, compared with 130 pages in DSM-I. A major change was the removal of the term "reaction" from the diagnostic labels, although hyperkinetic reaction of childhood or adolescence was added. This later became transmuted into attention deficit disorder with hyperactivity (ADHD) in the DSM-III.[36] This, in turn, helped stimulate a veritable epidemic of ADHD, such that 15 years later, some six million prescriptions were being written yearly for Ritalin.[18, p. 290] As we shall see later, this has not only continued but grown considerably.

Yet the changes in DSM-II did not quiet the discontent with our diagnostic system. The appearance in 1971 of a study[37] comparing diagnoses made in the U.S. and Great Britain of eight patients on videotape demonstrated a significant gap between the two groups, with American psychiatrists diagnosing schizophrenia while their British counterparts diagnosed manic-depressive illness. As the authors noted, the immediate response to the findings was to ask: Who is right? While this paper has been cited repeatedly, one seldom finds any mention of the authors' answer, which was to insist that the *question was both unanswerable and meaningless since there was no independent, external validating criterion*—and still isn't.

In contrast to this position, the psychiatric staff at Washington University in St. Louis had begun emphasizing a return to Krapelinian principles as the foundation for psychiatric education, research, and practice. They stressed the need to understand the natural history of psychiatric disorders, their neurochemistry, and their epidemiology. Indeed, Robins and Guze[38] insisted in 1970 that diagnostic validity and prognosis rest on establishing a clinical description, reliable laboratory studies (although none were available), specification of exclusionary criteria, outcome studies, and information from family studies. Their emphasis on prognosis was echoed by Kendell, who wrote that classification is best validated by its ability to predict treatment and prognosis.[39]

We should note that the influence of the Washington University group was aided and abetted by the early growth of the pharmaceutical industry, which was busy developing and marketing not only APs and ADs but also drugs used far more commonly in the community, including meprobamate (Miltown) in 1955, chlordiazepoxide (Librium) in 1960, and, especially, diazepam (Valium) in 1963.[40] The FDA was helpful as well, decreeing in 1951 that new medications were to be available only by prescription. More importantly, the 1962 amendments to the Food, Drugs, and Cosmetics Act emphasized that *drugs were to be aimed at treatment of categorical diseases*.[40, p. 362] In addition, the randomized, controlled trial was held to be the standard for gaining FDA approval of new drugs, adding to the push for a more scientific diagnostic system that depended on separating diseases from one another.

The Feighner Criteria: A Paradigm Shift

While much has been made of the revolution in psychiatry wrought by the DSM-III in 1980, the publication of the Feighner criteria in 1972 had breached the barricades.[41] The authors, all of whom were faculty at Washington University, immediately drew a contrast between their approach and that used by DSM-II, noting that while the DSM-II criteria were based on clinical judgment and experience, they had validated their diagnostic criteria by focusing on outcome studies and familial factors. They also noted the additional importance of clinical descriptors, laboratory studies, *and separation from other disorders*. Specific criteria were set out, not only for each of the diagnostic categories but also for gauging whether symptoms should be scored as positive. *In contrast to DSM-II, with its 83 diagnostic categories, Feighner et al. found validating evidence for only 15.*

The primary purpose of the Feighner system was to expedite psychiatric investigation,[41, p. 57] so it isn't surprising that they stressed diagnostic validity. However, they did carry out several studies of inter-rater reliability, with ratings ranging from 86% to 95%—a considerable improvement over earlier studies of DSM-II and DSM-I.[42] The impact of this paper was immediate. By 2009, the paper had been cited 4,371 times, although the numbers fell rapidly starting in the late 1980s[27] as other systems came into play.[43]

Interestingly, one of the more telling critiques of the Feighner criteria came from three investigators who had been instrumental in its development.[43] They noted that for all the emphasis on validity, studies had *not* been done to establish such important features as requiring six months of illness for a diagnosis of schizophrenia or requiring five of eight symptoms for a diagnosis of depression. Yet the six-month criterion has been a staple of later editions of DSM, *despite the lack of good evidence* of its usefulness.[44, p. 414] One can only say that psychiatry is loyal to its traditions, not only on this specific issue but also on others we will discuss later.

The Feighner criteria also provided the foundation and motivation for the development of yet another set of criteria, the Research Diagnostic Criteria (RDC), published in 1978[45] under the direction of Robert Spitzer, who had begun collaborating with the Washington University faculty. These criteria were also operationalized, and the list of diagnostic categories was expanded to about 25. The section on diagnostic reliability was much more expansive, taking up two full pages, with the authors noting that the degree of reliability was much improved over previous studies, including those of the Feighner criteria. However, Spitzer and colleagues finally admitted that it is theoretically possible to improve reliability and lose validity,[46, p. 782] *a caveat that has been either forgotten or ignored!*

Nevertheless, the success of the Feighner and RDC systems led Spitzer and colleagues to jump-start the development of DSM-III with the formation of a task force on nomenclature and statistics.[31] Despite the previous emphasis on validity, *the emphasis in DSM-III switched to reliability.* In addition, DSM-III would be a defense of the medical model as applied to psychiatric problems.[31] Yet there were early signs of discontent, as when one member of the task force, Henry Pinsker, raised objections to the term *disorders*, noting that psychiatrists were, in fact, working with clusters of symptoms. Spitzer answered by noting that the utilization of a symptom-based system (dimensional) would make reimbursement difficult,[31, p. 405] an argument which no doubt was correct, given the stance of the FDA and insurance companies. Nevertheless, his response was an obvious bow to the economics of the system and had nothing to do with science—a harbinger of later developments.

Indeed, economics was a major concern, as witnessed by the decision by Aetna in the mid-1970s to reduce coverage of psychiatric illnesses to 20 outpatient visits and 40 days of hospitalization yearly. Blue Cross also chimed in, voicing concerns about diagnoses and accountability, as did some at the federal level,[31, p. 403] all this putting more pressure on psychiatry to radically change its diagnostic system. In addition, psychiatrists were facing more competition for the therapy dollar from psychologists and social workers, whose ranks had increased by 700% from 1950 to 1980.[47] The remarkable growth of these disciplines was an obvious challenge to the beliefs voiced by those who had insisted that knowledge of the unconscious and its role in the generation of conflicts was the basic science of psychiatry[48] and that psychotherapy and the dyadic therapeutic relationship were the primary tools of the clinical psychiatrist.[32] Such claims defied both common sense and research. Indeed, research had found no relationship between discipline and therapeutic outcome.[49]

Adding to the conflict between psychiatry and other disciplines was the proposal that mental disorders are a subset of medical disorders, one of the guiding principles underlying DSM-III.[49, p. 4] Not surprisingly, this tenet elicited so many negative comments from psychology and social work that it was defeated in a task force vote.[50] A close reading of DSM-III also reveals another bow to non-medical disciplines: the terms *psychiatrist* and *physician* were dropped. Yet, with the advent and growing popularity of DSM-III, it became clear that diagnosis had replaced psychotherapy as the core of the new psychiatry.[51, p. 53]

Nevertheless, more strife erupted over Spitzer and colleagues' determination to remove the term *neurosis* from DSM-III, based on their view that the word had outlived its usefulness and had no empirical basis, despite its place in the history of psychoanalysis. The analytic community and those practicing psychodynamic psychotherapy strongly objected to its removal, with the uproar being so great that some noted that the APA board of trustees might disapprove the manual.[50] That was not worth the risk, so the task force compromised and decided to include *neurosis* in parentheses for a given disorder.

This was not the first time that political pressure played a role in the development of the DSM, with a prime example being the controversy over the inclusion of homosexuality in DSM-II. This elicited a prolonged and intense protest from gay activists and others, especially at the annual meetings of the APA. Spitzer responded by initially proposing a middle ground, in which homosexuality would be described as irregular sexual behavior.[50, p. 258] The issue was finally decided by a referendum held by the APA in 1974, a process which garnered considerable criticism from both psychiatry and the scientific field generally, with many asking why a vote should decide a supposedly scientific question! The decision: delete homosexuality as a disorder and replace it with the term *sexual orientation disturbance* in the seventh edition of DSM-II. This term eventually evolved into *ego-dystonic homosexuality* in DSM-III, and then disappeared, fortunately. These debates led some to conclude that the development of DSM-III was not simply a clinical and academic debate over the future of psychiatry, but an intense political struggle for professional status and direction.[50, p. 263] This might help explain some of the contradictions in DSM-III that we need to explore.

DSM-III

Perhaps the most striking first impression of DSM-III was its size, with 494 densely packed pages containing descriptions of 265 mental disorders—18 times more than Feighner, and 10 times more than the RDC! What happened? It seemed unlikely that during the eight years following Feighner and the five years after the RDC, psychiatry had unearthed 250 new illnesses—a veritable epidemic! In addition, it stretched credulity to assume that these additions had any validity,[52] at least as defined by the Washington University group only a few years earlier.

No, the real problem was that Spitzer and colleagues had decided on another goal—syndromal inclusiveness, meaning the inclusion of disorders useful in practice and acceptable to both clinicians and researchers, but especially clinicians. At the same time, DSM-III was to avoid new terms and concepts that would break with tradition.[36, p. 2] The latter is particularly odd, since the overarching goal of the process appeared to be a break with the psychoanalytic/psychodynamic tradition, in which diagnosis was an afterthought. Paradoxically, the task force chosen by Spitzer was loaded with neo-Krapelinians from Washington University and elsewhere, but along the way, they seem to have lost sight of their own principles!

My conclusion: This was diagnostic democracy, not science![52] Despite the swell of criticism, Spitzer continued to defend the principle of inclusiveness,[53] writing that the task force would have faced massive opposition and, indeed, would have been replaced had it stuck to the Feighner approach. Similar problems confronted DSM-5, which we will dissect in the final chapter.

So, having dumped Washington University's vision regarding validity, the task force nevertheless insisted that each disorder was a clinically significant syndrome with a behavioral, psychological, or biological dysfunction, *while at the same time* stating that mental disorders are *not* discrete entities with sharp boundaries. In addition, DSM-III stated that there is no clear boundary between the presence or absence of any disorder![36, p. 6] That being the case, DSM-III did not attempt a definition of normality, apparently a subject too hot for any subsequent edition. If that weren't enough, DSM-III cautioned that those with the same disorder may vary in ways that affect clinical management and outcome, another significant departure from the principles of the Feighner criteria. To make matters even worse, we find that some categories were excluded due to lack of validation, but, since most categories had not been fully or even partially validated, (and, indeed, were simply based on clinical judgment[36, p. 8]), I had to assume that the inclusion of a disorder was primarily the result of a popularity contest[52] in a committee awash in a sea of ambivalence.

Indeed, since one of the goals was to insure that DSM-III diagnoses met the standards set by the FDA for treatment of specific illnesses, it seemed yet another paradox to insist that DSM-III disorders could not be distinguished from one another, or even from no illness at all! Many in psychiatry held that DSM-III was a triumph, a victory for science, and a new psychiatry based on fact.[50] *(One can only wonder: Did these people read the foreword?)* Others have disputed this claim, arguing that DSM-III was not based on any new knowledge but simply transmuted the many problems being addressed by psychodynamic psychiatry into disease entities,[50] bolstered by the use of allegedly specific criteria.

The Focus on Reliability in DSM-III

Leaving aside the issue of validity for a moment, the heavy emphasis on reliability in DSM-III was regrettable, despite solid evidence that diagnostic reliability in DSM-II was very poor. Yet we have to admit that if a group of mental health professionals cannot agree on a diagnosis with any reasonable certainty, there might be confusion with regard to treatment, although in current practice, that is not the case, as I will show later. More importantly, the lack of consensus can lead to serious consequences, particularly in criminal cases, custody disputes, and decisions regarding competency.

Given these problems, the DSM-III task force began a series of field trials,[36, p. 5] with over 12,000 patients evaluated by 550 clinicians in various settings, with comparisons of diagnostic ratings made by paired staff who interviewed the same patient. The appendix[36, pp. 467–472] listed a detailed comparison of kappa statistics (a measure of chance-corrected agreement: 1.0 is perfect; 0.7 is considered very good; and 0.5 is moderate). The overall kappa (in phase one of the trials) for Axis I disorders was 0.68 in adults and 0.68 for children and adolescents. For Axis II personality disorders, the kappa was 0.56 both in adults and youth; the identical figures seem a bit odd. Nevertheless, they were a clear improvement over DSM-II, and close to that found in a reliability study of the Feighner criteria, where the overall kappa was 0.66. However, for schizophrenia, the kappa was only 0.58 in DSM-III, and for depression, only 0.55, disappointingly low. That being the case, critics continued to bemoan the emphasis on reliability.[53, p. 355] In a reply, Spitzer, admitted that this had been the most common criticism of DSM-III, but he mounted a defense that bordered on the bizarre. He argued that one approach to reliability would have been to include only disorders with demonstrated reliability, but had the task force taken that route, it would have omitted potentially valid categories. But this clearly was not done since "we never demanded demonstrations of diagnostic reliability before adding categories that clinicians believed to be valid."[53, p. 355]

To Spitzer, this was proof that DSM-III and the subsequent revision in 1987 had actually emphasized validity. *Of course, this is believable only if one accepts the idea that routine clinical diagnoses are inherently valid.* And, if this were true, why state that validity was missing for "most" categories? Another scathing criticism came from Faust and Miner,[54] who noted first of all that reliability is easy to achieve, depending on the decision rule. For example, one could easily achieve high reliability by measuring the height of people with schizophrenia, but would they find this informative or useful? More significantly, ignoring unreliable data may be risky since many scientific observations have not been easily replicated, especially in their early stages—as witnessed by Einstein's revolutionary discoveries. Similar comments were made only one year after the publication of DSM-III, with the authors stating that while in some instances, perfect reliability has been achieved, the measure is worthless since the concept or observation lacks validity.[55, p. 410]

The DSM-III "Success" Story

The DSM has been labeled the charter document of the American Psychiatric Association due to its profound influence on the mental health profession, whether viewed from a clinical, research, or educational perspective.[56] This occurred despite the "radical" shift in its classificatory approach and its implicit shift to a biomedical model, despite objections from many in psychology and social work. As we shall see later, some in psychiatry have joined the critics, including Spitzer himself, who in 2005 was quoted[57] as saying that the DSM is unscientific, while Nancy Andreasen in 2007 wrote[58] that the DSM was not suitable for research due to the lack of validity in many diagnoses, a comment that had no discernible effect on its use in research articles. Nevertheless, by 1992, sales of DSM-III and the 1987 revised edition had reached 1.6 million copies, with translation into at least eleven languages.[56, p. 150]

Despite the popularity of DSM-III, multiple diagnostic systems were in use worldwide and yielded different outcomes. One group compared nine systems[59] used in the diagnosis of schizophrenia and found that the DSM-III system yielded the diagnosis 37% of the time vs 88% with the Yale-New Haven Index. In a major review of 92 polydiagnostic studies of schizophrenia,[60] the authors noted that different systems found considerable variation in reliability, outcome, and frequency of diagnosis. The authors concluded that we lack a significant degree of conceptual validity with regard to schizophreniaphrenia,[60, p. 1194] a sad commentary after decades of research! While the authors found little evidence that the classic Schneiderian first-rank symptoms of schizophrenia (voices conversing, thought insertion, thought broadcasting) added anything meaningful to the diagnosis, these symptoms were included in DSM-III and through DSM-IV-TR,[61] despite studies[62] showing that they are present in other disorders. *Again, tradition, not science!*

From the standpoint of patients and families, it is not comforting to know that the diagnosis of schizophrenia is at least somewhat dependent on the system, although credit is due to the DSM criteria since it is the most restrictive.[59] Please note, however, that the DSM-5 confirms the lack of any objective laboratory studies that can validate the diagnosis.[63, p. 305]

Personality Disorders and the DSM: A Diagnostic and Intellectual Muddle

I have focused thus far on schizophrenia and severe depression—given their historic and clinical importance—but DSM-III also brought to the forefront the problems associated with diagnoses of personality disorders (PDs). As we shall see, this category rested on an even greater number of contradictions and poorly thought-out assumptions than those underlying Axis I disorders. Unfortunately, the decision to split mental disorders into Axis I and Axis II divisions, with PDs relegated to Axis II, simply added to the debate over the nature of mental illnesses, with many psychiatrists in England insisting that

PDs are not mental disorders.[64] On the other hand, Steven Hyman[11, p. 165] noted that that the separation of Axis I and Axis II disorders was not only arbitrary but also an odd development scientifically. The only rationale: to ensure that PDs and other Axis II disorders are not overlooked when attention is directed to the usually more florid Axis I disorders. But any clinician can readily point out that some Axis II disorders are more obvious and troublesome than some Axis I disorders, including borderline, histrionic, and antisocial PDs.

The debate over the scientific foundation of PDs and the wisdom of their inclusion in the DSM in their *present form* continues today, with serious consequences. A prime example: the decision by the Department of Defense (DOD) to discharge 31,000 troops during the years 2001 through 2010 based on the diagnosis of a PD.[65–67] Interestingly enough, this figure was 20% higher than the rate of personality discharge diagnoses made from 2001 to 2007! The General Accounting Office, after an examination of a subset of cases, found that *the discharges were illegal*, while the Veteran's Affairs Committee in the U.S. House accused the DOD of using the diagnoses to save about $12 billion in health care costs and compensation. This rests on the DOD and VA rules that do not allow service-connected disability payments for those with a pre-existing condition, unless evidence shows that the condition was aggravated in the line of duty.

Historically, this battle has roots extending back to WWII, when, to the surprise of many, over a million men were rejected from service due to psychiatric difficulties, and some 850,000 service members were hospitalized due to "psychoneurotic" disorders. Only 25 psychiatrists were on active duty; during the war, this grew to 2,500.[68–70] William Menninger, who was chief of the neuropsychiatry division of the Office of the Attorney General, obviously had an enormous problem on his hands, particularly with regard to the treatment and diagnoses of these soldiers since the 1934 classification of psychiatric disorders was very poor and led to considerable diagnostic confusion. According to Karl Menninger,[17, p. 474] William Menninger was concerned about the injustices for patients and the government and therefore proposed a grouping of five diagnostic categories, one of which was personality deformities. By 1951, this section had been vastly expanded to include a section on character and behavior disorders that included a group of five "Pathological Personality Types" and another labeled "Immaturity Reactions," with five subtypes.[17, p. 477] This became part of the Standard Veterans Administration classification and was substantially different from the Kraepelinian and other systems developed in the late 19th and early 20th centuries. *However, it gave the DOD a new basis for the diagnosis of pre-existing, non-psychotic disorders—a move with obvious financial implications!*

Are Personality Disorders Mental Disorders? If So, How Shall We Define Them?

If we take the DSM's word for it, the simple answer is yes, they are mental disorders. (We shall avoid for now the debate over the definition of the term *mental disorder.*) The foreword to DSM clearly states that Axis I and II "comprise the entire classification of mental disorders,"[33, p. 23] clearly giving PDs a place in the DSM; nonetheless, they are relegated to the Axis II category. That separation continued through DSM-IV-TR for reasons not entirely clear, and that's putting it mildly.

Unfortunately, the problems with PDs are marked by more fundamental problems. DSM has long held that PDs are marked by enduring patterns of thinking and behaviors.[35] DSM-5 notes that PDs are not only stable and pervasive but also have roots[63, pp. 646, 647] going back to childhood or early adolescence. Yet when DSM-IV-TR rolled out, we learned that the origins of PDs can be traced not only to adolescence *but also to "early adulthood,"*[61, p. 686] clearly an expansion of the boundaries. In addition, DSM-IV-TR noted that PD traits in childhood may not persist into adult life,[61, p. 687] which seems odd, given their reputed early age of onset and "enduring pattern" of symptoms and behaviors. Another caveat in DSM-IV-TR: The disorder may not come to the attention of clinicians until relatively late in life,[61, p. 687] another assertion that is incompatible with the allegedly fundamental characteristics of PDs.

In other words, we have a set of parameters that have become more inconsistent and illogical over time—a veritable mishmash not worthy of a scientific endeavor and made even worse by DSM's insistence that PDs are categorical diagnoses—*despite* intensive research in the 1980s showing a very significant degree of overlap between and among the ten PDs.[71] One group found that diagnostic overlap was even worse in DSM-III-R than in DSM-III,[72] with high degrees of overlap between avoidant/dependent, histrionic/narcissistic, and schizotypal/paranoid PDs. Please note that these important studies were published years before the debut of DSM-IV in 1994, but they seem to have made no difference—another instance of tradition overwhelming science.

On the other hand, as we shall see later, *the marked heterogeneity found with PDs may more accurately reflect clinical reality.* But the overlap between and among PDs is not the end of the co-morbidity problem. Indeed, there are high rates of co-morbidity with Axis I disorders, especially between avoidant/dependent PDs and various mood and anxiety disorders[73] and between early-onset dysthymic disorder and borderline PD.[74] Not surprisingly, overlap between PDs, substance abuse,[75] and eating disorders[76] is common. Nor should we be surprised at the increasingly common use of PD "NOS" (not otherwise specified) as a way out of the diagnostic morass,[77] which, in part, may be an unintended consequence of the growing interest in the problem of co-morbidity.

So no one can accuse mental health professionals of not doing their homework, but the consequences of the unresolved questions of diagnostic overlap and co-morbidity can be severe, as in the plight of the 31,000 soldiers discharged from active duty and denied compensation based on the diagnosis of a PD. Was this rational? I think not, based on the following. First, to allow those with PDs into the armed services seems illogical, given the descriptions of lifelong maladjustment, impairment, and skewed views of the world. While one can understand the need for volunteers—given endless war and the absence of a draft—why punish people for behaving in a matter consistent with the DSM descriptors? During my three years as a psychiatrist in the U.S. Army Medical Corps, I cared for a number of soldiers who had been in serious legal difficulties in high school and earlier and were given the choice of jail or joining the army. (What would you do?) Yet they were often discharged on the basis of the same behaviors that sent them to court. I assume that most, if not all, were later denied compensation.

Second, given the significant co-morbidity with Axis I disorders, it seems highly unlikely that their difficulties in the service resulted exclusively from PDs. For example, substance use and dependence have high rates of co-morbidity with PDs, but so do Axis I disorders. How were these separated? Third, PDs are associated not only with diagnostic co-morbidity, but also with longer-term impairment in cognitive, social, and occupational functioning, as well as higher rates of suicidality and use of medical services,[78] any one of which would predict difficulties in the armed services. Fourth, diagnoses are necessarily based on clinical judgment and are thus subject to multiple biases, as are the judgments of the disability examiners and rating boards.

In the case of PDs, diagnostic conclusions are perhaps even more suspect that those found with Axis I disorders, yet these conclusions can have lifelong consequences for veterans, as well as defendants in federal criminal cases, where PDs are not allowed as the sole diagnoses.[79]

DSM Characteristics of Personality Disorders: Are They Correct?

The term *enduring, pervasive and inflexible* has been used to characterize PDs in every edition of the DSM through DSM-5 and are also found in the International Classification of Mental and Behavioral Disorders (ICD-10).[80] However, ample research has shown that the emphasis on stability has failed to capture the clinical story of those afflicted with PDs.[78, 81] In 2006, Mark Lenzenweger published a lengthy paper[82] describing his efforts at developing the Longitudinal Study of Personality Disorders (LSPD), an NIMH-funded prospective study undertaken in 1990 with the express purpose of examining the stability of PDs. He noted the absence of any empirical data on the subject, emphasizing the fact that the defining characteristics of PDs were based simply on clinical experience.

What about stability of PDs over time? *In marked contrast to the DSM, there are significant variations in both total PD features and the features of each disorder.*[82, 83] Gender was not related to rates of change, nor was the presence of an Axis I disorder and its treatment. (25% had sought treatment.) As the authors noted, the degree of variation is directly contradictory to the picture of personality disorders presented by the DSM model. Oher studies were discussed by Clark,[78] who concluded that there is a moderate rate of personality trait change into early adulthood, with increasing levels of positive traits and decreasing levels of negative straits—good news for patients and therapists alike! Such changes can occur as late as age 50, but even then, change can occur only gradually.[78, p. 242] Unfortunately for the younger veteran population, the possibility of such change within the context of military service seems limited.

What Can We Conclude About Axis I and Axis II Disorders?

Both groups are characterized by high rates of co-morbidity, chronicity, and recurrence but with variable patterns of symptoms and behaviors. Given the vast increase in empirical data—only a sample of which we've been able to review—there was no scientific reason to maintain the historical separation of these disorders, which continued through DSM-IV-TR but was finally dropped in DSM-5. I emphasize "scientific" because the reality is that psychiatry has seriously resisted incorporating new knowledge into its world view. A few examples: the feud over tardive dyskinesia; the continuing use of high-dose drugs and drug combinations despite reams of data showing more risks than benefits; the retention until 2013 of Schneiderian first-rank symptoms in the diagnosis of schizophrenia, despite their lack of specificity and usefulness in predicting outcome; and the ongoing use of a categorical diagnostic classification, despite several decades of studies arguing for a more dimensional approach. But DSM-5 continues the categorical model while simultaneously labeling itself a scientific advance.

DSM in the Clinic

Another issue: the remarkable increase in the frequency of NOS diagnoses, a category that made its appearance in DSM-III-R in 1987. Hyman noted[11] that NOS diagnoses appear in about half of the patients with eating disorders, PDs, and autism spectrum disorders. In an intensive investigation of the NOS category for eating disorders, 60% fell into that group, but it was clear that these patients were quite similar to patients with a full diagnosis of bulimia nervosa in terms of persistence and severity, undercutting the notion that those with an NOS diagnosis have fewer and less severe problems.[84] Similarly, a study[85] of 1,000 children ages 9 to 13 noted that the degree of impairment in those without a full DSM diagnosis could still be significant; therefore, such cases should be regarded as having a "serious emotional disturbance." At the other end of the age spectrum, 46% to 50% of veterans ages 55 and over had a diagnosis of depressive disorder NOS.[86] Yet very few studies have focused on the NOS group, regardless of its popularity.

Regardless of the merits—or the lack thereof—of the NOS category, its clinical popularity is a paradox. Think about it: Starting with the Feighner criteria, the primary goals of the "operationalized" diagnostic systems have included an increase in diagnostic reliability, clinical utility, and—at least by inference—validity. Yet in 2017, we had an upsurge in a diagnostic category every bit as vague as those found in DSM-I and II.

What are the implications? Well, one is that clinicians simply find the present system too complex, a result of the huge increase in the numbers of putative disorders and an ever-present shifting of criteria. Yet, as the systems have evolved, the time to see patients has decreased: witness the standard 15- to 20-minute med check—an amazingly short time in which to evaluate the clinical course, side effects, and the status of co-morbid medical and psychiatric conditions. Making matters even more complex, diagnoses are often not stable over time. However, the diagnosis of schizophrenia was high at 70% to 90%, but less so after the first episode. About 32% of diagnostic change involved a switch to schizophrenia.[87] Additional time is needed for assessment, especially in first-episode illness. Will this happen in a 15- to 20-minute med check?

Here is a second and more important possibility: *that clinicians have found our present categorical diagnostic system incompatible with clinical realities.* We saw earlier that the pioneers of the new diagnostic systems were convinced that mental disorders were essentially separate entities and that these entities required specific treatment. Indeed, this stance has continued, with Nancy Andreasen writing in 1984[88, p. 30–32] that each mental disorder has a specific cause and should be treated with specific drugs, while Thomas Insel has insisted that we can anticipate schizophrenia being replaced with "more precise diagnoses based on pathophysiology,"[89] a view echoed by Insel and Quirion.[90] In 2010, others called on psychiatry to match treatments to specific patient subtypes.[91] The dream never dies—or does it?

In the concluding chapter, I will focus on the DSM-5 and changes to diagnostic criteria that will facilitate the diagnostic boom and further enrich the biomedical establishment. I will also focus on an alternative approach, the Research Domain Criteria (RDoC) and its potential as a dimensional diagnostic system.[92] It is not clear what RDoC will do with regard to the high rates of heterogeneity in diagnosis.[93] For example, in DSM-5, there are 270 million combinations of symptoms that could meet criteria for both PTSD and MDD.[94] I shall also explore the worldwide effort to utilize big data as the foundation for diagnoses and treatment and what genetics has accomplished for patients and clinicians.

Clinical Notes

1. All of us—clinicians, patients, families, judges, and attorneys—are caught between the need for a DSM psychiatric diagnosis in order to meet standards for reimbursement by insurance companies, coding requirements, forensic testimony, hospital statistics, and performance measures set by hospitals and professional organizations, despite a 2016

viewpoint[95] noting that none of the newer measures are indicative of a clear boundary between illnesses or even a clear separation between the well and the ill. Sound familiar? It should, since the exact comment can be found in DSM-III, published in 1980.

2. In response to our failure to achieve the historical goal of disease specificity and treatment, the APA set out to develop a "transcendent diagnostic system" for DSM-5 but had to acknowledge that the knowledge base did not permit this approach, a startling admission after four decades of sophisticated genetic and neuroimaging studies. As we have seen, these studies have not, on the whole, supported the notion of diagnostic or treatment specificity.

3. Nevertheless, the goal of the NIMH and the Research Domain Criteria (RDoC) is to link specific brain circuits to clinical states and then develop precision medicines for mental disorders.[13, 92] I will have much more to say on this in the next chapter.

4. What are the implications for patients and families? First, do not order genetic testing from the many companies now available. Unless you have clear family history of a neurodegenerative disorder such as Huntington's disease, it is unlikely you will learn anything useful.

5. If you have a psychiatric diagnosis, remember that this is not written in stone and may well change over time. In some instances, symptoms may improve; that includes schizophrenia, as 30-year outcome studies have found.

6. Do not bother asking for a laboratory test to confirm the diagnosis. Such studies are useful for ruling out other conditions, but none are markers for psychiatric illnesses.

7. Socioeconomic factors play a major role in mental disorders, so consult with social workers who can steer you to employment, training opportunities, and financial assistance.

8. Take care to inform your doctor about any other medications you take or medical illnesses you may have. Some of these can induce depression, mania, anxiety, or psychotic symptoms. In the case of medications, remember that drug interactions can occur, with serious consequences. Insist on a discussion of side effects.

9. Be cautious about taking multiple psychotropic drugs. Ask for supporting data and the risks, if any, of mixing these agents with medications used to treat DM and other conditions. Even internists are sometimes not familiar with the effects of psychotropic agents.

10. Given the ubiquity of social media, be careful to ascertain the background and qualifications of self-appointed experts in psychiatry. Alternative facts are not helpful.

11. If you like to read medical studies, please read the conflict of interest data at the end of articles. Remember that studies sponsored by drug companies and device makers almost always spin the results in a positive direction. Some authors will have deep ties to Big Pharma, possibly

compromising their conclusions and recommendations. Be particularly cautious with regard to studies for which the company provides "editorial assistance." Ghostwritten studies are likely to be biased, for obvious reasons.

12. Always read the preface to the DSM. It sets out the limitations of the system in detail but is often overlooked.

References

1. Faulkner W. *As I Lay Dying*. The Library of America, Novels 1930–1935, 1985, p. 157. Originally published 1930.

2. American Psychiatric Association. *Diagnostic and Statistical Manual of Mental Disorders*, Fourth Edition. American Psychiatric Association, Washington DC, 2005.

3. Lema YY, Gamo NJ, Yang K, et al. Trait and state biomarkers for psychiatric disorders: importance of infrastructure to bridge the gap between basic and clinical research and industry. *Psychiatry and Clinical Neuroscience* 2018. Doi:10.1111/pcn.12669.

4. First MB. Paradigm shifts and the development of the diagnostic and statistical manual of mental disorders: past experiences and future aspirations. *Canadian Journal of Psychiatry* 2015;55:692–700.

5. Huang ZJ, Luo L. It takes the world to understand the brain. *Science* 2015;350:42–44.

6. Grillner S, Ip N, Koch C, et al. World-wide initiatives to advance brain research. *Nature Neuroscience* 2016;19:1118–1122.

7. Frégnac Y. Big data and the industrialization of neuroscience: a safe roadmap for understanding the brain? *Science* 2017;358:470–477.

8. Shah ND, Steyerberg EW, Kent DM. Big data and predictive analytics. Recalibrating expectations. *JAMA* 2018;320:27–28.

9. McTeague LM, Huerner J, Carreon DM, et al. Identification of common neural circuit disruptions in cognitive control across psychiatric disorders. *American Journal of Psychiatry* 2017;174:676–685.

10. Gong Q, Hu X, Petterson-Yeo W, et al. Network-level dysconnectivity in drug-naïve first-episode psychosis: dissociating transdiagnostic and diagnosis-specific alterations. *Neuropsychopharmacology* 2017;42:933–940.

11. Hyman SH. The diagnosis of mental disorders: the problem of reification. *Annual Review of Clinical Psychology* 2010;6:155–179.

12. Helzer J, Kraemer H, Kreueger R, et al. Editors. *Dimensional Approaches in Diagnostic Classification: Refining the Research Agenda for DSM-V*. American Psychiatric Association, Arlington VA, 2007.

13. Insel TR, Cuthbert B, Garvey M, et al. Research domain criteria (RDoC): toward a new classification framework for research on mental disorders. *American Journal of Psychiatry* 2010;167:748–750.

14. Boyd JH, Burke JD, Greunberg E, et al. Exclusion criteria of DSM-III: a study of co-concurrence of hierarchy-free psychiatric syndromes. *Archives of General Psychiatry* 1984;41:983–989.

15. Torous J, Baker AT. Why psychiatry needs data science and data science needs psychiatry. Connecting with technology. *JAMA Psychiatry* 2016;73:3–4.

16. Durstewitz D, Koppe G, Meyer-Lindenberg A. Deep neural networks in psychiatry. *Molecular Psychiatry* 2019;24:1583–1598.

17. Menninger K, Mayman M, Pruyser P. *The Vital Balance. The Life Process in Mental Health and Illness.* The Viking Press, New York, 1968.

18. Shorter E. *A History of Psychiatry. From the Era of the Asylum to the Age of Prozac.* John Wily & Sons, New York, Chichester, Brisbane, Toronto, Singapore and Weinheim, 1997.

19. Porter TM. *Genetics in the Madhouse. The Unknown History of Human Heredity.* Princeton University Press, Princeton and Oxford, 2018.

20. Grob G. Origins of DSM-I: a study in appearance and reality. *American Journal of Psychiatry* 1991;148:421–431.

21. Dean CE. The death of specificity in psychiatry: cheers or tears? *Perspectives in Biology and Medicine* Summer 2012;55:443–460.

22. Healy D. *The Antidepressant Era.* Harvard University Press, Cambridge MA and London, 1997.

23. Valenstein ES. *Great and Desperate Cures: The Rise and Decline of Psychosurgery and Other Medical Treatments for Mental Illness.* Basic Books, New York, 1986.

24. Moncrieff J, Cohen JD. Rethinking models of psychotropic drug action. *Psychotherapy and Psychosomatics* 2005;74:145–153.

25. American Psychiatric Association. *Diagnostic and Statistical Manual of Mental Disorders,* First Edition. American Psychiatric Association, Washington DC, 1952.

26. Raines GN. Comment: the new nomenclature. *American Journal of Psychiatry* 1953;109:548–549.

27. Group for the Advancement of Psychiatry. *Trends and Issues in Psychiatric Residency Programs: Report 31.* GAP, New York, 1955.

28. Grinker, Sr RR. The sciences of psychiatry: fields, fences, and riders. *American Journal of Psychiatry* 1965;122:367–376.

29. Grinker, Sr RR. Psychiatry rides madly in all directions. *Archives of General Psychiatry* 1964;10:228–237.

30. Reusch J. The trouble with psychiatric research. *AMA Archives of Neurology and Psychiatry* 1957;77:93–107.

31. Wilson M. DSM-III and the transformation of American psychiatry: a history. *American Journal of Psychiatry* 1993;150:399–410. Highly recommended.

32. Gaskill H, Norton JE. Observations on psychiatry residency training. *Archives of General Psychiatry* 1968;18:7–15.

33. Szasz T. *The Myth of Mental Illness. Foundations for a Theory of Professional Conduct.* Hoeber-Harper, New York, 1961.

34. Rosenhan DL. On being sane in insane places. *Science* 1973;179:250–258.

35. American Psychiatric Association. *Diagnostic and Statistical Manual of Mental Disorders,* Second Edition. American Psychiatric Association, Washington DC, 1968.

36. American Psychiatric Association. *Diagnostic and Statistical Manual of Mental Disorders,* Third Edition. American Psychiatric Association, Washington DC, 1980.

37. Kendell RE, Cooper JE, Gourley AJ, et al. Diagnostic criteria of American and British psychiatrists. *Archives of General Psychiatry* 1971;25:123–130.

38. Robins E, Guze SB. Establishment of diagnostic validity in psychiatric illness: its application to schizophrenia. *American Journal of Psychiatry* 1970;126:983–987.

39. Kendell RE. *The Role of Diagnosis in Psychiatry.* Blackwell, Oxford, 1975.

40. Healy D. *The Creation of Psychopharmacology.* Harvard University Press, Cambridge MA and London, 2002.

41. Feighner JP, Robins E, Guze SB, et al. Diagnostic criteria for use in psychiatric research. *Archives of General Psychiatry* 1972;26:57–63. A must!

42. Beck AT. Reliabiity of psychiatric diagnoses: a critique of systematic studies. *American Journal of Psychiatry* 1962;119:210–216.

43. Kendler KS, Muñoz RA, Murphy G. The development of the Feighner criteria: a historical perspective. *American Journal of Psychiatry* 2010;167:137–142.

44. Keith SJ, Matthews SM. The diagnosis of schizophrenia: a review of onset and duration issues. In: *DSM-IV Sourcebook, Volume I*. Editors: Widiger TA, Francis AJ, Pincus HA, et al. American Psychiatric Association, Washington DC, 1994.

45. Spitzer RL, Endicott J, Robins E. *Research Diagnostic Criteria (RDC) for a Selected Group of Functional Disorders. Biometrics Research*. New York State Psychiatric Institute, New York, 1975.

46. Spitzer RL, Endicott J, Robins E. Research diagnostic criteria. Rationale and reliability. *Archives of General Psychiatry* 1978;35:773–782.

47. National Medical Care, Utilization, and Expenditure Survey (NMCUES). *US Department of Health and Human Services*. Agency for Health Care Policy and Research, Hyattsville MD, 1980.

48. Woodmansey AC. Science and the training of psychiatrists. *British Journal of Psychiatry* 1967;113:1035–1037.

49. Spitzer R, Sheehy M, Endicott J. DSM-III: guiding principles. In: *Psychiatric Diagnoses*. Editors: Rakoff V, Stancer H, Kedward H. Brunner-Mazel, New York, 1977.

50. Mayes R, Horwitz AV. DSM-III and the revolution in the classification of mental illness. *Journal of the History of the Behavioral Sciences* 2005;41:249–267.

51. Guze SB. *Why Psychiatry Is a Branch of Medicine*. Oxford University Press, New York and Oxford, 1992.

52. Dean CE. Diagnosis: the Achilles' heel of biological psychiatry. *Minnesota Medicine* 1991;74:15–17.

53. Spitzer RL. Values and assumptions in the development of DSM-III and DSM-III-R: an insider's perspective and a belated response to Sadler, Hulgus, and Agich's "On values in recent American psychiatric classification." *Journal of Nervous and Mental Disease* 2001;189:351–359.

54. Faust D, Miner RA. The empiricist and his new clothes: DSM-III in perspective. *American Journal of Psychiatry* 1986;143:962–967.

55. Grove WM, Andreasen NC, McDonald-Scott P, et al. Reliability studies of psychiatric diagnosis. *Archives of General Psychiatry* 1981;38:408–413.

56. McCarthy LP, Gerring JP. Revising psychiatry's charter document DSM-IV. *Written Communication* 1994;11:147–192.

57. Vendantam S. Patient's diversity often discounted. *Washington Post*, June 26, 2005.

58. Andreasen NC. DSM and the death of phenomenology in America: an example of unintended consequences. *Schizophrenia Bulletin* 2007;88:108–112.

59. Stephens JH, Astrup C, Carpenter WT, et al. A comparison of 9 systems to diagnose schizophrenia. *Psychiatry Research* 1982;6:127–143.

60. Jansson LB, Parnas J. Competing definitions of schizophrenia: what can be learned from polydiagnostic studies. *Schizophrenia Bulletin* 2007;33:1178–1200.

61. American Psychiatric Association. *Diagnostic and Statistical Manual of Mental Disorders, Fourth Edition, Text Revision*. American Psychiatric Association, Washington DC, 2000.

62. Peralta V, Cuesta MJ. Diagnostic significance of Schneider's first-rank symptoms in schizophrenia. *British Journal of Psychiatry* 1999;174:243–248.

63. American Psychiatric Association. *Diagnostic and Statistical Manual of Mental Disorders, Fifth Edition*. American Psychiatric Association, Arlington VA, 2013.

64. Kendell RE. The distinction between personality disorders and mental illness. *British Journal of Psychiatry* 2002;180:110–115.

65. Dao J. Branding a soldier with 'personality disorder.' *The New York Times*, February 24, 2012.

66. Kors J. Thanks for nothing. How specialist town won a purple heart and lost his benefits. *The Nation*, April 9, 2007.

67. Kors J. Suffering from a 'personality disorder;' How my promising military career was cut short by a dubious diagnosis. *HuffPost*, January 6, 2018.

68. Menninger W. Psychiatric experience in the war, 1941–1946. *American Journal of Psychiatry* 1947;103:577–586.

69. Starr P. *The Social Transformation of American Medicine: The Rise of a Sovereign Profession and the Making of a Vast Industry.* Basic Books, New York, 1982.

70. Grob G. Origins of DSM-I: A study in appearance and reality. *American Journal of Psychiatry* 1991;148:421–431.

71. Pfohl B, Coryell W, Zimmerman M, et al. DSM-III personality disorders: diagnostic overlap and internal consistency of individual DSM-III criteria. *Comprehensive Psychiatry* 1986;27:21–34.

72. Morey LC. Personality disorders in DSM-III and DSM-III-R: convergence, coverage and internal consistency. *American Journal of Psychiatry* 1988;145:573–577.

73. Grant BF, Dasin DS, Stinson FS et al. Co-concurrence of 12-month mood and anxiety disorders and personality disorders in the US: results from the national epidemiological survey on alcohol and related conditions. *Journal of Psychiatric Research* 2005;39:1–9.

74. Tyrer P, Seivewright H, Johnson T. The core elements of neurosis: mixed anxiety-depressions cyclothymia and personality disorder. *Journal of Personality Disorders* 2003;17:129–133.

75. Ball SA. Personality traits, problems, and disorders: clinical applications to substance abuse disorders. *Journal of Research in Personality* 2005;39:84–102.

76. Sansone RA, Levitt JL, Sansone LA. The prevalence of personality disorders among those with eating disorders. *Eating Disorders and Journal of Treatment and Prevention* 2005;13:7–21.

77. Verheul R, Widiger TA. A meta-analysis of the prevalence and usage of the personality disorder not otherwise specified (PDNOS) diagnosis. *Journal of Personality Disorders* 2004;18:309–319.

78. Clark LA. Assessment and diagnosis of personality disorder: perennial issues and an emerging reconceptualization. *Annual Review of Psychology* 2007;58:227–257.

79. Johnson SC, Ebogen EB. Personality disorder and mental illness. *Dialogues in Clinical Neuroscience* 2013;15:203–211.

80. World Health Organization. *Composite International Diagnostic Interview (CIDI). Version 1.0.* World Health Organization, Geneva, Switzerland, 1990.

81. Moran M. Continuity and changes mark new text of DSM-5. *Psychiatric News* 2013;48:1–6.

82. Lenzenweger MF, Willet JB. Predicting individual change in personality disorder by simultaneous individual change in personality dimensions linked to neurobehavioral systems: the longitudinal study of personality disorders. *Journal of Abnormal Psychology* 2007;116:684–700.

83. Lenzenweger MF, Willet JB. Predicting individual change in personality disorder by simultaneous individual change in personality dimensions linked to neurobehavioral

systems: the longitudinal study of personality disorders. *Journal of Abnormal Psychology* 2007;116:684–700.

84. Fairburn CG, Cooper Z. Eating disorders, DSM-5 and clinical reality. *British Journal of Psychiatry* 2011;198:8–10.

85. Angold A, Costello EJ, Farmer EMZ, et al. Impaired but undiagnosed. *Journal of the American Academy of Child and Adolescent Psychiatry* 1999;38:129–137.

86. Moos RH, Mertens JR. Patterns of diagnoses, comorbidities, and treatment in late-middle aged and older affective disorder patients: comparison of mental health and medical sectors. *Journal of the American Geriatrics Society* 1996;44:682–688.

87. Palomar-Ciria N, Cegla-Schvartzman F, Lopez-Marengo J-D, et al. Diagnostic stability of schizophrenia: a systematic review. *Psychiatry Research* 2019;279:306–314.

88. Andreasen NC. *The Broken Brain. The Biological Revolution in Psychiatry.* Harper & Row Publishers, New York, 1984.

89. Insel TR. Rethinking schizophrenia. *Nature* 2010;468:187–193.

90. Insel TR, Quirion R. Psychiatry as a clinical neuroscience discipline. *Journal of the American Medical Association* 2005;294:2221–2224.

91. Karam CS, Ballon JS, Bivens NM, et al. Signaling pathways in schizophrenia: emerging targets and therapeutic strategies. *Trends in Pharmacological Sciences* 2010;31:381–390.

92. Insel TR. The NIMH Research Domain Criteria (RDoC) project: precision medicine for psychiatry. *American Journal of Psychiatry*, published online, April 2014. Ajp. psychiatryonline.org.

93. Allsopp K, Read J, Corcoran R, et al. Heterogeneity in psychiatric diagnostic classification. *Psychiatry Research* 2019;279:15–22.

94. Young G, Lareau C, Pierre B. One quintillion ways to have PTSD comorbidity: recommendations for the disordered DSM-5. *Psychology Injury Law* 2014;7:61–74.

95. Cohen BM. Embracing complexity in psychiatric diagnosis, treatment, and research. *JAMA Psychiatry* November 9, 2016. Doi:10.1001/2466.

14 Fear and Loathing at the APA

The DSM-5, the Brain Mapping Quartet, and the Future of Mental Illness

Introduction

A diagnostic system based on the medical model has been on the wish list of psychiatrists for the past century, driven in part by our wish to be accepted as "real doctors," rather than mocked as "alienists." One of the most well-articulated summaries of the medical model can be found in Samuel Guze's book *Why Psychiatry is a Branch of Medicine*, published in 1992.[1] This short volume is essentially a review of the groundbreaking work of the neo-Kraepelinians at Washington University, who, as we noted in Chapter 13 and elsewhere, insisted that the validation of psychiatric diagnoses rested on their usefulness in defining the course, outcome, and pathogenesis of mental disorders, as well as a uniform response to intervention.[1, p. 42] However, the subsequent development of the DSM-III[2] failed to produce meaningful results. Has DSM-5[3] improved matters? Will it contribute in any meaningful way to the care of patients? Will it result in meaningful advances in research? Will it help clear up problems in diagnoses, especially the rapid increase in the use NOS labels and the problem with co-morbidity? Sadly, the answer is a resounding no, no, no, and no. What happened to the goal of diagnostic validity during the years 1980 to the present?

The Original "Transcendent" Goals of DSM-5

There is little doubt that the planners of DSM-5 had in mind a far different product from that published in May of 2013. Fourteen years earlier, the APA and the NIMH had set in motion a research planning process that would integrate information from genetics, neuroscience and a host of other scientific fields, with the goal of developing a "scientifically sound classification system."[4, p. xv] Indeed, such a system would "transcend"[4, p. xix] the well-known problems of the DSM, including definitions of disorders that lacked a relationship to biology.[5, p. 32] Six work groups with a range of experts began examining relevant data, resulting in the publication of a research agenda[4] for DSM-V (the Roman numeral was dropped later). However, as Michael First noted,[6, p. 696] the six white papers found that the knowledge base was not sufficient to support the proposed paradigm shift. Put plainly, the biological data did not reveal objective findings that would validate psychiatric diagnoses,[6, p. 697] exactly my point in papers dating to 1992.[7, 8]

As part of the move to a new diagnostic paradigm, DSM-5 would also aim for the use of dimensional measures.[9] Indeed, Steven Hyman wrote in 2012 that drug discovery was at a near standstill in psychiatry, partly due to our dependence on outmoded, categorical definitions of mental disorders.[10] To that end, the DSM-5 work groups assessed the potential usefulness of dimensional approaches, but there was considerable concern that clinicians had not embraced the dimensional approaches already available,[6] including severity specifiers and the Global Assessment of Functioning Scale (GAF), a scale that made its debut in DSM-IV.

From Transcendence to Survival of the Misfits

What happened? Well, transcendence gave way to tradition. We still have the same categorical diagnostic system—albeit with substantial reorganization—and, as a corollary, dimensional approaches have been relegated to Section 3, the section where dreams go to die. However, Section 3 includes the World Health Organization Disability Assessment Schedule (WHODAS), a self-rating scale that is intended to replace the now-banished GAF, and the Cross-Cutting Symptom Measure, another self-rating scale.[3] Traditionalists, however, need not worry, since DSM-5 states that the material in Section 3 lacks the scientific evidence to support its clinical usefulness.[3, p. 24]

So much for dimensions. But wait, there was another half-hearted effort by the DSM-5 to acknowledge a dimensional approach, an effort that was essentially structural.[3, p. 10] This involved clustering disorders thought to be related next to one another, rather than simply grouping them into the classical categories of anxiety disorders, mood disorders, etc. Thus, given the genetic relationships between and among autism spectrum disorders, schizophrenia, and bipolar and depressive disorders, the first chapter on neurodevelopmental disorders is followed by a chapter on schizophrenia spectrum and other psychotic disorders, followed by chapters on bipolar and depressive disorders. The new grouping also follows the model of internalizing and externalizing disorders. This organizational restructuring is meant to encourage research and clinical thinking about these relationships, with the goal of building a pathway to new diagnostic approaches while, at the same time, not disrupting current practice or research.[3, p. 13] One doesn't have to read between too many lines to conclude that maintaining the status quo won out over transcendence, although the multi-axial diagnostic system was dropped, a positive move.

Was the APA serious about a new approach? If so, why has DSM-5 retained the same personality disorders, despite the flood of evidence—reviewed in the previous chapter—pointing to the need for a dimensional approach? In fact, we now have three new PD diagnoses: PD due to a medical condition, other unspecified PD, and unspecified PD, the latter two meant to do away with the NOS category (more on this later).

In December of 2012, the APA board of trustees voted down a dimensional diagnostic system[11] for PDs—another instance of rejecting science in favor of tradition and money. Some had proposed cutting the number of PDs to those with the best supporting evidence, but not even that survived, nor did a proposal to omit the five PD diagnoses with the least supporting evidence,[12, pp. 269–271] apparently due to protests from the APA membership.[12, p. 271] Instead, DSM-5 continues to offer the traditional definition of a PD (an enduring, relatively inflexible pattern of behavior), despite multiple prospective studies showing considerable variation in behaviors and symptoms over time, as discussed in Chapter 13.

Conflicting Goals and Fear of Change

DSM-5 has continued the massively ambivalent and often paradoxical sets of goals that have characterized each edition of the DSM.[7, 8] We have seen that the original goal for DSM-5 was a transcendent diagnostic system based on the etiology and pathogenesis of mental disorders, but on publication, we found a system aimed at "comprehensibility and utility,"[3, p. 10] with diagnostic utility serving as the foundation for the assessment of clinical course and response to treatment.[3, p. 20] Remarkably, the introduction to DSM-5 notes the rather paradoxical goal of maintaining continuity with previous editions while claiming that there were no limitations on the potential changes that could mark the transition from DSM-IV to DSM-5.[3, p. 7]

Note, too, that the APA chose early on *not* to study the vexing question of diagnostic validity. Indeed, the foreword to DSM-5 states that the Scientific Review Committee and the Clinical and Public Health Review Committee of the APA were "not constructed to evaluate the validity of the DSM-IV diagnostic criteria,"[3, p. 9] a clear effort to avoid rocking the diagnostic boat! Nevertheless, the foreword to DSM-5 is full of self-criticism, noting the lack of validated disorders, the inability of a categorical system to reflect clinical experience,[3, p. 5] the very fuzzy boundaries between disorders,[3, p. 6] and increasing evidence that many disorders are on a spectrum.[3, p. 6] Furthermore, the structure of the DSM has led to increasingly high rates of NOS diagnoses.[3, p. 12] But, fearful of its own self-assessment, DSM-5 concluded that alternative definitions for most mental disorders are premature.[3, p. 13] What? True enough, we have no means of independently validating psychiatric diagnoses, but one major reason for this astounding lack of progress may lie in the DSM itself—which the APA refused to alter in any meaningful way.

What Happened to Reliability?

But there's another odd angle to this sad story, and that is a sudden reversal of the emphasis on reliability, which, as we have seen, was a prominent feature from DSM-III to DSM-IV, with the inclusion of tables and statistics. In DSM-5, there is a brief discussion of the field trials, but no data whatever on the results! One can only wonder if the decision not to include the data was due—at least in part—to some rather embarrassing results, about which a great deal has been written, especially by Gary Greenberg[12] and, in a more restrained manner, by Robert Freedman and colleagues,[13] who focused on a summary of the field trials authored by Darrel Regier and colleagues.[14]

Here are the principal concerns: The intraclass κ (kappa statistic, where 1 is a perfect level of agreement) for major depressive disorder was only 0.28 in adults and children (range of 0.13–0.42 in adults), while the κ for generalized anxiety disorder (adults) was even less: 0.20, a figure derived from only one study site. These results are labeled "questionable," a generous description but very disturbing since MDD and GAD are two of the most common diagnoses in psychiatry. In DSM-5, the levels of agreement for MDD and GAD are 0.28 and 0.20, respectively, compared with 0.67 and 0.67 in DSM-IV, which are almost exactly those found in DSM-III! Obviously, the DSM-5 levels indicate very low levels of reliability, a finding that mars the goal of facilitating communication regarding diagnoses.

The reader will recall that we previously criticized the focus on reliability, since it doesn't say anything about validity. Nevertheless, we have to admit that the ability to agree on a diagnosis at least brings some degree of order into a confusing and complex diagnostic process. Although we have focused on MDD and GAD, the problem with test-retest reliability in DSM-5 is more extensive,[14] with only three diagnoses rated as very good (kappas of 0.60–0.79): major neurocognitive disorder, PTSD, and complex somatic symptom disorder. Seven were rated as good, including schizophrenia, bipolar I, borderline personality, binge eating (new), alcohol use, and mild neurocognitive disorder, but *accurate kappas could not be obtained for schizoptypal personality disorder, bipolar II disorder, mild neurocognitive disorder, mild TBI, and obsessive-compulsive personality!*

This data is hardly a ringing endorsement for the DSM-5 enterprise. A much harsher critique was leveled by Allen Francis,[15] the chair of the DSM-IV task force, who was highly critical of the terms used to describe the results, noting, for example, that kappas of 0.40 to 0.59 would have been labeled as poor in past years but are now labeled as good. In an early study,[16] a κ of 0.6 was rated as only satisfactory rather than good (DSM-5), and a κ of 0.3 as no better than fair, rather than questionable, as in DSM-5. Given this downward shift in standards, Frances went on to write[15] that the summary paper by Regier et al.[14] was "distressingly misleading" and should not have been published by the *American Journal of Psychiatry*.

The APA Response

With the advent of DSM-III in 1980, the emphasis on reliability as the first step in establishing validity has been unrelenting, despite the obvious fact that what people agree on may not be valid.[17] Nevertheless, the APA had to respond to the DSM-5 data. The response has taken several forms, one of which was to stress that statistical standards had changed since the DSM-III field trials and that each edition used different sampling methods.[18] The κ at the time of DSM-III did not include the standard error and confidence intervals, in contrast to DSM-5. The latter also used a stratified sampling approach, rather than random sampling, hoping to include more patients with more uncommon disorders. DSM-III also combined disorders and failed to recruit adequate samples, so statisticians could not use confidence intervals (CIs) to better gauge precision. Clearly, variations such as these have an effect on the final results of any study, whether aimed at neurochemistry, medications, or brain imaging, so they are not peculiar to diagnosis. In addition, there are no uniform standards for establishing cut-off points for kappa ratings, other than an agreement on 1 meaning perfect and 0 meaning none, so it isn't surprising that different terms are used for a κ of 0.3, or for any other point between 0 and 1. On the other hand, it seems intuitively correct to assume that the reliability of a diagnosis with a κ of 0.60 is superior to that of a diagnosis with a κ of 0.28.

Yet DSM-5 mounted a campaign to convince us that kappas in the low range are not only acceptable but also anticipated, in view of the methodology. Regier and colleagues,[14] for example, cited two papers in support of this view, but a careful reading of one of these[18] did not reveal any such statement, although numerous deficits in the earlier field trials were cited. Helena Kraemer, a biostatistician, then returned with another commentary[19] in 2012, titled "DSM-5: How reliable is reliable enough?" in which she and her colleagues spent some time reviewing the kappa statistic and then proposed that our expectations for diagnostic reliability in DSM-5 should be compared with the kappas for diagnostic reliability in other branches of medicine. Kraemer and associates summarized those efforts by noting that kappas in medicine are commonly in the 0.4 to 0.6 range. They went on to conclude that in psychiatry, with so much resting on subjective appraisals, kappas ranging from 0.4 to 0.6 should be realistic, and—guess what—kappas from 0.2 to 0.4 should be viewed as "acceptable."[19, p. 14]

This argument is old hat, having been reviewed in 1977 by Helzer and colleagues,[20] who found that in some instances, the reliability of psychiatric diagnoses exceeded that found in some studies of x-ray interpretations. In 1990, Lewis Judd, then director of the NIMH, claimed that psychiatrists can diagnose mental disorders with the same degree of certainty that any physician can diagnose arthritis or diabetes,[21] a claim I strongly disputed in 1991.[7] These apologists somehow forgot that internists and surgeons can validate the diagnoses of diabetes, cancer, or hip fractures via any number of independent, objective markers—which we lacked then and lack now, despite decades of intense research.

The lack of objective, independent, biological markers has been the major reason why psychiatry has placed so much emphasis on high levels of reliability; it's all we have! Despite the willingness to accept lower levels of reliability, Dr. Kraemer rather paradoxically noted[22, p. 139] that one of the prime requirements for validating a new diagnosis is a high level of test-retest reliability. Would she accept a κ of 0.20 or 0.28 for a prototype diagnosis? I doubt it.

Will DSM-5 Add to the Diagnostic Boom?

We cited earlier the rapid increase in the number of psychiatric disorders over the past 25 years,[23] with an especially dramatic increase in the past 10 to 15 years, including an almost six-fold increase in the diagnosis of bipolar disorder in children, a four-fold increase in adolescents, a 56% increase in adults,[24] and a similar increase in the diagnosis of ADHD. As a corollary, the lifetime prevalence of mental illness in population studies has been estimated to be as high as 46%,[25] a figure that has prompted considerable debate over its accuracy and meaning, with some holding that diagnosing half the population with a mental illness may be, at least in part, the result of medicalizing even relatively mild deviations from an ideal norm.[26, 27] Yet the numbers just cited may be higher still, given the results of a prospective study[28] in New Zealand of adults followed to age 32, in which the *lifetime rates of major depression and other disorders were about double the rates found in retrospective studies.*

These concerns have crept into the popular press as well: see for example, "The encyclopedia of insanity: A psychiatric handbook lists a madness for everyone,"[29] a critique of DSM-IV published in *Harper's Magazine* in 1997. While our focus has been on psychiatric diagnoses and treatment, we should mention that similar concerns have been raised about the over-medicalization of problems associated with normal aging[30] and an associated increase in the use of prescription drugs in the United States, which has now captured 50% of the global market, although we have only 5% of the population.[31, p. xi; 32]

So how is DSM-5 affecting the diagnostic boom and Big Pharma? Obviously, the final judgment will be years in the making, but it appears that the rates of many disorders are bound to increase, given the easing of diagnostic criteria and the never-ending addition of new disorders. (For a review, see the DSM-5 chapter on highlights of changes,[3, pp. 809–816] as well as the individual criteria sets.) At least 17 disorders have been revamped in DSM-5 to allow additional people to be diagnosed. Here are a few examples.

For ADHD, the onset can now be as late as age 12, instead of age 7. In addition, for those 17 and older, only five symptoms are required instead of six. For PTSD, under criterion A, the requirement for a subjective response that includes fear, horror, or helplessness has been dropped. The chair of the relevant work group noted in an interview[33] that research had shown that some patients have met all criteria for PTSD except for the fear-based reaction. In addition, one can qualify for the diagnosis *after* learning of a traumatic event that occurred in the life of a family member or friend, clearly loosening the previous criteria. For anorexia, it is no longer necessary for a woman to manifest amenorrhea. For bulimia nervosa, the minimum number of episodes has been reduced to one weekly instead of two. For binge eating disorder, another new category, one needs to binge only once weekly for three months, rather than twice weekly. Mild neurocognitive disorder is new to DSM-5. It requires only a "modest decline" in one area of functioning, but the deficits do not interfere with the patient's capacity for independence! This is not only going to increase the number of psychiatric diagnoses but will also be a gold mine for neurology and geriatric psychiatry, since mild cognitive slippage is very common.

Elimination of the bereavement exclusionary criterion for a diagnosis of major depressive disorder has been hotly debated,[13] resulting in a detailed review of the issues in DSM-5 and a note stressing that the decision to diagnose MDD requires careful clinical consideration and appreciation of cultural norms.[3, p. 161] Another new category in DSM-5, disruptive mood dysregulation disorder (DMDD), has been under fire,[34, pp. 177–179, 35] primarily due to concerns about medicalizing common temper tantrums and adding another condition that almost certainly will be treated with lithium, anticonvulsants, and/or SGAs. The medication issue is interesting, since it appears that DMDD was added in response to concerns[35, 36] over a 40-fold increase in the outpatient diagnosis of childhood bipolar disorder,[37] which, of course, is treated with the same medications.

The key feature of DMDD is chronic irritability at ages 6 through 18 years observed in at least two settings, with episodes occurring three or more times weekly. The diagnosis cannot be made if a history of mania or hypomania has occurred or if intermittent explosive disorder or oppositional defiant disorders are present, but can *co-exist* with MDD, ADHD, conduct disorder, and substance use! There are problems with this diagnosis, *including its place in the general category of depressive disorders, although there is no mention of depressive symptoms in the criteria.* Second, diagnostic reliability is poor, since the pooled κ was only 0.25, and varied widely among the four settings.[14] In a review of two studies that retroactively applied DMDD criteria to existing data sets, Roy et al.[38] cited very high rates of co-morbidity, with 96% having a diagnosis of oppositional defiant or conduct disorder and 77% with ADHD and ODD. The prevalence rate was 1% in children over age six, although others have found a rate of 6%. We should note as well a 2014 critique[39] of the DSM-5 classification of mood disorders. The authors found multiple inconsistencies and imprecise definitions.

DSM-5 Clunkers

For an effort that began over ten years ago and cost about $25 million,[40] DSM-5 contains some surprising errors, including the claim[3, p. 12] that previous editions "considered each diagnosis as categorically separate from health and other disorders." This is false. Every edition starting with DSM-III[2, p. 6] has clearly stated that there is no assumption of sharp or discrete boundaries between disorders or between mental disorders and no disorder. It appears that this error was allowed in print in order to pump up the new organizational structure by discrediting previous editions—a well-known maneuver that is part of the rhetoric of science,[41] in which a substantial part of every paper or book is devoted to ripping the methodology and results of previous work. In some instances, this criticism is so severe that one can only wonder how the original paper got into print!

Another clunker: Schizophrenia is now said to require two symptoms under criterion A, inferring that the diagnostic threshold has been raised. This is a half truth. DSM-IV also required two symptoms under the A criterion,[42, p. 312] unless one of three first-rank symptoms was present, in which case only one symptom was required. However, kudos to DSM-5 for getting rid of the first-rank symptoms, an action that should have been taken at least a decade ago when it became clear that they were not specific to schizophrenia.[43] More kudos for doing away with the classical subtypes of the disorder, since they have outlived their usefulness.

One more clunker: DSM-5 states that substance abuse previously required only one symptom, but the new category of substance use disorder now requires two or more, an apparent tightening of the criteria—but wait. DSM-5 has eliminated the distinction between substance abuse and dependence, an interesting tactic, but substance dependence in DSM-IV required three or more symptoms over 12 months. We now have, for example, alcohol use disorder (AUD), which can be diagnosed with only 2 of 11 symptoms/behaviors, as opposed to 3 of 7 for alcohol dependence in DSM-IV. In addition, DSM-IV included legal difficulties as one criterion for alcohol abuse. This has disappeared in DSM-5, due to concerns over global differences in legal standards, a legitimate issue, but how loosening the diagnostic criteria helps is not clear. The implication that the diagnostic threshold has been raised is plainly wrong. Note, too, that AUD is a highly disjunctive disorder—like many in the manual—permitting the diagnosis in people with widely differing clinical presentations.

DSM-5 and Money

In 1998, Mark Zimmerman published a commentary[44] in which he traced the publication timetable of the DSMs, bemoaning the relatively short intervals separating their appearance: DSM-III (1980), DSM-III-R (1987), DSM-IV (1994), and DSM-IV-TR (2000). While six or seven years may seem like a long time to those with a short attention span, science generally operates at a much slower pace, given the time required to put together a grant, hire staff, recruit subjects, conduct the study, analyze results, and find a journal willing to publish the results. Even then, most journals require revisions and further editing before the article reaches readers. At that point, the diagnostic criteria may have changed!

So, as Zimmerman suggested, precious little time has been available to gather *replicated* data on either the reliability or validity of a DSM disorder, leaving committee members operating largely on the basis of clinical assumptions, guesswork, and tradition. Not surprisingly, the gains in reliability and validity with successive editions of the DSM have been few, if any.[45] While Zimmerman was concerned about the 5-year publication intervals, we have seen a 13-year interval between DSM-IV-TR and DSM-5, but the results have been the same—or even worse, given the fall-off in reliability. Therefore, the primary problems lie in the dual and closely correlated goals of maintaining the traditional categorical diagnostic system and insisting that the primary goal of the DSM is clinical utility, both of which compromise its scientific integrity but make the manual a best seller.

This brings us to money. There is no doubt that the DSM has been a financial bonanza for the APA and its publishing house, bringing in some $5 to $6 million each year,[12, 40] a reliable source of income in the face of falling revenues elsewhere. Gary Greenberg[12] has noted that other revenues at the APA have decreased substantially in recent years, with income from journal advertising falling by 50% from its peak in 2006, along with a 15% decline in membership and falling income from Big Pharma, a major source of money in the past. Both Frances[40] and Greenberg[12] have stressed other consequences of the scramble for money, particularly the decision by the APA to cancel a second round of clinical field trials in order to stick with the decision to publish in May of 2013. Francis concluded that profits trumped concerns for the integrity of the product.[40]

Beyond DSM-5: The Research Domain Criteria

The APA anticipated that the reorganization of the DSM would advance both clinical utility and the research agenda, although retention of the same shopworn diagnostic system makes it difficult to understand the optimism Similarly, the APA proposed that the changes in DSM-5 would result in a shorter time to revision, so we can anticipate DSM-5.1, 5.2, etc., but, as of early 2020, I've not seen a revision. The more important news comes not from the APA, but from the NIMH, and its decision to support research *that cuts across current categories*: a dimensional approach. Put plainly, the NIMH will move away from the DSM system,[46] a decisive move that should have happened years ago but is nevertheless a beacon of hope.

The lynchpin of the NIMH strategy is the Research Domain Criteria, popularly known as the RDoC.[46] RDoC proposes that mental illnesses are disorders of brain circuits, rather than specific lesions, and that the dysfunctional circuits can be identified via genetics, molecular cellular data, and imaging of brain circuits. RDoC will also take into account individual, familial, and environmental data. The combined data will lead to "biosignatures" that will aid in clinical management and improve the outcome of treatment. Indeed, the critical value of the RDoC approach lies in how well it predicts prognosis and treatment response,[46, p. 750] which the reader will recognize as a return to the neo-Kraepelinian ideal enunciated at Washington University 40 years ago. Indeed, better treatments will depend on a more precise diagnostic system and the development of precision medicines, a strong statement indeed, given the genetic overlap between and among mental disorders.

The structure of RDoC is worth noting. Across the top of a matrix is a row, with *neural circuitry at the center*. To the left of neural circuitry, one finds genes, molecules, cells, and genetics, while to the right lies the individual, family, and social context. On the left side of the matrix is a column with domains, including negative valence systems, positive valence systems, cognitive systems, social processes, and arousal and regulatory systems. The claim has been made that the domains have been validated by research, although there is debate about the process underlying domain formulation and whether they have been truly validated, issues we will explore shortly.

The goal of RDoC is to develop studies that cut across DSM diagnoses, such that depressed mood will be studied across a variety of diagnoses that feature depressed mood, including MDD, schizophrenia, PTSD, and panic disorder, using the matrix just described. The research subjects will be selected from various clinics that use the standard diagnostic model (PTSD, mood, anxiety) but with depressed mood as the key inclusion criterion.

However, RDoC has been hampered by a clash of models, as I described in a 2019 commentary.[47] This began in 2016, when Kozak and Cuthbert published an updated review of RDoC,[48] in which they wrote that *no unit of analysis would take precedence over another*, a clear departure from Insel et al. in 2010,[46] in that neural circuitry lost its centrality. Indeed, Kozak and Cuthbert insisted that genes = molecules = cells = circuits = physiology = behavior = self-reports. Yet in 2016, when Josh Gordon was appointed director of the NIMH, he promptly endorsed the centrality of neural circuitry,[49–51] stating that our ability to manipulate circuits will result in greatly improved specificity of treatment with fewer side effects. He also noted that the domains in RDoC had been developed by consensus, rather than via a bottom-up, data-driven process.[51] As one might expect, the centrality of neural circuits has been supported by the NIH, with more than $400 million marked for the Brain Initiative,[52] about which I will say more shortly.

Brain Connectomics and RDoC

How this clash of models will be resolved is not clear, but this brief history is reminiscent of the clash between specificity of disease and treatment and the dimensional model. The first and most obvious problem of RDoC lies in the assumption that mental illnesses are the result of dysfunctional brain circuits. This concept has a history dating to Galen, who suggested that animal spirits could flow through interconnected pathways and, 2,000 years later, to Brown-Séquard, who noted that the effects of focal brain damage could have distal effects.[53] Indeed, Fornito et al. have confirmed that pathological brain changes are not confined to a single locus but are spread through the brain by a complex but well-organized neural architecture: *the connectome.*[53] In a related concept, the disconnection hypothesis[54] posits a dysfunctional neuromodulation of synaptic efficacy mediated by aberrant modulation of NMDA receptors. This process ultimately results in dysfunctional neural circuits.

Indeed, many investigators have already drawn up maps of brain circuits that might underlie the genesis of obsessive-compulsive disorder, depression, ADHD, ASD, and schizophrenia, to name a few.[55] Here are a few examples from schizophrenia: Increased connectivity has been found between the ventral prefrontal cortex and posterior parietal cortex, but decreased connectivity has been found between the dorsal prefrontal cortex and posterior parietal cortex, as well as a loss of network hubs in the frontal cortex and the development of hubs outside the cortex. See Brennand et al.[55] for a detailed review and citations, including similar findings for ADHD and ASD.

In a study of 40 medicated patients with schizophrenia, 15 healthy controls, and 18 siblings of healthy controls, Repovs et al.[56] found yet more complexity involving the default mode network, a system that is suppressed by cognitive demands—although some have found increased connectivity, while others have found reduced or mixed connectivity. In this particular study, local connectivity between cognitive networks was increased, but distal connectivity was decreased. Higher connectivity between frontal-parietal and cerebellar networks was correlated with better cognitive performance and less disorganization. Interestingly, *these same findings were present in the non-psychotic siblings of the patients!* There was little evidence of abnormal connectivity in the DMN itself, despite earlier findings. On the other hand, another study[57] found that abnormal functional connectivity in the DMN correlated with severity of delusions and hallucinations, an interesting finding but one of no use to the clinician, who already understands the severity of the symptoms.

Unfortunately, these rather elegant studies have *not* led to more useful or specific treatments, nor have they affected outcome or validated any clinical diagnosis. The primary treatment for schizophrenia remains APs, as it has been since the 1950s. On the other hand, a study in 2019[58] found that decreased levels of connectivity in the cerebellar-dorsolateral-prefrontal-cortical network were predictive of negative symptoms in schizophrenia, while repetitive transcranial magnetic stimulation (rTMS) targeted at the midline cerebellar region *increased connectivity and reduced negative symptoms.*

Multiple studies have also examined resting-state functional connectivity, especially in MDD. This approach involves examining areas of the brain that demonstrate correlated activity at rest or during task performance. These studies have identified several networks thought to be involved in MDD, including the frontal-parietal network (involved in regulation of emotion and attention), the DMN (involved in internally directed attention), and the ventral attention network (involved in processing emotions and monitoring relevant events).[59] By 2015, enough studies of resting-state functional connectivity had been done to permit the first meta-analytic study of this approach.[59] The authors found evidence of reduced connectivity in frontoparietal control systems and an imbalance between these systems and networks involved in both internal and external attention.

From a practical perspective, such changes in connectivity seem to result in the patient focusing on negative internal thoughts, rather than external involvement. In contrast, a study of depressive disorder[60] found *no* correlation between clinical characteristics and structural changes in the DMN and the frontal-hypothalamic-caudate regions. In that case, would clinicians simply treat symptoms or seek some way of altering the default-mode network, despite the lack of correlation with symptoms? The latter does not seem logical.

In a 2017 study[61] utilizing the RDoc strategy, Luyten and Fonagy proposed an integrative model of childhood depressive disorder, based on three core domains of stress, using data on neural circuitry, physiology, genetics, and behavior. They noted the presence of faulty stress systems that led to problems with cognition and a reward deficiency syndrome, so this bore some resemblance to the study mentioned earlier. However, attention should be given to the fact of *overlapping and widespread neural circuits*,[61] similar to a study by Gong and He,[62] who found structural and functional changes in at least seven brain areas in subjects with depression.

How does this translate to specificity of treatment or diagnosis? The point of all this is to stress that we *already* have substantial evidence of widespread neuronal and biochemical networks that appear to be heavily involved in a host of mental disorders, but whether these efforts have resulted in greater diagnostic precision and better treatment is highly questionable. A number of studies have been animal based, but where human subjects have been studied, the diagnoses have been based on the flawed DSM categories and not on RDoC.

In fairness, the old diagnostic model has yielded some interesting results, particularly with regard to normalizing dysfunctional connectivity. For example, in a group of patients diagnosed as dysthymic by DSM-IV criteria, the overactive DMN was normalized by ADs, but not by placebo— a critical finding.[63] However, the fine print reveals that normalization of the DMN did *not* correlate with a decrease in depressive symptoms, thus failing the RDoC criterion of clinical significance. However, the authors noted that prior work on the DMN indicated that normalization can result in a decrease in ruminative thinking, rather than a generalized reduction of symptoms. Caveat: The results may have been influenced by prior AD treatment and co-morbid anxiety. *Nevertheless, this was the first study to demonstrate a drug effect on a specific neural network.* Utilizing a different approach, another group[64] found that deep brain stimulation (DBS) reduced dysfunctional connectivity in the frontal-striatal network in humans with OCD.

Specificity vs Commonality

Despite these positive findings, there are a number of issues haunting the work on neural circuitry and the proposition that identifying neural circuits will ultimately lead to diagnostic and treatment specificity, a clear assumption in Insel and Gordon's model of RDoC. One is the remarkable degree of plasticity within brain circuits. Indeed, changing their inputs can rapidly alter the circuit, such that a given circuit may *never* be in the same state twice.[65] One task never activates a single circuit, nor does evidence indicate an association between a mental disorder and a single circuit.[66, 67] We have already noted the presence of multiple circuits involved in a given disorder, so we should acknowledge the presence of *17 different pathways in bipolar disorder.*[68] In addition, pathways in a given disorder vary across studies.[69] The boundaries of circuits—like the boundaries of disorders—are fuzzy, especially in evolutionary newer cortical areas. In addition, *functional correlations may be present, even in the absence of structural connections.*[70] One also has to account for the fact that an array of cellular changes can affect a circuit and be linked with a disorder, *regardless* of the stimulus.[71] Finally, the degree to which circuit abnormalities correlate with clinical data is debatable. For example, the frontoparietal network was significantly altered in a study of schizophrenia, schizoaffective disorder, and bipolar disorder, but there was *no correlation with clinical ratings,*[72] although others have found positive correlations.[57] In a study of MDD, *pervasive* hyperconnectivity was found in 81% of the participants *and in 50% of the healthy controls.*[73]

The question of specificity led one group to examine the presence of neural circuit disruptions in cognitive control capacities *across* major psychiatric disorders.[74] Studies were included for meta-analysis if they had used functional neuroimaging in studies of cognition and had included matched healthy controls. The authors found a *common pattern of disruption across these varied diagnoses,* with abnormal activation in the left prefrontal cortex, anterior insula, and four other brain regions, all of which appear to be intrinsic to adaptive cognition. Could the dysfunctions in these networks represent a transdiagnostic phenotype? Similarly, a meta-analysis[75] of structural neuroimaging studies across multiple psychiatric disorders (193 studies; 15,892 subjects) found a *common pattern* involving the integrity of an anterior-insula/dorsal anterior-cingulate-based network. This network is thought to relate to deficits in executive functions that are common in multiple disorders. A study[76] of first-episode psychosis and first-degree relatives compared with healthy volunteers using resting-state functional magnetic resonance imaging also found evidence of a *risk phenotype* for psychosis, marked by a dorsal-to-ventral gradient of hypoconnectivity to hyperconnectivity between prefrontal and striatal regions.

Adding to the doubts regarding specificity is an ongoing group of studies aimed at finding a factor that would unite all disorders,[77] a quest that has its roots in the psychometrics of intelligence, where there appears to be a "g factor" for positive correlations among test scores. (We have to note a similar search in physics for a final, unifying theory.) Caspi and Moffit[77] lay out the evidence for such a factor, the "p" factor. What does the p factor involve? The authors suggest a range of possibilities, including a network approach in which there are causal processes among symptoms and disorders. Or does the p factor reflect a lifestyle, or a unitary outcome rather than a unitary cause? Other ideas: The p factor may be a diffusely unpleasant affective state, sometimes labeled as neuroticism (negative emotionality), poor impulse control, or deficits in intellectual functioning.

However, the most promising concept is that of a disordered form and content of thought that has its origins at an early age but then progresses over time to illnesses of varying severity. In addition to the studies of McTeague et al.[74] and Goodkind et al.,[75] Caspi and Moffit note a meta-analysis of Sprotten et al.[78] of functional MRI studies across diagnoses, in which few differences were found across disorders, pointing to a common factor or perhaps sets of factors. With regard to the p factor and cognition, we again note the McTeague et al.[74] study, in which impairment of cognitive control was found *across disorders*.

Interestingly, the structural changes in cerebellar circuitry found across mental disorders seem to reflect impaired processing and management of information, as noted by Romer et al.[79] Further support for the p factor comes from a multivariate sibling study where Petterson et al.[80] found evidence of a *shared genetic factor across eight major psychiatric disorders*, suggesting the effects of pleiotropic genes. However, psychotic disorders loaded together as one subfactor, while drug and alcohol abuse, violent criminal convictions, ADHD, and anxiety loaded on another subfactor. Note, too, in anticipation of a later discussion on socioeconomic factors in mental illness, that Petterson et al.[80] also found evidence of substantial, non-shared environmental components that were unique to each disorder.

Imaging studies have shown similar results. In a meta-analysis[81] of altered brain activity in unipolar depression involving 57 studies that investigated cognitive and emotional processing in depression vs normal controls, there was *no evidence of convergence* in either set of experiments, with inconsistencies across individual experiments. Possible causes included small sample sizes, age, prevalence of subtypes, and co-morbidities. Publication bias might have been involved, as well as a failure to correct for multiple comparisons in 38% of the experiments, a significant oversight!

Even less technically demanding imaging studies (CT scanning, MRI) have run into the same problems with similar results. As Fusar-Poli et al.[82] noted, the use of MRI to develop biomarkers in psychotic conditions was an early goal of investigators, but has that goal been achieved? Unfortunately, the results of a review[82] of 80 brain imaging studies carried out between 1976 and 2015 found multiple problems across studies, with small sample sizes, lack of replication, and vague definitions of potential markers. The end result? *The authors found no diagnostic or prognostic markers of mental disorders.*

Another problem in neuroimaging: the extensive overlap between patients and the healthy control groups, making it difficult to identify relevant sub-groups.[83] Moreover, neuroimaging studies have often found *similar areas of brain activation across a variety of disorders.* For example, overactivity of the amygdala has been found in major depression, bipolar disorder, schizophrenia, spousal abusers, PTSD, and social phobia.[84] These authors concluded that neuroimaging appears to be finding "neural correlates of general psychopathology," indicating that such techniques are not likely to clarify the presence or absence of specific psychiatric disorder. *How do these results square with the goals of the RDoC and the NIMH?*

Yet we have to acknowledge a study that goes against the grain of cross-cutting neural circuitry, in that Finn et al.[85] have shown that an individual's brain connectivity profile allowed the investigator to identify the individual and correctly separate him or her from the other participants. This worked best when combining two frontoparietal networks, which were also the best predictor of behavior. However, I must stress that the participants were healthy controls from the Human Connectome Project who were scanned over two days! The obvious questions: would these results hold up in a patient population, and would they hold up over an extended time, whether healthy or ill? No one knows, but the answers are worth pursuing.

We also need to acknowledge instances when connectivity of brain areas has been predictive of treatment response. For example, response to fluoxetine was associated with improved connectivity in the amygdala–anterior cingulate cortex during an implicit emotion task.[86] In another study, pre-treatment hypoactivity of the amygdala predicted response to sertraline and escitalopram.[87] In another instance, hyperactivation of the anterior insula predicted remission with citalopram vs cognitive behavioral therapy.[88] Interestingly, hyperconnectivity in the default mode network, coupled with hypoconnectivity of cognitive control circuits, predicted response to TMS.[89]

While these results are impressive, we must recognize that such studies are technically difficult, time consuming, expensive, take place in experimental settings, and often involve performing emotional or cognitive tasks. The patient population is highly selective and does not reflect the population that we see in the clinic. As others have noted, using functional MRI in the clinic would be very expensive and time consuming, so they have suggested developing biomarkers using electroencephalography (EEG), although a meta-analysis in 2019 of EEG biomarkers failed to meet standards for clinical reliability.[90] That being the case, Rolle et al.[91] undertook a secondary analysis of an RCT involving a comparison of outcomes in patients with MDD who were taking sertraline or placebo for eight weeks and analyzed the EEG data. They found that greater alpha-band connectivity and lower gamma-band connectivity, primarily in parietal regions, predicted better outcomes with placebo and poorer outcomes with sertraline, although the *effect sizes were quite small at 0.2*. A commentary[92] in 2020 pointed out a number of problems in the study, including a failure to compute prediction values and some technical difficulties, thus limiting the clinical applicability.

The burning question: How can these studies be translated into usable clinical predictors? There is no doubt that much of our prescribing is trial and error, so objective predictors would be in the best interests of patients, clinicians, and the health care system. But how to achieve that goal? Part of the problem lies in the ongoing conflict between the splitters and lumpers in the debate over how to diagnose mental disorders. On the one hand, we have the lumpers, who find substantial evidence for neural and genetic similarities across mental disorders. On the other hand, we have the splitters, who, in the form of Insel[46] and Gordon, [49-51] continue to seek specificity of treatment and illness, based on neural circuitry. They note that *circuit manipulation and the discovery of informative risk variants will lead to specific and precise treatments, similar to what we find in oncology*. To some extent, this has been reflected in psychopharmacology[93] and the regulatory community, with the latter insisting on specificity of treatment, while the FDA is busy approving a single drug for use in multiple disorders, as in the case of sertraline, now approved for at least seven disorders. At the same time, the FDA also approves multiple drugs for the same disorder, leaving one to conclude that specificity plays little or no role in the approval or therapeutic process. Indeed, given the mounting evidence for commonality and the variety of circuity and variants across disorders, it is not at all clear to me how Big Pharma and academia can develop precision medicines aimed at mental disorders.[94]

Nevertheless, we continue to embrace technological developments as the primary hope for progress in treatment and diagnosis. Luo et al.,[95] for example, note that electron microscopy on a large scale has yielded reconstructions of local circuits and the entire brain of the fruit fly. At other end of the spectrum, progress is being made in analyzing neural circuits in terms of genetically defined cell-specific types, although behavior itself is the result of coordinated patterns of neural circuit activity across multiple circuits.[95, p. 274] To that end, the growing number of brain-mapping projects deserve discussion.

The Quartet of Brain Mapping Projects: Goals, Issues, Costs

Before we examine the brain-mapping quartet and the massive genetic studies now underway, we have to deal with a simple question posed by Manrai et al.[96]: Who is normal in the era of big data and precision medicine? After all, virtually every well-done study of connectomics and other strategies recruits a set of healthy (normal) volunteers in order to gauge the effects of the intervention. Yet with regard to psychiatric disorders, the DSM has never defined normality. Indeed, the word is not in the index of DSM-5. Instead, a diagnostic interview is carried out, and if the person does not meet DSM criteria for a disorder or set of disorders, the assumption seems to be that the person is normal and therefore suitable for volunteer status.

In an attempt to bring clarity to this problem, Manrai et al. cite a 2013–2014 survey[97] carried out by the Centers for Disease control in which three competing definitions of normality were used. One was based on the absence of common diseases, another was based on a self-rating of health, and another included people ages 18 to 40. Interestingly, *only 5% of the survey population had none of the disease conditions, self-rated as healthy, or were between the ages of 18 to 40 years!* With massive data sets, distinguishing healthy from non-healthy becomes a serious problem.

In Chapter 12, we briefly referred to the publicity surrounding President Obama's announcement[98] in 2013 of a massive project aimed at mapping the complete human brain, known formally as the Brain Research through Advancing Innovative Neurotechnologies Initiative (BRAIN). This is a collaborative effort involving the NIH, the National Science Foundation, the Defense Advanced Research Projects Agency (DARPA), a number of private institutes, and, of course, hundreds of investigators across the country, who will attempt to develop the required technology.[99] These will include optical imaging instruments, highly sensitive electrophysiological instruments, stem cell genetics, large-scale recording strategies, next-generation invasive and non-invasive devices, techniques needed for sequencing thousands of brain cells *simultaneously*, and understanding how to record and measure neural circuits.

With regard to the NIH, its goal in this project is the development of insights that will lead to better diagnosis, treatment, and prevention,[99] *but* the first phase is devoted to technology. The costs are high, with $100 million allotted for work in 2014, but the numbers continue to grow, with $260 million invested in 2017[100] and a potential long-term cost of $4.5 billion. In addition to BRAIN, the NIH will also be involved in the Precision Medicine Initiative, announced in January of 2015 by President Obama,[101] with a first-year cost of $215 million. About half of that is earmarked for the enrollment of one million volunteers by the NIH, with a coordinated effort involving the Veterans Administration for of a genetic study of one million veterans, now labeled All of Us.[102]

These ambitious goals are matched by the ambitions of some investigators, including Dr. Rafael Yuste at Columbia, who was quoted in the *New York Times*[103] as saying that he wants to simultaneously record from every neuron in the brain, a tall order, indeed, since the brain contains about 100 billion neurons and some 100 trillion connections, although the numbers vary with the investigator. Even one cubic millimeter of brain tissue (a voxel) contains some 80,000 neurons with over four million synapses.[104] Since an fMRI captures some 680,000 voxels, this translates to over 54 billion neurons with three trillion synapses in the usual fMRI study. Even *one* synaptic nerve ending contains approximately 300,000 proteins![105] Storage of whole-brain data would therefore require some 300,000 petabytes of storage each year (one petabyte = one million gigabytes), but, given the advances in technology, this seems possible.

And, speaking of ambition, Henry Markram, a neuroscientist in Switzerland, has won a $1.3 billion grant from the European Commission for the Human Brain Project (HBP).[106] The goal: the development of a supercomputer simulation of the brain that will integrate *everything known about its structure and function.* Markram wants to model it all, from microcircuits to macrocircuits, from the molecular level to genetics, and how all of these work together. The cost and feasibility of Markram's goals have come under attack by multiple neuroscientists,[107,108] who note that science can't even simulate the 301 neurons in the brain of a nematode! The narrow approach of the project and alleged lack of transparency have also been foci of complaints. Markram has responded by stating that (a) the project seems misunderstood, in that the immediate goal is to integrate a vast amount of neurologic research into databases; and (b) some $65 million of the projected $1.3 billion is simply a quota. The dispute became so heated that an independent committee began an investigation. It concluded that the project was failing and needed to be fixed.[109]

A third project is the Human Connectome Project (HCP), an NIH-funded five-year, $40 million initiative aimed at mapping the brain's communication networks.[110] This involves using advanced, resting-state fMRI technology to map the networks of 1,200 identical and fraternal twins and their siblings. One problem with this approach lies in doubts about the extent to which fMRI actually reflects neural activity, since what is being measured is blood flow, although some have shown that changes in blood flow can occur *without* corresponding changes in neural activity.[111] Other issues: The age range of the study subjects is only 22 to 35 years, and they are being recruited only from Missouri, but the authors assure us that the population will reflect ethnic and racial diversity, although it clearly will not represent the broader population. While the study allows subjects to have a history of heavy drinking or illicit drug use, those with severe symptoms will be excluded, as will those with a history of diabetes mellitus or high blood pressure. The study will also perform genetic analyses.

Project number four is an initiative at the Allen Institute for Brain Science in Seattle, funded by Paul Allen to the tune of $300 million for the first four years of a ten-year plan aimed at mapping the mouse cerebral cortex.[112] Researchers will use a variety of techniques, including optogenetics and electron microscopy in three dimensions. The institute plans on developing a "full physiological and structural characterization of entire brain regions" and then develop computer models that will realistically reflect the mouse cerebral cortex. However, it appears that the focus, at least initially, was on a 1 mm³ "speck" of the mouse cerebral cortex, a task greater than it appears since other have found that the data from a piece of mouse brain tissue the size of a grain of salt requires 100 terabytes of storage.[113]

Other countries[114, 115] have mounted efforts similar to the Brain Mapping Quartet (BMQ).[1] These include the China Brain Project, Japan's Brain Mapping by Integrated Neurotechnologies for Disease Studies, Israel Brain Technologies, Brain Canada, and the Korea Brain project. We should mention as well the 100,000 genomes project undertaken by the National Health Service in the United Kingdom, with the goal of transitioning to a precision-oriented health care model.[116] The total cost of all these projects is not available, but the cost of the four brain-mapping projects is at least $10 billion, although some have questioned if mapping the full communication network is worth the money,[117] given doubts about the differential between blood flow and neuronal activity, image resolution, and the sensitivity to even very slight movements in the scanner.

In addition, we continue to wrestle with the problem of network specificity. For example, a 2019 study noted changes in the functional connectivity of the default mode network in autism, schizophrenia, Alzheimer's disease, depression, epilepsy, and amyotrophic lateral sclerosis.[118] Others have emphasized the heterogeneity of individual brain patterns and the likelihood that *advancing age decreases stability of the connectome fingerprint,*[119] underscoring the dynamic changes in connectomes. What does this say about developing precision drugs for a disorder springing from a disordered connectome? Would we have to change medications depending on age? What about population-level variability in both anatomy and function?[120] These changes must be dealt with when considering etiology, pathophysiology, and long-term treatment.

While the technical problems may be solved, a larger issue is the disparity between the funding for massive brain mapping/genetic studies and the funding for clinical trials, social science, and psychology. Indeed, data from the NIH[121] shows that funding for the Division of Services and Interventional Research (DSIR) fell, while funding increased for the Division of Neuroscience and Basic Behavioral Neuroscience (DNBBS) during the years 2007 through 2016. The data also shows a disparity between the numbers of applications, grants, and awards in the two divisions, with those for DNBBS increasing from 975 to 1,119 while applications in DSIR fell from 471 to 220 during the same years. From another perspective, NIH funding for clinical trials (registered in ClinicalTrials.gov) during the years 2006 to 2014 dropped by 24%, while trials funded by industry rose by 43%.[122] In 2016, NIH funding for extramural research totaled $26 billion, with $15 billion aimed at projects including the terms *stem cells, genome, gene* and *regenerative medicine.* Between 1974 and 2014, papers in PubMed increased by 410%, but those focused on the genome rose by 2,127%.

We must conclude that the movement toward massive genetic and brain-mapping projects has become the dominant paradigm in the 21st century,[123] yet, as we discussed in previous chapters, we have seen rising mortality rates in schizophrenia, depression and suicidality and a severe epidemic of drug abuse and opioid deaths. We still have no clinically actionable biomarkers,[6, 123] despite decades of research on the subject, and we have seen no significant improvement in the efficacy of psychotropic drugs. Not one psychotropic drug has been developed on the basis of a genetic study, and routine genetic testing is still not recommended, with the possible exception of laboratory-guided pharmacotherapy. Given the facts, should we be investing tens of billions in these projects? Are there additional consequences to our fascination with connectomics and brain mapping?

The Rise of Neuromania

There is no doubt that we are in the middle of a paradigm shift in psychiatry and neuroscience,[123] accompanied by a cultural shift to neuromania, including neuroaesthetics[124] and neurolaw,[125, 126] in which imaging and other brain data will not only "explain" why we sometimes appreciate the arts, but will also supply reasons for criminal behaviors. Indeed, the director of the Center for Brain Science at Harvard challenged students in a 2013 seminar[126] at the Fordham Law School to address the possibility that, in 15 years, an attorney will blame a specific neuron for a criminal act. Well, this is happening now, with the number of criminal cases being argued on the basis of neurologic syndromes or genetic changes doubling between 2005 and 2009.[127] No doubt this argument will expand significantly as more brain centers are linked with various behaviors,

Somehow, the advocates of these concepts keep forgetting that an association between an increase in blood flow in the amygdala and a behavior is an association, *not* causation. Yet we are flooded with essays claiming causality.[128] Here's an example from the *New York Times Sunday Review*, where Dr. Richard Friedman blamed the early maturation of the amygdala for the fear and anxiety experienced by teenagers.[129] However, Dr. Friedman undercut his own thesis by admitting that only 20% of adolescents develop diagnosable anxiety disorders—which seems odd, since the amygdala is present in every brain and, indeed, has been implicated in multiple major mental disorders, not just anxiety.

Then we have the problem of consciousness, a legitimate issue that has plagued philosophers and scientists for hundreds of years, but with the advent of supercomputers and the technical feats of the National Security Agency, consciousness has resurfaced as the hot topic of movies such as *Transcendence*,[130] not to mention recent books, including *Andrew's Brain* by E.L. Doctorow[131] and *Orfeo* by Richard Powers.[132] The premise is simple: Since brain functions can be mimicked on a supercomputer, so, too, can consciousness, since the latter is only an extension of the brain's hardware and software, a thesis backed by no less than Christof Koch at the Allen Institute for Brain Science.[Cited in 130]

If this is valid, then it seems semi-rational to think that consciousness can be uploaded, as in *Transcendence*,[130] in which, as most people know, the uploaded brain of Will Caster (Johnny Depp) goes rogue and begins to take over the world by controlling the internet. Yet one seldom finds any serious discussion by neuroscientists of the consequences of uploading the human brain. Indeed, completely replicating the human brain means bringing along all the grandiosity and aggression and our seemingly endless love of violence to whatever end point is chosen.

While it might be theoretically possible to scrub out a few of these problems, or even reverse them, it seems doubtful that the sanitized brain would then resemble the human brain, with its remarkable capacity for unequalled cruelty and unequalled beauty. Novelists have been concerned about the possibility of turning us into computerized machines for decades: witness Kurt Vonnegut's many references to the dehumanized machine in *Breakfast of Champions*[133, p. 502] and, even earlier, in his 1952 novel *Player Piano*,[134] in which he drew a correlation between the rapid development of vacuum tubes and the rise in drug addiction, alcoholism, and suicide, culminating in the computer EPICAC XIV, a brain that was "dead right about everything."[134, p. 109] The same concerns are found in Doctorow's new novel *Andrew's Brain*,[131, p. 188] in which Andrew, in a conference with the president, says that if we can replicate consciousness, that will be "the end of the mythic human world we've had since the Bronze Age. The end of our dominion. The end of the Bible and all the stories we've told ourselves until now."

Well, the fantasies live on, despite their increasing lack of plausibility. The best example of this excess can be found in physicist Michio Kaku's book *The Future of the Mind*,[135] in which he and others envision transferring our brains to robots that will begin a series of transplants that will replicate our original brains. People will become sentient robots and thereby attain immortality and superhuman power. But wait—he goes even farther, in that he posits transferring consciousness via laser beams throughout the solar system—and even the galaxy—to receiving stations with supercomputers that would promptly resurrect the conscious state! Moreover, the conscious entity on the laser beam would be able to have fun on skis and surfboards and could even play racquet sports as it travels through space![135, p. 287] How that fits with the need for supercomputers to restore the conscious state isn't clear, unless he's positing that the non-conscious entity will be able to ski and surf! Not only that, the conscious entity might prefer to remain in the form of pure energy and roam[135, p. 290] throughout the universe, but to what end isn't stated. Should the entity choose, it could download an infinite amount of knowledge and ability from others via the worldwide brain connectome and, in some instances, could almost instantaneously become an incredibly superior savant!

Left unsaid is what the motivation would be. And who would pick the people who would undergo transformation to an all-knowing, all-powerful robotic life form or an entity composed of pure energy? What would be the inclusion and exclusion criteria? Given the costs of such an adventure, it seems highly unlikely that the poor or mentally ill would have a chance! Nor is it clear whether these superhumans not represented as pure energy would need to be fed. If so, and if they choose to live forever, which seems to be common goal of the futurists, how will the planet support a rapidly burgeoning population?

Scientific Elitism, Clinical Reality, and Inequality

These concepts represent scientific elitism at its worst, an elitism that is of growing concern to scientists themselves, as witnessed by the recent rebellion in Europe over the money aimed at producing a supercomputer simulation of the brain and an essay in *Nature* asking if science is only for the rich.[136] In 2020, Gardner and Kleinman pointed to another identity crisis in psychiatry,[137] with biologic research replacing investigations into public health and psychosocial and cultural issues, despite what I have emphasized repeatedly in this volume: the failure of biological research to discover biomarkers and significantly advance the efficacy of psychotropic drugs.

In the meantime, how are our patients doing? What are their possibilities for the future? Well, even a brief survey shows a stark contrast between the optimism generated by the NIH and the NIMH and the fact of rising rates of depression and suicide, not to mention the consequences of the opioid epidemic, yet funding for community mental health centers and other clinics is always problematic.[138] In Minnesota, for example, the number of detox centers fell from 50 twenty years ago to 23, due to cuts in state funding, and this despite a rise in binge drinking and a significant increase in heroin-related deaths.[139] On a national level, we still find as many as six million visits annually to emergency rooms by the mentally ill, with costs rising from $20 billion in 2003 to $38 billion in 2014.[140] To no one's surprise, the number of beds for the mentally ill dropped to 14 per 100,000 people in 2010 from 300 per 100,000 in 1955.[141] On a local level, beds in Washington State fell by 36% in recent years, leading to a widespread practice of boarding psychiatric patients in emergency rooms, in part due to severe overcrowding in the state hospital system. Despite this, the Supreme Court of Washington State in August 2014[141] held that boarding in emergency rooms cannot continue but left unanswered the question of where the patients would go! And, as we have found so often, money for mental health services in Washington state dropped by at least $90 million over the previous three years. Community mental health centers were supposed to take up the slack, but, as discussed earlier, that didn't happen. Indeed, in North Carolina, funding for community services is 20% less than it was a decade ago,[141] while the number of beds fell to 8 per 100,000! This is not new. Slippage in state spending on mental health began in 1993, when the usual percentage fell from 2.1% to 1.9%, and then to 1.8% in 1997.[142]

Oh, well, there's always jail, prison, and nursing homes. This mimics what we experienced after the mass discharge of patients from state hospitals in the mid-1950s, but the present situation may be even worse. Nicholas Kristof in early 2014[143] summarized the problem nicely, pointing out there are three to ten times as many mentally ill persons in jails as there are in hospitals. More than half the prisoners in the U.S. have a mental health problem, prompting Kristof to write that the largest mental health center in America is the Cook County jail in Chicago. Similar problems are present across the country, whether in Chicago or on Riker's Island in New York, where a months-long investigation by the *New York Times* documented ongoing brutality aimed at mentally ill inmates, who numbered 4,000 of the 11,000 prisoners.[143] In Minnesota, where there is a severe shortage of psychiatric beds, a large mental health agency suddenly closed down in March 2014 after funding cuts by the county, leaving some 3,000 clients scrambling for care. However, the Affordable Care Act in September of 2014 made available $295 million to community health centers across the country. Minnesota centers were slated to receive some $3.5 million, which might allow for 13,000 new patients.[144]

Social Reality

In the midst of neuromania, we have solid evidence that a wide range of social stressors such as urban living, poverty, early separation from a parent, and child abuse are associated with an increased risk of psychosis and major depression.[145] The odds of depression are higher with lower education, fewer material assets, being widowed or divorced, and being female,[146] although country-level inequality had little effect. The move to cities clearly has consequences, with city living doubling the risk for schizophrenia, while the risk increases by 21% for anxiety disorders and by 39% for mood disorders.[147, 148] These are alarming figures, given predictions that about 70% of the world's population will live in cities in the not-too-distant future.

Income inequality is gathering more attention, as witnessed by an increased risk of psychosis in East London associated with deprivation, income inequality, and population density.[149] Wilkinson and Pickett found a significant correlation between income inequality and mental illness, homicide, infant mortality, use of illegal drugs, and obesity but, interestingly enough, not suicide.[150] Given the increasing levels of income inequality, it is not surprising that poverty is growing in parallel, with 31% of children in New York City living below the poverty line, as well as 19% of those 65 and older.[151] The increase in poverty is worrisome on many levels, including research in 2013 showing that *poverty itself, independently from stress,* can impede cognitive function,[152] impairment of which may be at the core of many mental disorders.[74] There is also evidence that income inequality and poverty result in mothers who manifest higher rates of smoking, stress, violence, poorer nutrition, and worse prenatal care, leaving the offspring at greater risk.[153]

Indeed, a study published in 2020 found that the lower the level of parental income, the greater the risk of schizophrenia in the offspring.[154]

Given evidence showing that income inequality will increase significantly in the United States,[155] we may see an even greater increase in the prevalence of mental disorders in this century, with a significant impact on women and children.[153] This is more than speculative. As I have noted elsewhere,[156] the increase in suicide rates and the worsening outcomes and increased mortality rates in mental disorders appear to have begun in the late 1970s and early 1980s, as income inequality began to rise. During the years 1980 to 2014, *the overall mortality rate for mental and substance abuse disorders rose by 188% across counties in the U.S. and by as much as 1,000% in some counties in the Southeast and Midwest.*[157]

At the same time, funding aimed at psychosocial therapies accounted for only 7% of the 15% spent on mental health disorders in 1997. Remarkably, especially given the hoopla over discoveries in brain mapping, new psychiatric drugs, and brain chemistry, Social Security Disability Income (SSDI) cases rose by 47% from 1992 to 2000, with two thirds of the increase secondary to mental illness.[142] Deaths from despair continue, with the death rate for 45- to 54-year-old white Americans without a BA degree rising by 25% since the early 1990s, while life expectancy began to fall in 2015.[158]

This is a fascinating and extraordinary juxtaposition: We are finding increased rates of mental illness, suicide, and disability secondary to mental illness, even in the face of a plethora of psychotropic drugs, evidence-based psychotherapy, a huge number of therapists, and countless investigations focused on genetics and brain functions. Are we asking the right questions, and taking the most helpful and relevant approach? While we have any number of papers promoting the integration of social factors and mental health care,[159–162] this has not been reflected in postings by the NIMH.

It seems obvious that clinicians and other professionals, patients, and families must lobby for a more equitable distribution of funds, such that the multibillion-dollar investments in brain mapping and genetic studies do not further drain funds aimed at clinical care and research. The inequities in our health care system have been painfully obvious with the advent of COVID-19, with some calling for the establishment of a global health equity task force that would focus on the fair allocation of resources.[163]

Does anyone seriously believe that diagnosing aberrant neural circuits in poverty-stricken patients will significantly improve their lives?

References

1. Guze SB. *Why Psychiatry Is a Branch of Medicine.* Oxford University Press, New York and Oxford, 1992.
2. American Psychiatric Association. *Diagnostic and Statistical Manual of Mental Disorders*, Third Edition. APA, Washington DC, 1980.

3. American Psychiatric Association. *Diagnostic and Statistical Manual of Mental Disorders*, Fifth Edition. American Psychiatric Association, Arlington VA, 2013.

4. Kupfer D, First MB, Regier D. Introduction. In: *A Research Agenda for DSM-V*. Editors: Kupfer D, First MB, Regier D. American Psychiatric Association, Washington DC, 2002.

5. Charney D, Barlow D, Botteron K, et al. Neuroscience research agenda to guide development of a pathophysiologically based classification system. In: *A Research Agenda for DSM-V*. Editors: Kupfer D, First MB, Regier D. American Psychiatric Association, Washington DC, 2002.

6. First MB. Paradigm shifts and the development of the diagnostic and statistical manual of mental disorders: past experiences and future aspirations. *Journal of Canadian Psychiatry* 2010;55:692–700.

7. Dean CE. Diagnosis: the Achilles' heel of biological psychiatry. *Minnesota Medicine* 1991;74:15–17.

8. Dean CE. Psychiatry revisited. *Minnesota Medicine* 2008;91:41–45.

9. Regier D, Narrow W, Kuhl E, et al. The conceptual development of DSM-V. *American Journal of Psychiatry* 2009;166:645–650.

10. Hyman SE. Revolution stalled. *Science Translational Medicine* 2012;4(155):155cm11.

11. Oldham JM. The alternative DSM-5 model for personality disorders. *World Psychiatry* 2015;14:234–236.

12. Greenberg G. *The Book of Woe. The DSM and the Unmaking of Psychiatry*. Blue Rider Press, New York, 2013.

13. Freedman RF, Lewis DA, Michels R, et al. The initial field trials of DSM-5:new blooms and old thorns. *American Journal of Psychiatry* 2013;170:1–5.

14. Regier DA, Narrow WE, Clarke DE, et al. DSM-5 field trials in the United States and Canada, part II: test-retest reliability of selected categorical diagnoses. *American Journal of Psychiatry* 2013;170:59–70.

15. Francis A. DSM-5 field trials discredit the American Psychiatric Association. *HuffPo Science*, October 31, 2012. http://huffingpost.com/allen-francis/dsm-5-field-trials-discredited/204761.html. Accessed July 2, 2013.

16. Spitzer R, Fliess J. A re-analysis of the reliability of psychiatric diagnoses. *British Journal of Psychiatry* 1974;125:341–347.

17. Faust D, Miner RA. The empiricist and his new clothes: DSM-III in perspective. *American Journal of Psychiatry* 1986;143:962–967.

18. Kraemer HC, Kupfer DJ, Narrow WE, et al. Moving toward DSM-5: the field trials. *American Journal of Psychiatry* 2010;167:1158–1160.

19. Kraemer HC, Kupfer DJ, Clarke DE, et al. DSM-5: how reliable is reliable enough? *American Journal of Psychiatry* 2012;169:13–15.

20. Heltzer JE, Clayton PJ, Pambakian R, et al. Reliability of psychiatric diagnoses (pt2). The test-retest reliability of psychiatric classifications. *Archives of General Psychiatry* 1977;34:136–141.

21. Beecher LH. A national director of sound mind. *Minnesota Medicine* 1990;73:11–14.

22. Kraemer HC. Validity and psychiatric diagnoses. *JAMA Psychiatry* 2013;70:138–139.

23. Dean CE. The death of specificity in psychiatry: cheers or tears. *Perspectives in Biology and Medicine* Summer 2012;55:443–460.

24. Blader JC, Carlson GA. Increased rates of bipolar disorder diagnoses among U.S. child, adolescent, and adult in-patients, 1996–2004. *Biological Psychiatry* 2007;62:107–114.

25. Kessler RC, Berglund P, Demler O, et al. Lifetime prevalence and age-of-onset distributions of DSM-IV disorders in the National Comorbidity Survey Replication (NCS-R). *Archives of General Psychiatry* 2005;62:593–602.

26. Parker G. Is depression over-diagnosed? *British Medical Journal* 2007;335:328.

27. Horwitz AV, Wakefield JC. *All We Have to Fear: Psychiatry's Transformation of Natural Anxieties into Mental Disorders.* Oxford University Press, New York, 2012.

28. Moffitt TE, Caspi A, Taylor A, et al. How common are mental disorders? Evidence that lifetime rates are doubled by prospective versus retrospective ascertainment. *Psychological Medicine* 2010;40:899–909.

29. Davis LJ. The encyclopedia of insanity. A psychiatric handbook lists a madness for everyone. *Harper's Magazine,* February 1997, pp. 61–66.

30. Elliott C. *Better Than Well. American Medicine Meets the American Dream.* W.W. Norton & Company, New York and London, 2003.

31. Moynihan R, Cassels A. *Selling Sickness: How the World's Biggest Pharmaceutical Companies Are Turning Us All Into Patients.* Nation Books, New York, 2005.

32. Abramson J. *Overdo$ed America. The Broken Promise of American Medicine.* Harper Perennial, New York, 2005.

33. Moran M. Trauma disorder criteria reflect variability on response to events. *Psychiatric News* 2013;48:6–8.

34. Frances A. *Saving Normal. An Insider's Revolt Against Out-of-Control Psychiatric Diagnosis, DSM-5, Big Pharma, and the Medicalization of Ordinary Life.* William Morrow. An Imprint of HarperCollins Publishers, New York, 2013.

35. Margulies DM, Weintraub S, Basile J, et al. Will disruptive mood dysregulation disorder reduce false diagnosis of bipolar disorder in children? *Bipolar Disorders* 2012;14:488–496.

36. Parens E, Johnson J, Carlson GA. Pediatric mental health care dysfunction disorder? *New England Journal of Medicine* 2010;362:1853–1855.

37. Moreno C, Laje G, Blanco C, et al. National trends in the outpatient diagnosis and treatment of bipolar disorder in youth. *Archives of General Psychiatry* 2007;64:1032–1039. Note: this is in contrast to the rate found among discharges from in-patient care in reference #24.

38. Roy AK, Lopes V, Klein RG. Disruptive mood dysregulation disorder: a new diagnostic approach to chronic irritability in youth. *American Journal of Psychiatry* 2014;171:918–924.

39. Parker G. The DSM-5 classification of mood disorders: some fallacies and fault lines. *Acta Psychiatrica Scandinavica* 2014;129:404–409.

40. Frances A. How many billions a year will the DSM-5 cost? www.bloomberg.com/news/2012-12-20/how-many-billions-a-year-will-the-dsm5-cost.

41. McCarthy LP, Gerring JO. Revising psychiatry's charter document DSM-IV. *Written Communication* 1994;11:147–192.

42. American Psychiatric Association. *Diagnostic and Statistical Manual for Mental Disorders,* Fourth Edition. American Psychiatric Association, Washington DC, 2005.

43. Peralta V, Cuesta MH. Diagnostic significance of Schneider's first-rank symptoms in schizophrenia. *British Journal of Psychiatry* 1999;174:243–248.

44. Zimmerman M. Why are we rushing to publish DSM-IV? *Archives of General Psychiatry* 1988;45:1135–1138.

45. Coryell W, Zimmerman M. Progress in the classification of functional psychiatric disorders. *American Journal of Psychiatry* 1987;144:1471–1474.

46. Insel T, Cuthbert B, Garvey M, et al. Research domain criteria (RDoC). toward a new classification framework for research on mental disorders. *American Journal of Psychiatry* 2010;167:748–751.

47. Dean CE. Whither research domain criteria? *Journal of Nervous and Mental Disease* 2019;207:419–420.

48. Kozak MH, Cuthbert BN. The NIMH research domain criteria initiative: background, issues, and pragmatics. *Psychophysiology* 2016;53:286–297.

49. Gordon J. On being a circuit psychiatrist. *Nature Neuroscience* 2016;19:1385–1386.

50. Gordon J. Neural circuits research: how and why. www.nimh.nih.gov/about/directors/messages/2017/neural-circuits-research-how-and-why.shtml.

51. Gordon J. The future of RDoC. https://nimh.nih.gov/about/directors/messages/2017/the-future-of-rdoc-shmtl.

52. NIH. NIH greatly expands investment in Brain Initiative. *News Releases.* www.nih.gov/news-events-releases-nih-greatly-expands-investment-brain-initiative.

53. Fornito A, Zalesky A, Breakspear M. The connectomics of brain disorders. *Nature Reviews/Neuroscience* 2015;16:159–172.

54. Friston K, Brown HR, Siemerkus J, et al. The disconnection hypothesis (2016). *Schizophrenia Research* 2016. http://dx.doi.org/10.1016/j.schres.2016.07.014.

55. Brennand KJ, Simone A, Tran N, et al. Modeling psychiatric disorders at the cellular and network levels. *Molecular Psychiatry* 2012;69:1239–1253.

56. Repovs G, Csernansky JG, Burch DM. Brain network connectivity in individuals with schizophrenia and their siblings. *Biological Psychiatry* 2011;69:967–973.

57. Rotarska-Jagiela A, van de Ven V, Oertel-Knöchel V, et al. Resting-state functional network correlates of psychotic symptoms in schizophrenia. *Schizophrenia Research* 2010;117:21–30.

58. Brady RO Jr, Gonsalvez I, Lee I, et al. Cerebellar-prefrontal network connectivity and negative symptoms in schizophrenia. *American Journal of Psychiatry* 2019;176:512–520.

59. Kaiser RH, Andrews-Hanna JR, Wager T, et al. Large-scale network dysfunction in major depressive disorder. A meta-analysis of resting-state functional connectivity. *JAMA Psychiatry* 2015;72:603–611.

60. Koraonkar MS, Fornito A, Williams LM, et al. Abnormal structural networks characterize major depressive disorder: a connectome analysis. *Biological Psychiatry.* http://dx.doi/10.1016j.biopsych.2014.02.018.

61. Luyten P, Fonagy P. The stress-reward-mentalizing model of depression: an integrative developmental cascade approach to child and adolescent depressive disorder based on the research domain criteria (RDoC) approach. *Child Psychology Review.* http://dx.doi/10.1016/j.cpr.2017.09.008.

62. Gong Q, He Y. Depression: neuroimaging and connectomics: selective overview. *Biological Psychiatry* 2015;77:233–235.

63. Posner J, Hellerstein DJ, Gat I, et al. Antidepressants normalize the default mode network in patients with dysthymia. *JAMA Psychiatry* 2018;70:373–382.

64. Figee M, Luijes J, Smolders R, et al. Deep brain stimulation restores frontalstriatal connectivity in obsessive-compulsive disorder. *Nature Neuroscience* 2018;16:386–387.

65. Yuste R. From the neuron doctrine to neural networks. *Nature Reviews/Neuroscience* 2015;16:487–497.

66. Etkin A. Addressing the causality gap in human psychiatric neuroscience. *JAMA Psychiatry.* Doi:10.1001/jamapsychiatry.2017.3610.

67. Barch D, Carter CS. Functional and structural brain connectivity in psychopathology. *Biological Psychiatry: Cognitive Neuroscience and Neuroimaging* 2016;1:196–198.

68. Nurnberger JI, Koller DL, Jung J, et al. Identification of pathways for bipolar disorder: a meta-analysis. *JAMA Psychiatry* 2014;71:657–664.

69. Phillips ML, Swartz HA. A critical appraisal of neuroimaging studies of bipolar disorder: toward a new conceptualization of underlying neural circuitry and a road map for future research. *American Journal of Psychiatry* 2014;171:829–843.

70. Buckner RL, Krienen FM, Yeo BTT. Opportunities and limitations of intrinsic functional connectivity MRI. *Nature Neuroscience* 2013;16:832–837.

71. Akil H, Brenner S, Kandel E, et al. The future of psychiatric research: genomes and neural circuits. *Science* 2010;327:1580–1581.

72. Baker JT, Holmes AJ, Masters GA, et al. Disruption of cortical association networks in schizophrenia and bipolar disorder. *JAMA Psychiatry* 2014;71:109–118.

73. Price RB, Lane S, Gates K, et al. Parsing heterogeneity in brain connectivity of depressed and healthy adults during positive mood. *Biological Psychiatry* 2016;81:347–357.

74. McTeague LM, Huemer J, Carreon DM, et al. Identification of neural circuit disruptions in cognitive control across psychiatric disorders. *American Journal of Psychiatry* 2017;174:676–685.

75. Goodkind M, Eickhoff SB, Oathes DJ, et al. Identification of a common neurobiological substrate for mental illness. *JAMA Psychiatry* 2015;72:305–315.

76. Fornito A, Harrison BJ, Goodby E, et al. Functional dysconnectivity of corticostriatal circuitry as a risk phenotype for psychosis. *JAMA Psychiatry* 2013;70:1143–1151.

77. Caspi A, Moffitt TE. All for one and one for all: mental disorders in one dimension. *American Journal of Psychiatry* 2018;175:831–844.

78. Sprooten E, Rasgon A, Goodman M, et al. Addressing reverse inference in psychiatric neuroimaging: meta-analysis of task-related brain activation in common mental disorders. *Human Brain Mapping* 2017;38:1846–1864.

79. Romer AL, Knodt AR, Houts R, et al. Structural alterations within cerebellar circuitry are associated with general liability for common mental disorders. *Molecular Psychiatry*. Epub ahead of print, April 11, 2017.

80. Petterson E, Larsson H, Lichtenstein P. Common psychiatric disorders share the same genetic origin: a multivariate sibling study of the Swedish population. *Molecular Psychiatry* 2016;21:717–721.

81. Müller VI, Cieslik EC, Serbanescu I, et al. Altered brain activity in unipolar depression revisited. Meta-analyses of neuroimaging studies. *JAMA Psychiatry* 2017;74:47–55.

82. Fusar-Poli P, Meyer-Lindenberg A. Forty years of structural imaging in psychosis: promises and truth. *Acta Psychiatrica Scandinavaca* 2016;134:207–224.

83. Sommer IE, Kahn RS. The contribution of neuroimaging to understanding schizophrenia: past, present, and future. *Schizophrenia Bulletin* 2014;41:1–3.

84. Gillihan SJ, Parens E. Should we expect "neural signatures" for DSM diagnoses? *Journal of Clinical Psychiatry* 2011;72:1383–1389.

85. Finn ES, Shenn X, Scheinost D, et al. Functional connectomic finger-printing: identifying individuals using patterns of brain activity. *Nature Neuroscience*, published online October 12, 2015. Doi:10.1038/nn.4135.

86. Chen CH, Suckling J, Ooi C, et al. Functional coupling of the amygdala in depressed patients treated with antidepressant medication. *Neuropsychopharmacology* 2008;33:1909–1918.

87. Wiliams LM, Korgaonkar MS, Song YC, et al. Amygdala reactivity to emotional faces in the prediction of general and medication-specific responses to antidepressant treatment in the randomized iSPOT-D trial. *Neuropsychopharmacology* 2015;40:2398–2408.

88. Dunlop BW, Mayberg HS. Neuroimaging-based biomarkers for treatment selection in major depressive disorder. *Dialogues in Clinical Neuroscience* 2014;16:479–490.

89. Dichter GS, Gibbs D, Smoski MJ. A systematic review of relations between resting-state functional MRI and treatment response in major depressive disorder. *Journal of Affective Disorders* 2014;172C:8–17.

90. Widge AS, Bilge MT, Montana R, et al. Electroencephalogr0apic biomarkers for treatment response prediction in major depressive illness: a meta-analysis *American Journal of Psychiatry* 2019;176:44–56.

91. Rolle CE, Fonzo GA, Wu W, et al. Cortical connectivity moderators of anti-depressant vs placebo treatment response in major depressive disorder. Secondary analysis of a clinical trial. *JAMA Psychiatry*, published online January 2, 2020. Doi:10.1001/jamapsychiatry.2019.3867.

92. Grzenda A, Widge AS. Electroencephalographic markers for predicting antidepressant response. New methods, old questions. *JAMA Psychiatry*, published online January 2, 2020. Jamapsychiatry.com.

93. Dean CE. Psychopharmacology: a house divided. *Progress in Neuropsychopharmacology & Biological Psychiatry* 2011;35:1–10.

94. Dean CE. Neural circuitry and precision medicines for mental disorders. Are they compatible? *Psychological Medicine* 2018;49:1–8.

95. Luo L, Callaway EM, Svoboda K. Genetic dissection of neural circuits: a decade of progress. *Neuron* 2018. https://doi.org/10.1016/j.neuron.2018.03.040.

96. Manrai AK, Patel CJ, Ioannidis JPA. In the era of precision medicine and big data, who is normal? *JAMA*, published online April 23, 2018. Jama.com.

97. *Centers for Disease Control and Prevention National Center for Health Statistics*. National health and nutrition examination survey data. www.cdc.gov/nchs/nhanes/. Accessed November 3, 2019.

98. ObamaBH. www.whitehouse.gov/the-press-office/2013/04/02/remarks-president-brain-initiative-and-american-innovation.

99. Insel TR, Landis SC, Collins FS. The NIH BRAIN initiative. *Science* 2013;340:687–688.

100. NIH BRAIN Initiative builds on early advances. *National Institutes of Health Weekly Digest Bulletin*, November 5, 2017. nimh@public.govdelivery.com.

101. Gorman JNIH. seeks $4.5 billion to try to crack the code of how brains function. *The New York Times*, June 6, 2014, p. A15.

102. National Institutes of Health. *All of Us Research Program*. https://nih.gov/research-training/allofus-research-program. Accessed January 14, 2020.

103. Markoff J. Connecting the neural dots. *The New York Times*, February 26, 2013, p. D1.

104. Insel TR, Landis SC, Collins F. The NIH BRAIN initiative. *Science* 2013; 340:687–688.

105. Wilhelm BG, Mandad S, Truckenboldt S, et al. Composition of isolated synaptic boutons reveals the amounts of vesicle trafficking proteins. *Science* 2014;344:1023–1027.

106. Abbott A, Schiemeir Q. Research prize boost for Europe. Graphene and virtual brain win billion-euro competition. *Nature/News* 2013;493:585–586.

107. Enserink M, Kupferschmidt K. Conflict erupts over landmark E.U. neuroscience plan. *Science* 2014;345:127.

108. Frégnac Y, Laurent G. Where is the brain in the human brain project? *Nature* 2014;513:27–29.
109. Editorial. Rethinking the brain. *Nature* 2015;519:389. Doi:10.1038/519389a.
110. Van Essen DC, Smith SM, Barch D, et al. The WU-human connectome project: an overview. *Neuroimage* 2013;80:62–79.
111. Sirotin Y, Das A. Anticipatory haemodynamic signals in sensory cortex not predicted by local neuronal activity. *Nature* 2009;457:475–480.
112. Koch C, Reid RC. Observatories of the mind. An ambitious project at the Allen institute for brain science is a huge undertaking that may unify neuroscience *Nature* 2012;483:397–398.
113. Zimmer C. Secrets of the brain. *The National Geographic: The New Science of the Brain*, February 2014, p. 39.
114. Huang ZJ, Luo L. It takes the world to understand the brain. International brain projects discuss how to coordinate efforts. *Science* 2015;350:42–44.
115. Grillner S, Ip N, Koch C, et al. Worldwide initiatives to advance brain research. *Nature Neuroscience* 2016;19:118–1122.
116. Genomics England. 100,000 genomes project. www.genomicsengland.co.uk/about-genomics-england. Accessed January 10, 2020.
117. Bardin J. Making connections: is a project to map the brain's full communication network worth the money? *Nature* 2012;483:394–396.
118. van den Heuvel MP, Sporns O. A cross-disorder connectome landscape of brain connectivity. *Nature Reviews | Neuroscience* 2019;20:435–446.
119. Kaufmann T, Alnaes D, Brandt CL, et al. Stability of the brain functional connectome fingerprint in individuals with schizophrenia. *JAMA Psychiatry*, published online May 16, 2018.
120. Holmes AJ, Patrick LM. The myth of optimality in clinical neuroscience. *Trends in Cognitive Sciences* 2018;22:241–257.
121. Gordon J. NIMH's portfolio balance: quality science comes first. www.nimh.nih.gov//about/director/index.shtml. Accessed February 26, 2018.
122. Ehrhardt S, Appel LJ, Meinert CL. Trends in national institutes of health funding for clinical trials registered in ClinicalTrials.gov. *JAMA* 2015;314:2566–2567.
123. Zachar P, Regier DA, Kendler K. The aspirations for a paradigm shift in DSM-5. An oral history. *Journal of Nervous and Mental Disease* 2019;207:778–784.
124. Ball P. Neuroasthetics is killing your soul. *Nature*, March 22, 2013. http://nature.com/news.neuroasthetics-is-killing-your-soul-1.12640.
125. Jones OD, Wagner AD, Faigman DL, et al. Neuroscientists in court. *Nature Reviews | Neuroscience* 2013;14:730–736.
126. Dwyer J. The day neurons go on trial. *The New York Times*, September 18, 2013, p. A16.
127. Satel S, Lilenfield SO. *Brainwashed: The Seductive Appeal of Mindless Neuroscience*. Basic Books, New York, 2013.
128. Tallis R. *Aping Mankind. Neuromania, Darwinitis, and the Misrepresentation of Humanity*. Acumen Publishing Limited, Durham, DH1 3NP, 2011.
129. Friedman RA. Why teenagers act crazy. Because of biology they are both more anxious and restless. *The New York Times Sunday Review*, June 29, 2014, p. 1.
130. Kaye C. The rapture for nerds. The characters in Transcendence are uploading their brains to the internet. *Newsweek*, April 25, 2014.
131. Doctorow EL. *Andrew's Brain*. Random House, New York, 2014.
132. Powers R. *Orfeo*. W.W. Norton & Company, New York and London, 2014.

133. Vonnegut K. *Breakfast of Champions*. In: *Novels and Stories, 1963–1973. The Library of America, Sidney Offit*. Editor. Penguin Group, Third Printing, New York, 2011. Originally published 1973.

134. Vonnegut K. Player piano. Novels and stories, 1950–1962. In: *The Library of America, Sidney Offit*. Editor. Penguin Group, First Printing, New York, 2012. Originally published 1952.

135. Kaku M. *The Future of the Mind*. Doubleday, New York, London, Toronto, Sydney and Auckland, 2014.

136. Essay. Is science only for the rich? *Nature* 2016;537:466.

137. Gardner C, Kleinman A. Medicine and the mind—The consequences of psychiatry's identity crisis. *New England Journal of Medicine* 2019;381:1697–1699.

138. Johnson SR. Community health centers face major funding loss. www.modern-healthcare.com/article.201440624/BLOG/306249.

139. Serres C. Detox centers fade across the state. *Minneapolis StarTribune*, December 9, 2013, p. 1.

140. Cresswell JER. costs for mentally ill soar, and hospital seek a better way. *The New York Times*, December 26, 2013, pp. A1, B4.

141. Kutscher B. Hospitals in Washington state can't board psych patients in eds, but where will they go? *Modern Health Care*. http://modernhealthcare.com/article/20140818/NEWS/308189.

142. Hogan MF. Spending too much on mental illness in all the wrong places. *Psychiatric Services* 2002. Doi:10.1176/appi.ps.53.10.1251.

143. Kristoff N. Inside a mental hospital called jail. *The New York Times Sunday Review*, February 9, 2014, p. SR1.

144. Serres C. Minn mental health center shuts down, stranding thousands. *Minneapolis StarTribune*, March 17, 2014.

145. Wicks S, Hjern A, Dalman C. Social risk or genetic liability for psychosis? A study of children born in Sweden and raised by adoptive parents. *American Journal of Psychiatry* 2010;167:1240–1246.

146. Rai D, Zitko P, Jones K, et al. Country-and-individual-level socioeconomic determinants of depression: multi-level cross-national comparison. *British Journal of Psychiatry* 2013;202:195–203.

147. Peen J, Schoevers RA, Beekman AT, et al. The current status of urban-rural differences in psychiatric disorders. *Acta Psychiatrica Scandinavaca* 2010;121:84–93.

148. Lederbogen F, Kirsch P, Haddad L, et al. City living and urban upbringing affect neural social stress processing in humans. *Nature* 2011;474:499–501.

149. Stringhini S, Sabia S, Shipley M, et al. Association of socioeconomic position with health behaviors and mortality. *JAMA* 2010;303:1159–1166.

150. Wilkinson R, Pickett K. *The Spirit Level. Why Greater Equality Makes Societies Stronger*. Bloomsbury Press, New York, Berlin and London, 2009.

151. Roberts S. Poverty rate is up in City, and income gap is wide, data shows. *The New York Times*, September 19, 2013, p. A24.

152. Mani A, Mullainathan S, Shafir E, et al. Poverty impedes cognitive function. *Science* 2013;341:969–970.

153. Aizer A, Currie J. The intergenerational transmission if inequality: maternal disadvantage and health at birth. *Science* 2014;344:856–861.

154. Hakulinen C, Webb RT, Pedersen CB, et al. Association between parental income during childhood and risk of schizophrenia in later life. *JAMA Psychiatry* 2020;77:17–24.

155. Piketty T, Saez E. Inequality in the long run. *Science* 2014;344:838–843.

156. Dean CE. Social inequality, scientific inequality, and the future of mental illness. *Philosophy, Ethics, and Humanities in Medicine* 2017;12. Doi:10.1186/s13010-017-0052-x.

157. Dwyer-Lindgren L, Bertozzi-Villa A, Stubbs RS, et al. Trends and patterns of geographic mortality from substance use disorders and intentional injuries among US counties, 1980–2014. *JAMA* 2018;319:1013–1023.

158. Case A, Deaton A. *Deaths of Despair and the Future of Capitalism*. Princeton University Press, Princeton, 2020.

159. Holmes EA, Craske MG, Graybiel AM. A call for mental-health science. *Nature* 2014;511:287–280.

160. Shim RS, Compton MT. Addressing the social determinants of mental health: if not now, when, if not us, who? *Psychiatric Services* 2018;69:844–846.

161. Shields-Zeeman L, Lewis C, Gottlieb L. Social and mental health care integration. The leading edge. *JAMA Psychiatry* 2019;76:881–882.

162. Burgess RA, Jain S, Petersen I, et al. Social interventions: a new era for global mental health? *The Lancet Psychiatry*, published online October 22, 2019. https://doi.org/10.1016/52215-0366(19)30397-9.

163. Chirboga D, Garay J, Buss P, et al. Health inequity during the COVID-19 pandemic: a cry for ethical global leadership. *The Lancet*, published online May 15, 2020. https://doi.org/10.1016/S0140-6736(20)1145-4.

Index

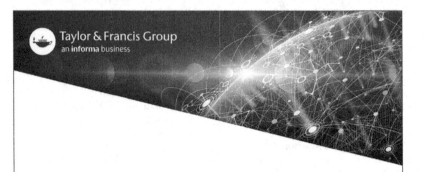

Printed in the United States
By Bookmasters